Stefan Stübinger · Florian Klämpfl
Michael Schmidt · Hans-Florian Zeilhofer
Editors

Lasers in Oral and Maxillofacial Surgery

Springer

Editors
Stefan Stübinger
Hightech Research Center of Cranio-Maxillofacial Surgery
University Hospital of Basel
Allschwil
Switzerland

Florian Klämpfl
Institute of Photonic Technologies
Friedrich-Alexander University Erlangen-Nürnberg
Erlangen
Germany

Michael Schmidt
Institute of Photonic Technologies
Friedrich-Alexander University Erlangen-Nürnberg
Erlangen
Germany

Hans-Florian Zeilhofer
Hightech Research Center of Cranio-Maxillofacial Surgery
University Hospital of Basel
Allschwil
Switzerland

Clinic for Oral and Cranio-Maxillofacial Surgery
University Hospital of Basel Oral and Maxillofacial Surgery
Basel
Switzerland

ISBN 978-3-030-29603-2 ISBN 978-3-030-29604-9 (eBook)
https://doi.org/10.1007/978-3-030-29604-9

This Springer imprint is published by the registered company Springer Nature Switzerland AG
The registered company address is: Gewerbestrasse 11, 6330 Cham, Switzerland

Preface

In 2020, the laser will celebrate its 60th anniversary. While in the beginning, it was a solution looking for a problem; it is meanwhile widely spread in industry, science, medicine, in offices, or even at home. It is used to weld car bodies, to prove the existence of gravitational waves, to treat eyes, or to measure distances. These are only a few examples of its applications. This wide use results from its unique properties. It is a light source which can be focused on a very small spot; it is typically highly monochromatic, and there are lasers which produce pulses with a duration in the fs second regime. These pulses are among the shortest events created by humans. Light, which takes only a second to travel almost eight times around the earth, travels less than the diameter of a human hair during the duration of these pulses. While for a long time these so-called ultrafast lasers were used only in scientific laboratories, they have found these days their way into application, even medical application. Today, they are used in fs-Lasik systems to carry out the flap cut during refractive cornea surgery, which is probably the most famous application of lasers in medicine. Refractive cornea surgery is only possible with a laser. It requires high precision. The error must be in the range of micrometers or less. This is only possible by an automated system, even the most capable surgeon cannot work with such precision. And a laser is the perfect tool for automated processes as it works contact free. This is an advantage which is also taken by car manufactures when they weld car bodies with lasers or one by speakers using a laser pointer to emphasize important parts of slides projected on a wall. Working contact free however has not only advantages regarding automation it also has medical advantages during surgeries not limited to eye surgery. Applying no force reduces the damage to surrounding tissues, after the surgery fewer edemas develop, and it is easier to maintain sterility during surgery. Besides this, studies showed also that the healing process after a surgery is quicker than in the conventional surgery. However after all these advantages, one cannot neglect the disadvantages of using a laser for surgery. First of all, lasers are expensive. Even the example of the laser pointer proves this. A simple wooden stick for pointing costs less than a laser pointer. But advantages of the laser pointer count in this case. Second, lasers require safety measures; this does not apply to a laser pointer, but it is easily understandable that a laser which can ablate tissue is highly dangerous for the human eye. This applies even to lasers which cannot ablate tissue but which exceed a certain power limit. Third, a laser used for surgery requires new skills of surgeons. The techniques they trained and learned using traditional instruments over years do not apply anymore to lasers, so they start again from the beginning in this case. But these disadvantages can be overcome, and one can benefit from the advantages a laser provides. This is also one of the points where this book tries to help. It will help physicians and engineers to understand how to take advantage of lasers especially in the area of maxillofacial applications and to give an impression of what can be done with lasers in this area today.

The book is split into two parts. The first part covers the physical fundamentals. It cannot replace more detailed studies in physics or even a good book about laser physics, optics, or laser tissue interaction, but it should help the reader without previous knowledge to understand the second part of the book which covers a broad range of applications. The first part itself is divided into four chapters. After this introduction, one chapter offers a brief revision of the necessary physical fundamentals so the understanding of the following two chapters is easier. The third chapter gives an introduction to lasers, their design, and function with regard to the systems normally used in maxillofacial surgery. The fourth chapter describes the basics of how these lasers interact with tissue, so it lays the foundation for the second part.

Overall, the second part covers five major clinical and technical topics. Firstly, different laser treatment regimes of skin and mucosa are presented. Thereby, the authors set a clear focus on the usage of lasers for cancer therapy and oral rehabilitation. The second key aspect addresses the application of various laser wavelengths for hard tissue ablation. Besides enamel and dentin, state-of-the-art and innovative developments in laser bone surgery are also described. The third part summarizes special applications of lasers in oral and cranio-maxillofacial surgery. The goal is to provide the reader with current and approved clinical procedures of surgical and non-surgical laser applications. In this respect, two chapters also give an overview of implementing laser light for diagnostic or planning issues. The fourth part gives an insight into current research and future trends in laser technology. Novel and advanced potentials and scopes for manufacturing processes are discussed. Finally, the book closes with a chapter on general laser safety.

We hope that you enjoy this first edition of *Lasers in Oral and Maxillofacial Surgery* and that it becomes a trusted partner in your clinical and educational experience. It is hoped that the information and techniques included in the present work will provide clinicians with sufficient knowledge to help them achieve successful and sustainable results and provide their patients with satisfaction and comfort as a result of the treatment.

Erlangen, Germany — Florian Klämpfl
Allschwil, Switzerland — Stefan Stübinger

Contents

Part I

Laser Fundamentals

Physical Fundamentals

1

Florian Klämpfl

Contents

Abstract

The chapter gives a short introduction into the physical fundamentals of light propagation and the interaction of light with matter. The chapter is neither a strict scientific description nor does it replace a textbook. It should only help the reader to understand the book more easily, and it should be a starting point for further studies.

Keywords

Physical fundamentals of light
Light propagation · Light-matter interaction

1.1 Prequel

This chapter tries to summarize important physical fundamentals to enable the reader to understand the remainder of this book. However, it cannot replace a good textbook on optics or describe these fundamentals in a strict scientific manner. For this, the bibliography of the chapter contains several references: [1–3].

F. Klämpfl (✉)
Institute of Photonic Technologies,
Friedrich-Alexander University Erlangen-Nürnberg,
Erlangen, Germany
e-mail: florian.klaempfl@fau.de

S. Stübinger et al. (eds.), *Lasers in Oral and Maxillofacial Surgery*,
https://doi.org/10.1007/978-3-030-29604-9_1

Light is a physical phenomenon that is fundamental to human life. For example, the energy from the sun is transferred to the earth by light, and furthermore, approximately 80% of the information input to humans is by light through the eyes. Due to this, for several millennia, humans have been thinking about the nature, behavior, and properties of light.

1.2 Basic Properties of Light

Over time, several models have been developed, which allow to explain light. The simplest model uses the so-called geometrical optics.

1.2.1 Geometrical Optics: Light as Rays

Geometrical optics assumes that light consists of rays. This means that light starts at a certain point and propagates in a straight line until it hits a surface that absorbs it or changes its direction. Geometrical or ray optics can be used to explain phenomena of light reflection or refraction, so the basic behavior of optical elements like lenses, mirrors, or prisms can be explained. However, effects like diffraction or polarization cannot be described by ray optics, neither is there a good explanation for the idea of "color" in terms of ray optics. To explain these effects, a different model is needed, which describes light as waves.

1.2.2 Wave Optics

The base of wave optics is the *Maxwell equations* [4]. This is a set of partial differential equations that describe the behavior of electromagnetic fields, and as light is an electromagnetic field, light propagation can be described by the Maxwell equations. Making a few assumptions (nonconducting medium, no space charges), two equations can be derived from the Maxwell equations, which are similar to wave equations, and thus, light can be described as a wave. Two equations are needed because light consists of both an electric field/wave and a magnetic field/wave in terms of wave optics. These two waves oscillate perpendicular to each other as well as to the propagation direction of light, so light is a traversal wave: it oscillates perpendicular to its propagation direction. As the electric and magnetic radiation fills the whole space, they are also called fields. Thus, in terms of wave optics, light consists of an electric field and a magnetic field, which both contribute to the behavior of light. Both fields are vector fields, i.e., at each point, the field has not only a value but also a direction.

The remainder of this chapter will concentrate on the electric field because the electric field/wave is often better suited for an explanation for the behavior of light. Besides this, the direction of the electric field also defines the polarization of a light wave. A light wave with linear polarization has an electric field where the vectors of the field always point in the same direction. Another important property is the wavelength of light: it is a physical unit associated with its color. By dividing the speed of light by its wavelength, one gets the associated frequency of the light wave.

While wave optics covers many effects, some effects cannot be explained by it. One example is the photoelectric effect: by irradiating matter with light, it is possible to break away electrons. If this effect is present, it shows a threshold regarding the wavelength: above a certain wavelength, it does not happen, not even at higher intensities.

1.2.3 Photons

This photoelectric effect can be explained by assuming that light consists of particles, so-called photons. A photon has a certain energy depending on its wavelength. If this energy exceeds the energy needed to break the bonding of an electron to its atom, the electron can be released from the atom when the photon is absorbed by the atom. This effect is hard to explain by ray or wave optics. So in this case, it is useful to assume that light consists of photons.

In general, it cannot be said that a certain model of light is the best model for all purposes. It depends on the application and/or the effect that shall be explained which model is the most useful.

1.3 Light Propagation

When working with light or lasers, it is important to be able to influence the direction of the light. The simplest means to change the direction of light is a mirror. It reflects the incoming light back following the law that the angle of incident equals the angle of reflection. This is illustrated by Fig. 1.1: $\Theta_1 = \Theta_2$.

A mirror typically consists of a substrate that defines its shape and a highly reflective coating that is responsible for reflecting the light. The simplest case of a mirror is a plane mirror. A plane mirror does not change the angle between the rays of a beam of light; a parallel beam reflected by a plane mirror stays a parallel beam. Plane mirrors are, for example, used to guide a laser beam from the laser source to the processing/treatment area. If the angle between the rays of a beam of light needs to be changed, a curved mirror can be used. For example, a curved mirror with a concave, spherical shape can be used to focus a parallel beam into a small spot.

Another phenomenon that can be used to change the direction of light is refraction. Refraction happens when light propagates from one medium to another where it has a different propagation speed. The propagation speed of light in a medium is described by the index of refraction. The refractive index is a factor that describes how much faster the light propagates in vacuum than in the medium at hand. So, to get the velocity of light in a medium, the speed of light in vacuum must be divided by the refractive index. Typical values for the refractive index of glasses and tissue are around 1.5. The change in direction by refraction is described by Snell's law; see Fig. 1.2. It says that the refractive index of the medium where the light beam comes from (n_1) multiplied by the sine of the angle of incident (θ_1) is equal to the refractive index of the medium where the light goes to (n_2) multiplied by the sine of the angle of the refracted light beam (θ_2) or written as a formula $n_1 \bullet \sin \theta_1 = n_2 \bullet \sin \theta_2$.

So, when light propagates from air to glass, it is always refracted toward the normal surface. In case that light propagates perpendicular to the surface of the interface from one medium to the other, refraction does not change its direction. The effect of refraction is used by lenses to change the direction of light. Almost any optical system makes use of lenses; the human eye uses lenses for imaging, cameras typically use lenses for imaging, and laser system uses lenses for focusing the laser beam into a small spot. A lens is made out of a material that is transparent with regard to the wavelength at hand. It has two optically relevant surfaces with a defined shape,

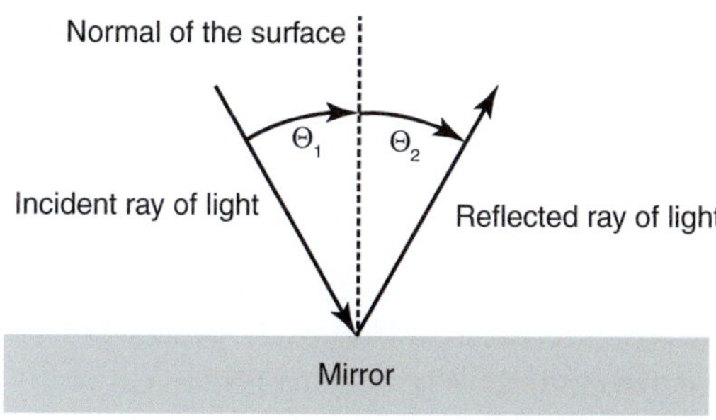

Fig. 1.1 Principle of a plane mirror

Fig. 1.2 Snell's law

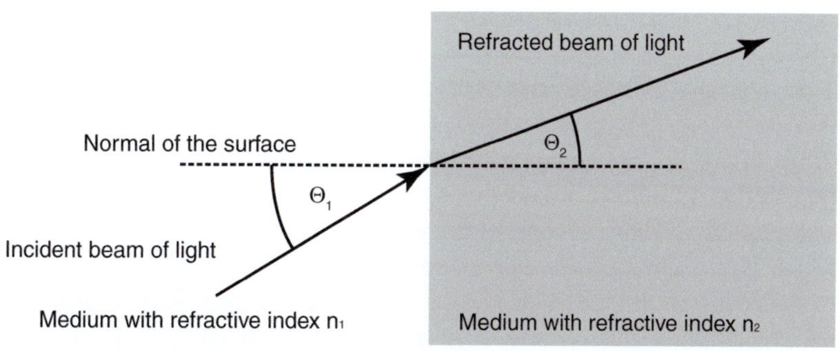

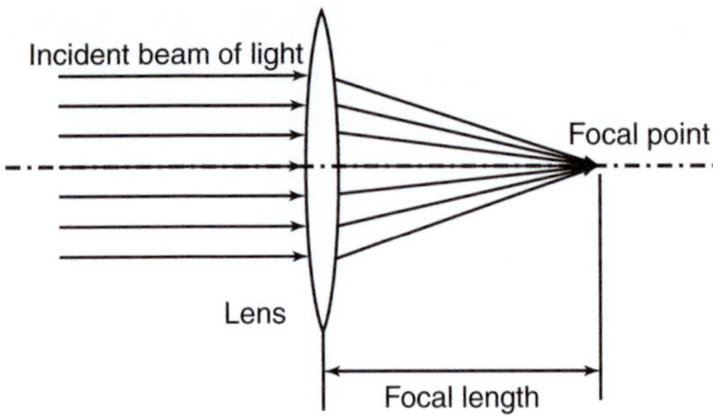

Fig. 1.3 Focal length of a lens

which define the properties of the lens. Those surfaces can be plane, spherical, or aspherically curved, and they can be concave or convex; what shape the surfaces have depends on the purpose of the lens. The shape of the surface together with the refractive index of the lens material defines one important property of a lens: its focal length. The focal length is the distance at which a parallel beam of light is focused by the lens into a single spot. This is illustrated in Fig. 1.3.

This property of a lens is used, for example, to focus a laser beam into a single spot. However, a real lens does not work as well as the drawing suggests. It has aberrations. For example, if the surface is spherical, not all rays meet in one point, and the outer rays are focused at a shorter focal length. This property is called spherical aberration. Another aberration is wavelength dependent. The refractive index of a material is not constant with the wavelength; this effect is called dispersion. Due to dispersion, light of different colors is refracted less or more. While for a lens this effect is not desired, it is used by prisms to split up light into its components depending on the wavelength.

1.4 Light-Matter Interaction

When discussing the behavior of light, it is not only necessary to have a model of light, but it is also necessary to have a model of the objects with which light is interacting. For matter, different models exist at different levels of detail. For the understanding of this chapter, it is sufficient to know that matter consists of atoms, and these atoms consist of a nucleus that is positively charged and of electrons that are negatively charged. This simple model allows already to explain sufficiently well phenomena like the absorption of light by matter or certain types of scattering. The electric field of the light wave accelerates the electrons, and they start to oscillate with the frequency of the incident light wave. Depending on the material and the incident frequency, the energy is transferred to the lattice of the material, so the lattice starts to vibrate, which means the material is heated. It could also be that, by the movement of the electrons, the energy is reemitted—as by an antenna where also moving charges are responsible for the emission of a wave. If a charge moves back and forth emitting energy/a wave, this is called a Hertzian dipole. The emitted field and the resulting wave of a Hertzian dipole have a very characteristic appearance: in the direction of the oscillation vector, the *dipole moment vector*, no electric field is emitted. In all other directions, lines of the electric field form a plane with the dipole moment vector. So the direction of the electric field vector does not change over time at a given location, so the emitted light is linearly polarized.

1.5 Scattering of Light

When light interacts with matter, different effects happen: for example, the light might be reflected, absorbed, refracted, or scattered. All these effects happen in tissue. When talking about light propagation in the tissue, scattering is one of the dominant effects. Scattering means that incident light changes its direction when hitting a *scattering center*. In the simplest case, nothing else happens. This is *elastic scattering*. However, it is also possible that the light changes not only its direction but also its wavelength. This is *inelastic scattering*.

1.5.1 Elastic Scattering

Elastic scattering is something that can be experienced daily. Elastic scattering is the reason why the sky is blue, but it is also the reason why clouds or milk appear white. It is the reason why a finger appears to glow red when it is irradiated even with a low-power (class 1) red laser pointer. In case of the blue sky, the molecules of the atmosphere are the scattering centers; in case of the cloud, it is the small water droplets a cloud consists of. In case of tissue, scattering centers are the cells or parts of them. While scattering is an interesting effect, it is something that is unwelcome when doing diagnostics or therapeutics with light: the incident light does not only reach the tissue at which it is aimed; it might also affect the surrounding tissue, or in case of diagnostics, the received light is not only received by the target structure but also by other structures. While the effect cannot be avoided, understanding it helps to deal with it. The most suitable model to describe elastic scattering in light is *Mie theory* [5]. It is an approach to solve the Maxwell equations in the environment of spherical particles. While understanding this theory involves a lot of mathematics, the overall approach can be easily understood and some conclusions can be drawn from it. Mie theory assumes that the incident wave is absorbed by dipole structures in the particle. Those dipoles remit the wave again. The number of dipoles that absorb the wave depends on the size of the particle. So, the bigger the particle, the more dipoles are involved. The radiations of the dipoles interfere, so interference patterns appear inside the reemitted radiation. Furthermore, as a dipole emits in all directions, the light wave is deflected from its incident direction. However, this happens not in one fixed direction, but in all directions with different intensities. The detailed angular intensity distribution depends on several parameters like wavelength, size of the particle, refraction index of the particle, and refraction index of the environment. For example, the shorter the wavelength is, the more deviation happens, or the bigger the particle is, the less the light is deflected. Significant elastic scattering happens only if the particle has a size in the magnitude of the wavelength or below. When the particles are very small, the deviation is the highest: in this case, only one dipole is excited, and in this case, the intensity of the scattered light follows exactly the characteristics of a dipole. This happens, for example, if the scattering centers are only single molecules. This type of scattering is called Rayleigh scattering. While it can be also described by Mie theory, it has a separate name due to historic reasons: it was discovered and investigated independently of Mie theory, and it took some time until it was understood that both types of elastic scattering can be described by the same mathematical model. The effect that the red laser pointer makes the whole fingertip glow is mostly Mie scattering.

1.5.2 Inelastic Scattering

When the light changes not only its direction but also its "color," i.e., its wavelength, it is called inelastic scattering. Several mechanisms and types for inelastic scattering are known. For medical applications, two types are the most important ones: Raman scattering and fluorescence. In case of Raman scattering, the wavelength can be increased or decreased, i.e., the photons can gain or lose energy. The energy difference is left or comes from the scattering center. Those are atoms or molecules that might change their vibrational state. Raman scattering is something that happens normally together with Rayleigh scattering. However, the intensity of the Raman scattered light is magnitudes lower than that of the Rayleigh scattered light, so it is something that is not experienced in daily life. Raman scattering can only be measured with an appropriate setup. In case of Raman scattering, the scattered light is not limited to one wavelength or a small band, but the scattered light has a rather broad spectrum with certain peaks. This spectrum is very characteristic of the matter of the scattering center, and it can be considered as a fingerprint of the material. So, Raman scattering can be used for the identification of materials.

Fluorescence is very similar to Raman scattering. However, the wavelength of the scattered light is always longer, i.e., the photon energy is lower. In case of fluorescence, the incoming photon is absorbed by a resonant transition of the molecule or atom, which enters an excited state.

After a short time (~nanoseconds), the excited particle returns through several intermediate levels to the ground state by releasing the absorbed energy of the photon again. Part of this energy is released or emitted as a photon. As this photon must have a lower energy than the incident photon, the wavelength of the scattered light is shorter. Fluorescence is something that can be experienced daily. For example, neon tubes use this effect to generate white light. But fluorescence also has its application in medicine: in diagnostics, it is used by fluorescence microscopy. Furthermore, photodynamic therapy takes advantage of it to generate highly reactive molecules and treat certain diseases.

References

1. Träger F, editor. Springer handbook of lasers and optics. New York: Springer; 2012.
2. Hecht E. Optics. London: Pearson; 2016.
3. Pedrotti FL, Pedrotti LM, Pedrotti LS. Introduction to optics. Cambridge: Cambridge University Press; 2017.
4. Maxwell JC. A dynamical theory of the electromagnetic field. Philos Trans R Soc Lond. 1865;155:459–512.
5. Mie G. Beiträge zur Optik trüber Medien, speziell kolloidaler Metallösungen. Ann Phys. 1908;330:377–445.

An Introduction to Laser

2

Gholamreza Shayeganrad

Contents

Abstract

For a better understanding of the special advantages of laser light in oral and maxillofacial surgery, we need to know the principle of generation of laser light and the properties that distinguishes it from conventional light or other energy sources, as well as, how a laser works and the different types of lasers that can be used in medical applications. Light theory branches into the physics of quantum mechanics, which was conceptualized in the twentieth century. Quantum mechanics deals with behavior of nature on the atomic scale or smaller.

This chapter briefly deals with an introduction to laser, properties of laser light, and laser-beam propagation. It begins with a short overview of the theory about the dual nature of light (particle or wave) and discusses the propagation of laser beam, special properties of laser light, and the different types of lasers that are used in medical applications.

Keywords

Laser principle · Coherence · Gaussian beam optics · Laser medicine · Laser surgery

G. Shayeganrad (✉)
Optoelectronic Research Centre, University of Southampton, Southampton, SO17 1BJ, UK
e-mail: g.shayeganrad@soton.ac.uk

S. Stübinger et al. (eds.), *Lasers in Oral and Maxillofacial Surgery*,
https://doi.org/10.1007/978-3-030-29604-9_2

2.1 Introduction

Light is electromagnetic radiation within a certain portion of the electromagnetic spectrum that includes radio waves (AM, FM, and SW), microwaves, THz, IR, visible light, UV, X-rays, and gamma rays. The primary properties of light are intensity, brightness, wave vector, frequency or wavelength, phase, polarization, and its speed in a vacuum, $c = 299, 792, 458$ m/s. The speed of light in a medium depends on the refractive index of the medium, which is c/n. Intensity is the absolute measure of power density of light wave and defines the rate at which energy is delivered to a surface. Brightness is perceptive of intensity of light coming from a light source and depends on the quality of the light wave as well. The frequency of a light wave determines its energy. The wavelength of a light wave is inversely proportional to its frequency. The wave vector is inversely proportional to the wavelength and is defined as the propagation direction of the light wave. Phase cannot be measured directly; however, relative phase can be measured by interferometry. A light wave that vibrates in more than one plane like sunlight is referred to as unpolarized light. Such light waves are created by electric charges that vibrate in a variety of directions. Depending on how the electric field is oriented, we classify polarized light into: linear polarization, circular polarization, elliptical polarization, radial and azimuthal polarization. We say a light wave is linearly polarized if the electric field oscillates in a single plane. If electric field of the wave has a constant magnitude but its direction rotates with time at a steady rate in a plane perpendicular to the direction of the wave, it is called a circular polarized wave. In general case, electric field sweeps out an ellipse in which both magnitude and direction change with time, which is called elliptical polarized wave. Radially and azimuthally polarized beams have been increasingly studied in recent years because of their unique characteristic of axial polarization symmetry, and they can break the diffraction limit with a strong longitudinal electromagnetic field in focus [1–3]. The unpolarized light can be transformed into polarized light by wire grid, polaroid filter, molecular scattering, birefringent materials, retarder waveplates, reflection at Brewster's angle, polarizing cubes, total internal reflection, optical activity, electro-optic effect, or liquid crystals.

The understanding of light refers to the late 1600s with raising important questions about the dual nature of light (particle or wave). Sir Isaac Newton held the idea that light travels as a stream of particles. In 1678, Dutch physicist and astronomer Christiaan Huygens believed that light travels in waves. Huygens' principle was the successful theory to introduce the appearance of the spectrum, as well as the phenomena of reflection and refraction, which indicated that light was a wave. Huygens suggested that the light waves from point sources are spherical with wavefronts, which travel at the speed of light. This theory explains why light bends around corners or spreads out when shining through a pinhole or slit rather than going in a straight line. This phenomenon is called diffraction. Huygens stated that each point on the wavefront behaves as a new source of radiation of the same frequency and phase. Although Newton's particle theory came first, the wave theory of Huygens better described early experiments. Huygens' principle predicts that a given wavefront in the present will be in the future.

None of these theories could explain the complete blackbody spectrum, a body with absolute temperature $T > 0$ that absorbs all the radiation falling on it and emits radiation of all wavelengths. In 1900, Max Planck proposed the existence of a light quantum to explain the blackbody radiation spectrum. In 1905, Albert Einstein individually proposed a solution to the problem of observations made on photoelectric phenomena. Einstein suggested that light is composed of tiny particles called "photons," and each photon has energy of $h\nu$, where $h = 6.63 \times 10^{-34}$ J/s is Planck's constant and ν is the frequency of photons.

In 1924, de Broglie proposed his theory of wave–particle duality in which he said that not only photons of light but also particles of matter such as electrons and atoms possess a dual character, sometimes behaving like a particle and sometimes as a wave. He gave a formula, $\lambda = h/p$, to connect particle characteristics (momentum, p) and wave characteristics (wavelength, λ). Light as well as particle can exhibit both wave and particle properties at the same time. Light waves are also called electromagnetic waves because they are made up of both electric (E) and magnetic (H) fields. Electromagnetic radiation waves can transport energy from one location to another based on Maxwell's equations. Maxwell's equations describe the electromagnetic wave at the classical level. Light is a transverse wave and electromagnetic fields E and H are always perpendicular to each other and oscillate perpendicular to the direction of the traveling wave. The particle properties of light can also be described in terms of a stream of photons that are massless particles and traveling with wavelike properties at the speed of light. A photon is the smallest quantity (quantum) of energy that can be transported.

In 1803, Thomas Young studied the wave properties of light by interference of light through shining two narrow slits separated equally from the center axis. The light emerging from the double-slit spreads out according to Huygens' principle, and the interference pattern appears after overlapping two wavefronts as shown in Fig. 2.1. The two beams exiting from the two slits are electromagnetic waves and can be described by $A_0\sin(2\pi\nu t)$ and $A_0\sin(2\pi\nu t + \delta)$, respectively, where A_0 is the field amplitude, ν is the frequency of light, t is the time, and $\delta = d{\bullet}\sin(\theta)$ is the path difference between the two beams at angle θ.

2.2 Physics of Laser

Although there are many different types of lasers, most lasers follow similar operation principle. The Light Amplification by Stimulated Emission of Radiation (LASER) was developed by Theodore Maiman first [4]. Since then, laser have found a wide range of different scientific and technical applications from the industrial to applied and fundamental research including information technology, consumer electronics, medicine, industry, military, law enforcement, and research. The invention of the laser in 1960 dates from the nineteenth century, when Albert Einstein explained the concept of "stimulated emission of radiation" in a paper delivered in 1916 and German physicist Max Planck proposed the quantum theory of light in 1900. As mentioned before, Planck assumed energy should be composed of discrete packets, or quanta, in the form of photons. According to Planck's radiation law, when an oscillator changes from an energy state E_2 to a state of lower energy E_1, a photon

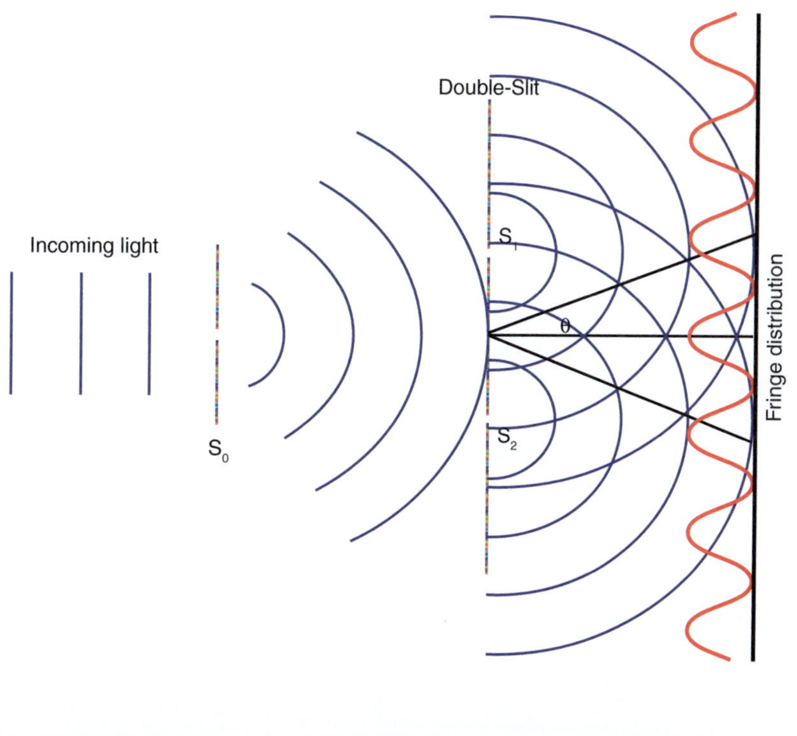

Fig. 2.1 Thomas Young's double-slit interference experiment

with discrete amount of energy $E_2 - E_1 = h\nu$ emits.

The Danish physicist Niels Bohr expanded the quantum theory to help explain the structure of atoms called Bohr's model. In Bohr's model, the nucleus of an atom is surrounded by orbiting electrons that are confined to specific energy states depending on the chemical structure of the atom. In other words, electrons can only occupy certain energy states, which are fingerprints of each atom. An electron can absorb a photon and thereby can be pushed into a higher energy state, called absorption. When an electron is in an exited state, it is inherently unstable and will spontaneously drop to the lower energy states by releasing a photon, called spontaneous emission. The underlying principle of the laser phenomenon stimulated emission is purely a quantum effect. Einstein postulated that emission would be triggered by other photons, in which, an incoming photon of a specific frequency can interact with an excited electron causing it to drop to a lower energy state and release two photons with specific properties, including identical phase, frequency, polarization, and similar direction of propagation. The process of absorption, spontaneous emission, and stimulated emission is depicted in Fig. 2.2.

Notice that the root of the invention of laser lies in fundamental physics research, specifically, a 1917 paper by Albert Einstein on the quantum theory of radiation or stimulated emission, but it was a paper on laser theory published in 1958 by two physicists, Charles Townes and Arthur L. Schawlow, which spurred the race to make the first working laser. According to the Einstein principle, there is an equal probability that a photon will absorb or emit. Thereby, according to the

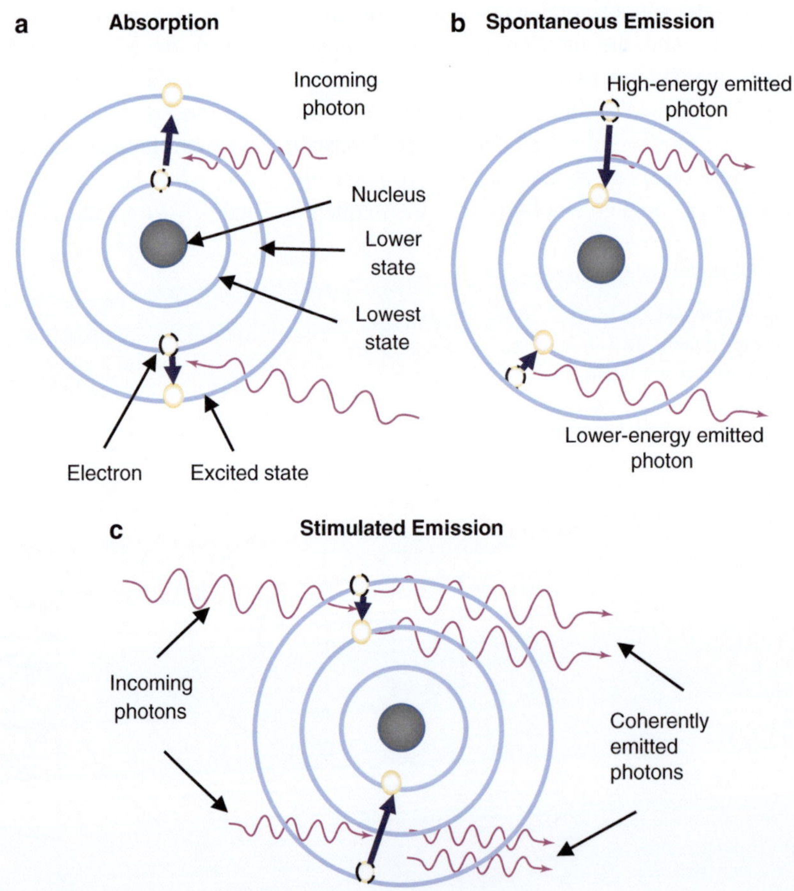

Fig. 2.2 Schematic of absorption (**a**), spontaneous emission (**b**), and stimulated emission (**c**) of two photons with different frequencies

Boltzmann distribution that when there are more atoms in the ground state than in the excited states and light is incident on the system of atoms, in thermal equilibrium, the probability of absorption of energy is much higher than emission. However, in the case that more atoms are in an excited state than in a ground state and strike with photons of energy similar to the excited atoms, many of atoms will induce the process of stimulated emission, whereby a single excited atom would emit a photon identical to the interacting photon. Under the proper conditions, a single input photon can result in a cascade of stimulated photons, and thereby amplification of photons will result. All of the photons generated in this way are in phase, traveling in the same direction, and have the same frequency as the input photon.

As shown in Fig. 2.3, a laser requires three major parts: (1) gain medium (e.g., gas, solid, liquid dye or semiconductor); (2) pump source (e.g., an electric discharge, flashlamp, or laser diode); and (3) the feedback system, e.g., optical resonator. For instance, in the case of the first invented laser, the gain medium was ruby, and the population inversion was produced by intense broadband illumination from a xenon flashlamp. However, in the case of diode-pumped lasers, the population inversion is produced by laser diode that benefits from higher total conversion efficiency. Laser wavelength emission is determined by the gain medium and the characteristics of the optical resonator (see, for example, [5–12]). It is noticeable that some high-gain lasers do not use an optical oscillator and work based on amplified spontaneous emission (ASE) without needing feedback of the light back into the gain medium. Such lasers emit light with low coherence but high bandwidth.

For optical frequencies, population inversion cannot be achieved in a two-level system. In 1956, Bloembergen proposed a mechanism in which atoms are pumped into an excited state by an external source of energy. A lasing medium consists of at least three energy levels: a ground state E_1, an intermediate (metastable) state; E_2, with a relatively long lifetime, t_s, and a high energy pump state; and E_3, as shown in Fig. 2.4. To obtain population inversion, t_s must be greater than t_3, the lifetime of the pump state E_3. Note

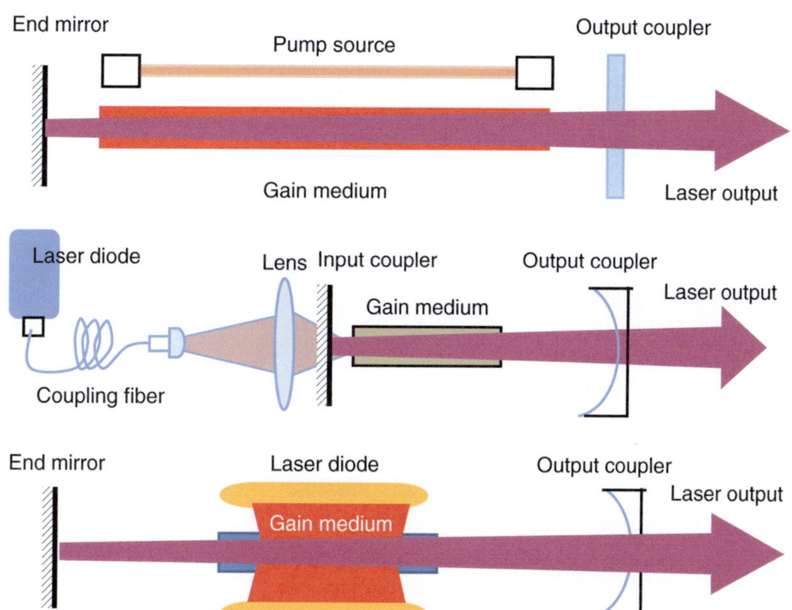

Fig. 2.3 Schematic diagram of a typical laser (top) flashlamp pumped, (middle) laser-diode end-pumped, and (bottom) laser-diode side-pumped configurations, showing the three major parts: (1) laser gain medium, (2) pump source, and (3) optical resonator

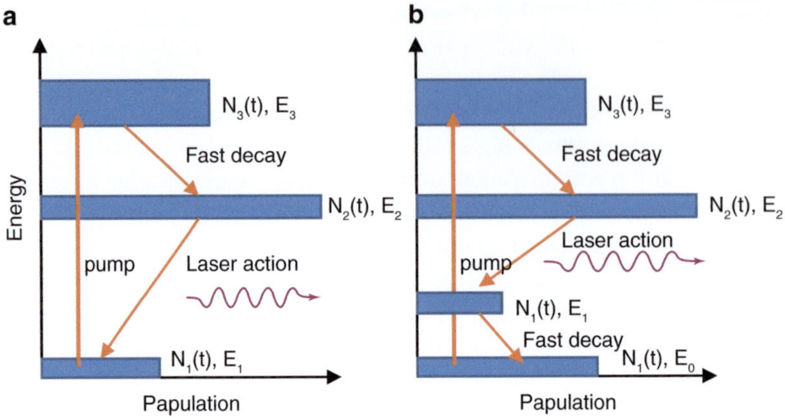

Fig. 2.4 Schematic diagram of three-level laser (**a**) and four-level laser (**b**)

that a characteristic of the three-level laser material is that the laser transition takes place between the excited laser level E_2 and the final ground state E_1, the lowest energy level of the system. The three-level system has low efficiency. The four-level system avoids this disadvantage.

Figure 2.4 compares schematically the three-level and four-level laser systems. In three-level lasers, initially, all atoms of the laser material are in the ground state level E_1. The pump radiation rises the ground state atoms to a short-lived pump state E_3. Atoms from this state undergo fast decay (radiationless transition) to a metastable state E_2. In this process, the energy lost by the electron is transferred to the lattice. A population inversion takes place between ground state and the metastable state where the lasing transition occurs. In general, the "pumping" level 3 is actually made up of a number of bands, so that the optical pumping can be accomplished over a broad spectral range. If pumping intensity is below laser threshold, atoms in level 2 predominantly return to the ground state by spontaneous emission. While, when the pump intensity is above laser threshold, the stimulated emission is the dominated processes compared with spontaneous emission. The stimulated radiation produces the laser output beam.

In the case of four-level lasers, the pump excitation extends again by radiation from the ground state (now level E_0) to a broad absorption band E_3. As in the case of the three-level system, the atoms so excited will transfer fast radiationless transitions into the intermediate sharp level 2. The electrons return to the fourth level E_1, which is situated above the ground state E_0, by the emission of a photon to proceed the laser action. Finally, the electrons return to the ground level E_0 by radiationless transition. In a true four-level system, the terminal laser level E_1 will be empty. To qualify as a four-level system, a material must possess a relaxation time between the terminal laser level and the ground level, which is fast compared to the fluorescence lifetime, t_s. In addition, the terminal laser level E_1 would be far above the ground state E_0 so that its thermal population can be considered as negligible. In a kind of situation, where the lower laser level is so close to the ground state that an appreciable population in that level occurs in thermal equilibrium at the operating temperature, the laser called quasi-three-level laser. As a consequence, the unpumped gain medium causes some reabsorption loss at the laser wavelength same as three-level lasers.

The purpose of the resonator is to provide the positive feedback necessary to cause oscillation. The resonator has mirror at the ends so that photons are reflected back and forth and are constantly renewing the process of stimulated emission as they strike more of the excited atoms in the laser medium. The mirrors also align the photons so that they force to travel in the same direction. Typically, one will be a high reflector (HR) and the other will be a partial reflector (PR). The latter is called output coupler that allows some of the light to transmit out of the resonator to produce the laser output beam. The buildup of oscillation is triggered by spontaneous emission. The produced photons by spontaneous emission are reflected by the mirrors back into the laser medium and amplified by stimulated emission. Other optical devices, such as prism, Q-switch modulators, filters, etalon, and lens, may be placed within the optical resonator to produce a tunable laser, pulsed laser, and narrow bandwidth laser or shape the laser beam.

If the gain medium has a homogeneous (Lorentzian) gain profile, as the oscillating intensity grows and the population of excited atoms depletes by causing sufficient stimulated emission, photons oscillating at ν_0 can emit from all atoms in the medium, and oscillation at frequency ν_0 can suppress oscillation at any other frequency under the gain profile. Generally, the oscillation will build up with frequency, which has maximum emission probability. However, in an inhomogeneously broadened gaseous medium, the additional oscillation at frequencies far away from ν_0 is also possible.

2.3 Laser Light Properties

The laser happens when stimulated-emission process is dominant compared with absorption and spontaneous emission. It means, in laser, stimulated emission leads to the unique characteristics, e.g., (1) coherence, (2) divergence and directionality, (3) monochromatic, and (4) brightness. These properties differentiate laser light from ordinary light and make it very interesting for a range of applications.

2.3.1 Coherence

Coherence of electromagnetic radiation means maintaining a constant phase difference between two points of wavefront of the wave in space (spatial coherence) and in time (temporal coherence). Coherence is one of the most important concepts in optics and is strongly related to the ability of light to exhibit interference effects. Temporal coherence is related to the intrinsic spectrum bandwidth of the light source, while spatial coherence can be affected by size of the light source. Laser radiation has high spatial and temporal coherence compared with ordinary light sources. In ordinary light sources like bubble lamp, sodium lamp, and torchlight, the electron transition from higher energy level to lower energy level occurs in spontaneous process. In other words, electron transition in ordinary light sources is random in time. In these sources, no phase relation exists between the emitted photons, and the phase difference between different atoms changes in time. Thus, the photons emitted by an ordinary light source are out of phase as illustrated schematically in Fig. 2.5.

In contrast to incoherent sources, in laser, a phase relation between electron transitions exists. In other words, in laser, electron transition occurs in specific time. Therefore, the emission of laser is in phase in space and time as illustrated schematically in Fig. 2.5. In laser, the stimulated emission process produces coherence light. Because of the coherence, a large amount of power can be concentrated in a narrow space. For a light source with a Gaussian emission spectrum, the coherence length can be obtained as follows:

$$l_c = c\tau_c = \sqrt{\frac{2\ln 2}{\pi n}}\frac{\lambda^2}{\Delta\lambda} = \sqrt{\frac{2\ln 2}{\pi n}}\frac{c}{\Delta v} \quad (2.1)$$

where c is the speed of light, n is the refractive index of the medium, λ is the central wavelength, and $\Delta\lambda$ is the full-width half-maximum (FWHM) of the emission peak in wavelength spectrum. The light sources with a small $\Delta\lambda$ such as lasers are highly temporally coherent, while the light sources with a large $\Delta\lambda$ such as white light lamps are

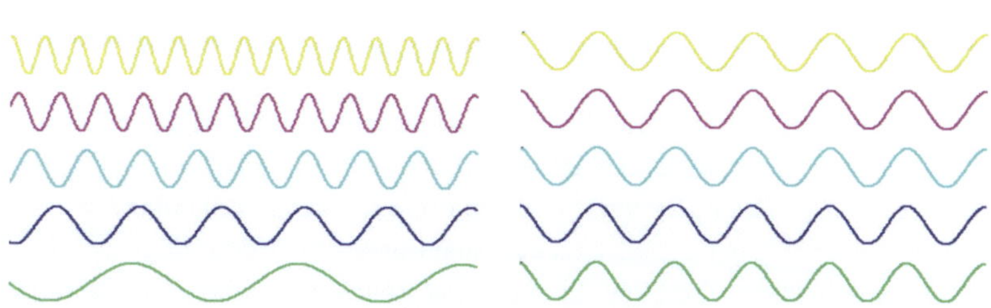

Fig. 2.5 Schematic of incoherent (left) and (right) coherent light waves

Table 2.1 Comparing the coherence length and coherence time of some medical laser systems and ordinary sources

Source	$\Delta\nu_c$ (THz)	τ_c	$l_c = c\tau_c$
Filtered sunlight (400–800 nm, $\lambda_0 = 550$ nm)	374	1.8 fs	0.32 μm
InGaAs ($E_g = 0.9$ eV, $\lambda_0 = 1300$ nm)	6.2	0.11 ps	17.7 μm
Low-pressure sodium lamp ($\lambda_0 = 589$ nm)	0.5	1.33 ps	0.399 mm
Single-mode He-Ne laser ($\lambda_0 = 633$ nm)	1×10^{-6}	0.66 μs	198 m
CO_2 laser ($\lambda_0 = 10.6$ μm)	40×10^{-6}	0.16 ns	4.8 m
Ruby laser ($\lambda_0 = 694$ nm)	0.36	1.85 ps	0.555 mm
Nd:YAG ($\lambda_0 = 1064$ nm)	0.18	3.7 ps	1.11 mm
Nd:Glass ($\lambda_0 = 1059$ nm)	9	73.8 fs	22.2 μm
Dye laser (Typ. R6G $\lambda_0 = 570$–610 nm)	100	6.6 fs	1.98 μm

temporally incoherent. The coherence length and coherence time of some medical optical sources and ordinary sources are compared in Table 2.1.

There is not a single universal technique to measure laser linewidth or coherence length. Temporal coherence can be measured by the Michelson interferometer, while spatial coherence can be measured by Young's double-slit experiment. The van Cittert-Zernike theorem states that the spatial coherence area, A_c, is given by the following:

$$A_c = \frac{d^2\lambda^2}{\pi D^2} \tag{2.2}$$

where D is the diameter of the light source, and d is the distance away. The spatial coherence area is large for sources with small diameter and large wavelength.

2.3.2 Divergence and Directionality

The propagation and directionality of radiation is described by diffraction theory. Maximum intensity of radiation is limited by the angle of divergence. In conventional light sources, photons emit and travel in random direction. Therefore, the radiation from these light sources has a large divergence angle. However, in laser, the optical resonator leads to travel all photons in the same direction with low beam divergence, which results in a high directionality. In contrast, the collimated light waves from a laser diverge little over relatively great distances. For example, a laser beam can be pointed at the moon, which is ~4×10^5 km away from earth. For diffraction-limited laser radiation with wavelength λ and diameter D, the divergence angle is given from diffraction theory by the following:

$$\theta_d = 1.22\frac{\lambda}{D} \tag{2.3}$$

If a free-aberration positive lens is used for focusing a laser light, the radius of the central lobe behind the lens on the focal plane is $a \approx f\cdot\theta_d \approx 1.22f\cdot\lambda/D$, where f is the focal length of the lens. For a multimode beam, TEM_{pl}, the minimum diameter of the focal spot is given by the following:

$$a = 1.22\frac{\lambda f(2p+l+1)}{D} \tag{2.4}$$

2.3.3 Monochromaticity

Monochromatic light means a light containing a single color or frequency. In ordinary light sources, the emitted photons have many different energies, frequencies, wavelengths, or colors with a wide spectrum bandwidth. However, in laser, stimulated emission leads all the emitted photons to have the same energy, frequency, or wavelength. Therefore, laser radiation has a very narrow spectrum bandwidth. This means that the radiation emitted by the laser is nearly monochromatic. This purity is unique to laser light in contrast to all other light sources which are of mixed wavelengths. Monochromaticity enables great precision when a laser is used for medical or surgical purposes because components of human tissue preferentially absorb electromagnetic energy of specific wavelengths. Further, monochromatic aspect of lasers is essential for temporal coherence.

According to the Heisenberg's uncertainty principle, if the momentum of a particle is precisely known, it is impossible to know the position precisely and vice versa. This relationship also applies to energy and time. It means one cannot measure the precise energy of a system in a finite amount of time. Uncertainties in the products of "conjugate pairs" (momentum and position, and energy and time) are as below:

$$\Delta x \Delta p \geq \frac{\hbar}{2} \tag{2.5a}$$

$$\Delta t \Delta E \geq \frac{\hbar}{2} \tag{2.5b}$$

where Δ refers to the uncertainty in that variable and $\hbar = h/2\pi$ is reduced Planck's constant in which h is Planck's constant. For a monochromatic light with $\Delta E \approx 0$, Heisenberg's uncertainty principle results to $\Delta t \rightarrow \infty$. It means a perfectly monochromatic source (if it existed!) would give an infinitely long wavetrain which is uniformly distributed over the infinite constant-phase planes.

2.3.4 Brightness

The brightness is characterized by a light source that takes into account the power that can convey into the laser spot. It is defined as the power emitted per unit area and unit solid angle as follows:

$$B = \frac{p}{A.\Omega} \tag{2.6}$$

where P is power, $A = \pi D^2/4$ is area of laser spot, and Ω is solid angle defined as below:

$$\Omega = 2\pi\left(1 - \cos\theta\right) \approx \pi\theta^2 \tag{2.7}$$

Maximum brightness is obtained if $\theta = \theta_d$. From Eqs. (2.6) and (2.3), maximum brightness can be simplified as follows:

$$B = \frac{4p}{\pi^2 \left(1.22\right)^2 \lambda^2} \tag{2.8}$$

One can see that maximum brightness is proportional to the inverse square of the center wavelength of radiation. Notice that in an ordinary light source, the light spreads out uniformly in all directions, while, in laser, the light due to *directionality* spreads in small region of space. Thereby, laser light has greater intensity and brightness when compared to the ordinary light.

2.4 Gaussian Beam Optics

In most laser applications, it is necessary to know the propagation characteristics of laser beam. The propagation of a laser beam is a paraxial solution of the Maxwell's equations. In general, laser beam propagation can be approximated by assuming that the laser beam has a Gaussian intensity profile. A Gaussian beam has a radially symmetrical distribution whose electric field variation is given by the following:

$$E\left(r,z\right) = E_0\left(z\right)\exp\left[-r^2 / w^2\left(z\right)\right] \tag{2.9}$$

with a Gaussian intensity distribution in a cross-sectional plane at z, r as follows:

$$I\left(r,z\right) = I_0\left(z\right)\exp\left[-2r^2 / w^2\left(z\right)\right] \tag{2.10}$$

where $I_0(z)$ is the beam peak intensity in a cross-sectional plane at z. Many lasers emit beams with a Gaussian profile. The fundamental transverse mode, or TEM_{00} mode, is a perfect Gaussian beam. In most cases, the laser output beam deviates from TEM_{00} mode. When a Gaussian beam propagates into an optical medium like lens, a Gaussian beam is transformed into another Gaussian beam characterized by a different set of parameters.

A simple and commonly used measure to evaluate laser beam propagation is the beam propagation ratio M-square factor M^2, which compares the propagation properties of a real beam to those of a perfect diffraction-limited Gaussian beam. In other words, the $M^2 \geq 1$ describes the deviation of a laser beam from a perfect Gaussian beam. For a perfect laser beam, $M^2 = 1$. Most gas lasers have $M^2 \approx 1$. Although most solid-state lasers have an M^2 value between 1.1 and 1.5, some lasers, such as flashlamp pumped lasers and high-power solid-state lasers, have an M^2 value over 10.

A Gaussian beam can be fully described with the use of the complex beam parameter, q, and ABCD matrix. It facilitates the study of Gaussian beams in the presence of optical elements such as lenses, spherical mirrors, etc. The general form of the complex beam parameter, q, can be written in terms of two real parameters, R and w, as follows:

$$\frac{1}{q(z)} = \frac{1}{R(z)} - i\frac{\lambda M^2}{n\pi w^2(z)} \tag{2.11}$$

where $R(z)$ is the radius of curvature of beam wavefront and $w(z)$ is the spot radius of the beam at z. For the Gaussian beam, spot radius w is considered the radius where $I = I_0/e^2$. At focusing point, a Gaussian beam achieves a minimum spot size (called waist with radius w_0) when the wavefront becomes a plane ($R = \infty$). Therefore:

$$\frac{1}{q_0} = -i\frac{\lambda M^2}{n\pi w_0^2} \tag{2.12}$$

The transformation of a Gaussian beam can be described by the following:

$$q_2 = \frac{Aq_1 + B}{Cq_1 + D} \tag{2.13}$$

where A, B, C, and D are the elements of the $ABCD$ transform matrix characterizing the optical medium. From $ABCD$ matrix of free space ($A = 1$, $B = z$, $C = 0$, $D = 1$) with thickness of z, the value of q at z away from the waist in free space are given by the following:

$$q = q_0 + z \tag{2.14}$$

or we can obtain the following equation by applying Eq. (2.13) and considering $ABCD$ matrix of a thin lens with focal length f ($A = 1$, $B = 0$, $C = -1/f$, $D = 1$) as follows:

$$\frac{1}{q_2} = \frac{1}{q_1} - \frac{1}{f} \tag{2.15}$$

Figure 2.6 illustrates propagation characteristics of a Gaussian beam showing spherical wave-

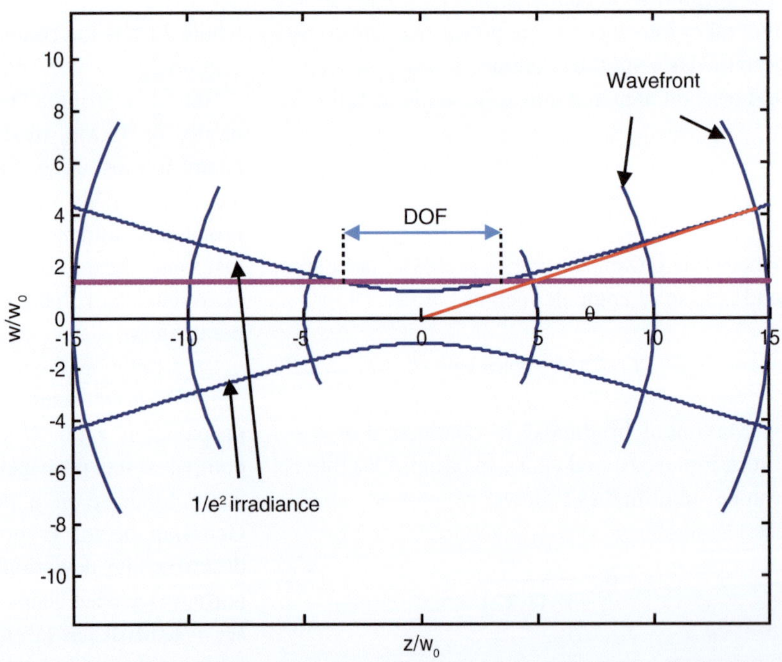

Fig. 2.6 Propagation characteristics of a Gaussian beam with parameters $w_0 = 50$ μm, $\lambda = 2.94$ μm, and $M^2 = 15$, showing spherical wavefronts. DOF is depth of focus

fronts. Once again, a Gaussian beam does not come to a focus at a point but rather achieves a minimum spot size w_0 where the wavefront becomes a plane. From Eqs. (2.11)–(2.14), one can obtain the following:

$$w(z) = w_0 \left[1 + \left(\frac{M^2 \lambda z}{n\pi w_0^2} \right)^2 \right]^{1/2} \tag{2.16}$$

$$R(z) = z \left[1 + \left(\frac{n\pi w_0^2}{M^2 \lambda z} \right)^2 \right] \tag{2.17}$$

Equations (2.16) and (2.17) can be simplified in the following forms:

$$w(z) = w_0 \left(1 + \frac{z^2}{z_R^2} \right)^{1/2} \tag{2.18}$$

$$R(z) = z \left(1 + \frac{z_R^2}{z^2} \right) \tag{2.19}$$

where:

$$z_R = \frac{n\pi w_0^2}{\lambda M^2} \tag{2.20}$$

is the Rayleigh length that reflects the distance from the waist to the place where the spot size increases by a factor of $\sqrt{2}$.

The divergence of a Gaussian laser beam in the depth of focus (DOF) is negligible, and it can be considered as parallel beam. The DOF or confocal parameter is twice the Rayleigh length:

$$\text{DOF} = \frac{2n\pi w_0^2}{\lambda M^2} \tag{2.21}$$

The parameter $w(z)$ approaches a straight line for $z >> z_R$. The angle between this straight line and the central axis of the beam is called far-field divergence:

$$\theta \simeq \frac{\lambda M^2}{\pi w_0} \tag{2.22}$$

The angle θ is inversely proportional to the beam waist w_0 and proportional to the M-square factor M^2 and the wavelength λ.

As mentioned in Sect. 2.2, according to the gain material, lasers can be divided into solid-state, gas, dye (liquid), or semiconductor. In the following, the commonly used lasers with typical applications and wavelengths are listed in each type.

2.5 Solid-State Lasers

The first functional laser was invented by Maiman in 1960. It was a ruby laser in visible region (694.3 nm) pumped by a xenon flashlamp; the first laser was used in medicine in 1960 by Leon Goldman, the "father of laser medicine," who tried to lighten tattoos by aiming a ruby laser at the pigmented skin until the pigment granules broke apart. In 1963, Charles Campbell used a ruby laser to treat a detached retina. In 1980s, the Nd:YAG flashlamp pumped laser was developed. Soon after, novel laser diode-pumped solid-stare lasers with different gain medium were constructed. So far, continuous-wave (CW) or pulsed solid-state lasers from different crystals, mainly Nd^{3+} doped, such as Nd:YAG, Nd:YLF, Nd:YVO_4, (Er, Nd):YAG, (Ho, Nd):YAG, Nd:$GdVO_4$, Nd:LYSO, Nd:YAP, Nd:YAB, Nd:Mgo:$LiNbO_3$, Nd:GSAG, Nd:$LuVO_4$ Nd:$YAIO_3$, Ti:sapphire, Yb:KGD$(WO_4)_2$, and Nd,La:SrF_2, with different laser emission wavelength has been demonstrated (see, for instance, [6, 7, 13–20]). In ref. [21] influence of length of gain medium and pump beam quality on performance of the laser and required design parameters has been investigated. The active ion of Nd^{3+} has mainly three allowed transitions of $^4F_{3/2} \rightarrow {}^4I_{9/2}$, $^4F_{3/2} \rightarrow {}^4I_{11/2}$, and $^4F_{3/2} \rightarrow {}^4I_{13/2}$, corresponding to the emitting wavelengths around 0.9, 1.06, and 1.3 μm, respectively, which makes it possible to achieve single- and multi-wavelength operations of an Nd^{3+} laser through a proper design of the laser. The capability of a laser can be extended by multiple wavelength engineered emission. Notice that dual- or multi-wavelength simultaneously emission laser sources have been used in different scientific and technical applications in optical coherence tomography (OCT) [22, 23],

Table 2.2 The most important solid-state lasers with wavelength and typical applications

Laser type	Wavelength(s)	Applications
Ruby	694.3 nm	Pulsed holography, tattoo removal and cosmetic dermatology, high-speed photography, hair removal
Nd:YAG	1.064 μm, (1.32 μm, 946 nm)	Material processing, laser target designation, glaucoma surgery, dentistry, research, pumping other lasers, cataract surgery, water vapour remote sensing, underwater communication
Erbium-doped glass/fiber	1.53–1.56 μm	Optical amplifiers for telecommunications
Ho:YAG	2.1	Surgery, dentistry, material processing, arthroscopic surgery, remote sensing
Er:YAG	2.94 μm, 1.53–1.56 μm	Surgery, resurfacing of human skin, oral surgery, dentistry, osteotomy, removal of warts, soft tissue
Er,Cr:YSGG	2.790 μm	Surgery, dentistry, soft tissue
Tm:YAG	2.01 μm	Remote sensing, material processing, optical communication, dentistry

optical testing [24], atom interferometry [25], spectroscopy [26], THz radiation generation [27, 28], and remote sensing [29–31]. Table 2.2 summarizes the most important solid-state lasers with their wavelength emission and typical applications.

2.6 Gas Lasers

The gas lasers can be basically categorized into three distinct families: (i) the neutral gas laser, (ii) the ionized gas laser, and (iii) the molecular gas laser. Table 2.3 summarizes the most important gas lasers with their wavelength and typical applications. He-Ne laser is the first invented gas laser in 1960 by Ali Javan. This laser radiates in a continuous regime CW and uses electric discharge excitation in a neutral gaseous environment. It soon became the first commercial laser with a power of 1 mW. The argon laser operating in the visible and ultraviolet spectral regions was invented in 1964 by William Bridge. CO_2 laser was developed by Kumar Patel in 1964 at Bell Laboratories. The CO_2 laser operates both pulsed and CW mode in the middle infrared region on rotational-vibrational transitions of carbon dioxide at 10.6 and 9.4 μm wavelengths. It is one of the most powerful and efficient lasers available.

Table 2.3 The most important gas lasers with wavelength and typical applications

Laser type	Wavelength(s)	Applications
He-Ne laser	632.8 nm	Interferometry, holography, spectroscopy, barcode scanning, laboratory testing, aiming beam
Ar^+ ion laser	454.6 nm, 488.0 nm, 514.5 nm	Retinal phototherapy (for diabetes), plastic surgery, dermatology, lithography, confocal microscopy, spectroscopy pumping other lasers
CO_2 laser	10.6 μm, (9.4 μm)	Material processing (cutting, welding, etc.), dentistry, osteotomy, vaporization and coagulation, gynecology
Excimer laser	193 nm (ArF), 248 nm (KrF), 308 nm (XeCl), 353 nm (XeF)	Ultraviolet lithography for semiconductor manufacturing, surgery, skin treatment, material processing, lithography, nanofabrication, LASIK

2.7 Semiconductor Lasers

Semiconductor lasers or diode lasers are a special type of solid-state lasers. They are portable, compact, and efficient with wavelength versatility and reliable benefits. This type of laser can be operated in a CW or pulsed mode. The frequency of the emitted photons depends on the gain material composition. Typical operation wavelengths of different diode lasers are summarized in Table 2.4. Diode lasers were developed very soon after solid-state and gas lasers. The first laser

Table 2.4 Typical operation wavelength of different diode lasers

Laser type	InP	InGaN/GaN	GaSb based	InGaAsP	Quantum cascade laser (QCL)	Vertical-cavity surface-emitting laser (VCSEL)
Wavelength(s)	375–488 nm	630–980 nm	1.5–4 μm	1.0–2.1 μm	Mid-IR to Far-IR	650–3500 nm

Table 2.5 The medical applications of diode lasers in terms of wavelength

Application	Wavelength (nm)									
Dentistry			430–470					810–980		
Surgery				630–635				800–1500		
LLLT			465	630		652	660–690			
PDT	405	410–430		630	635	652	660–690	753		
Hyperthermia tumors								940, 980	1064	
Cosmetic treatment								810		
Tumor ablation								800–980		
Blood oximetry				630						
Ecology										1500–4000
Acne treatment										1450–1470

emission from a semiconductor GaAs was obtained in 1962 by Robert N. Hall at General Electric and by Marshall Nathan at IBM TJ Watson Research Center.

The principle operation of semiconductor lasers is different from gas and solid-state lasers. It is based on recombination "electrons" and "holes." Forward electric bias across the p-n junction of gain medium creates an area with an excess of electrons and holes that recombine with the release of photons. This recombination can be stimulated by a positive feedback induced by an optical resonator. The optical gain is directly proportional to the injection current through the junction and also to the reciprocal value of the size of the active region. The maximum emission wavelength of semiconductor lasers is given by the following:

$$\lambda_{\max} = \frac{hc}{E_g + kT/2} \approx \frac{hc}{E_g} \tag{2.23}$$

with the spectral bandwidth of:

$$\Delta v = \frac{1.8kT}{h} \tag{2.24}$$

where T is the absolute temperature in Kelvin, and $k = 1.38\ 9\ 10^{-23}$ J/K is the Boltzmann constant. These equations show that the peak wavelength is inversely proportional to the bandgap energy E_g, and bandwidth is proportional to the absolute temperature.

Semiconductor diode lasers are used in different medical applications such as photodynamic therapy (PDT), photodynamic detection (PDD), optical coherence tomography (OCT), nonsurgical treatment of varicose veins, dentistry and soft-tissue oral surgery, cosmetic treatments, blood oximetry, low-level laser therapy (LLLT), tumor ablation, ecology, coagulation, and hair removal. Some typical applications of semiconductor lasers in terms of wavelength are summarized in Table 2.5.

It is noticeable that light-emitted diodes (LEDs) are an optical semiconductor device that emits incoherent light when voltage is applied. Their high reliability, high efficiency, and lower overall system cost compared with lasers and lamps make these devices very affordable and attractive to both consumer and industrial segments. LEDs are now used in a large number of diverse markets and applications. LEDs do not carry the same eye safety concerns or warnings that laser diodes do. But LEDs cannot be made into extremely small, highly collimated, and optically dense spots. In applications where extremely high power density within a small area is required, a laser is almost always required.

References

1. Dorn R, Quabis S, Leuchs G. Sharper focus for a radially polarized light beam. Phys Rev Lett. 2003;91(23):233901.
2. Zhan Q. Cylindrical vector beams: from mathematical concepts to applications. Adv Opt Photon. 2009;1(1):1
3. Youngworth KS, Brown TG. Focusing of high numerical aperture cylindrical-vector beams. Opt Express. 2000;7(2):77.
4. Maiman TH. Stimulated optical radiation in ruby. Nature. 1960;187:493–4.
5. Shayeganrad G, Mashhadi L. Dual-wavelength CW diode-end-pumped a-cut Nd:YVO4 laser at 1064.5 and 1085.5 nm. Appl Phys B Lasers Opt. 2012;111:189–94.
6. Shayeganrad G, Huang Y-C, Mashhadi L. Tunable single and multiwavelength continuous-wave c-cut Nd:YVO4 laser. Appl Phys B Lasers Opt. 2012;108:67–72.
7. Shayeganrad G. Actively Q-switched Nd:YVO4 dual-wavelength stimulated Raman laser at 1178.9 nm and 1199.9 nm. Opt Commun. 2013;292:131–4.
8. Zapata-Nava OJ, Rodríguez-Montero P, Iturbe-Castillo MD, Treviño-Palacios CG. Grating cavity dual wavelength dye laser. Opt Express. 2011;19:3483–93.
9. Liu X, Yang X, Lu F, Ng J, Zhou X, Lu C. Stable and uniform dual-wavelength erbium-doped fiber laser based on fiber Bragg gratings and photonic crystal fiber. Opt Express. 2005;13:142–7.
10. Guo L, Lan R, Liu H, Yu H, Zhang H, Wang J, Hu D, et al. 1319 nm and 1338 nm dual-wavelength operation of LD end-pumped Nd:YAG ceramic laser. Opt Express. 2010;18:9098–106.
11. Yao B, Tian Y, Li G, Wang Y. InGaAs/GaAs saturable absorber for diode-pumped passively Q-switched dual-wavelength Tm:YAP lasers. Opt Express. 2010;18:13574–9.
12. Yoshioka H, Nakamura S, Ogama T, Wada S. Dual-wavelength mode-locked Yb:YAG ceramic laser in single cavity. Opt Express. 2010;18:1479–86.
13. Shayeganrad G, Mashhadi L. Dual-wavelength CW diode-end-pumped a-cut Nd:YVO4 laser at 1064.5 and 1085.5 nm. Appl Phys B Lasers Opt. 2012;111:189–94.
14. Luo CW, Yang YQ, Mak IT, Chang YH, Wu KH, Kobayashi T. A widely tunable dual-wavelength CW Ti:sapphire laser with collinear output. Opt Express. 2008;16:3305.
15. Qin Z, Qiao Z, Xie G, Yuan P, Ma J, Qian L, Jiang D, Ma F, Tang F, Su L. Femtosecond and dual-wavelength picosecond operations of Nd,La:SrF_2 disordered crystal laser. IEEE Photon J. 2017;9:1502007.
16. Li W, Hao Q, Ding J, Zeng H. Continuous-wave multi-wavelength diode-pumped Yb:GYSO laser. J Opt A Pure Appl Opt. 2008;10:095307.
17. Li CY, Bo Y, Xu JL, Tian CY, Peng QJ, Cui DF, Xu ZY. Simultaneous dual-wavelength oscillation at 1116 and 1123 nm of Nd:YAG laser. Opt Commun. 2011;284:4574–6.
18. Brenier A. Tunable THz frequency difference from a diode-pumped dual-wavelength Yb3+:KGd(WO4)2 laser with chirped volume Bragg gratings. Laser Phys Lett. 2011;8:20–524.
19. Xu B, Wang Y, Cheng Y, Lin Z, Xu H, Cai Z, Moncorgé R. Diode-pumped CW laser operation of a c-cut Nd:YAlO3 crystal on low-gain emission lines around 1.1 um. IEEE Photon J. 2015;7:1503407.
20. Shayeganrad G. Tunable single- and dual-wavelength nanosecond Ti:Sapphire laser around 765 nm. Appl Phys B. 2018;124(8):162.
21. Shayeganrad G, Mashhadi L. Efficient analytic model to optimum design laser resonator and optical coupling system of diode-end-pumped solid-state lasers: Influence of gain medium length and pump beam M2 factor. Appl Opt. 2008;47:619–27.
22. Mao Y, Chang S, Murdock E, Flueraru C. Simultaneous dual-wavelength-band common-path swept-source optical coherence tomography with single polygon mirror scanner. Opt Lett. 2011;36:1990–2.
23. Chang S, Mao Y, Flueraru C. Dual-source swept-source optical coherence tomography reconstructed on integrated spectrum. Int J Optics. 2012;2012:565823.
24. García-Arellano A, Granados-Agustín F, Campos-García M, Cornejo-Rodríguez A. Ronchi test with equivalent wavelength. Appl Opt. 2012;51:3071–80.
25. Ménoret V, Geiger R, Stern G, Zahzam N, Battelier B, Bresson A, Landragin A, Bouyer P. Dual-wavelength laser source for onboard atom interferometry. Opt Lett. 2011;36:4128–30.
26. Shibata S. Dual-wavelength spectrophotometry. Angew Chem Int Ed Eng. 1976;15:673–9.
27. Saha A, Ray A, Mukhopadhyay S, Sinha N, Datta PK. Simultaneous multi-wavelength oscillation of Nd laser around 1.3 lm: a potential source for coherent terahertz generation. Opt Express. 2006;29:4721–6.
28. Maestre H, Torregrosa AJ, Fernández-Pousa CR, Rico ML, Capmany J. Dual-wavelength green laser with a 4.5 THz frequency difference based on self-frequency- doubling in Nd3+ –doped aperiodically poled lithium niobate. Opt Lett. 2008;33:1008–10.
29. Shayeganrad G, Parvin P. DIAL–phoswich hybrid system for remote sensing of radioactive plumes in order to evaluate external dose rate. Prog Nucl Energy. 2008;51:420–33.
30. Fredriksson KA. DIAL technique for pollution monitoring: improvements and complementary systems. Appl Opt. 1985;19:3297–304.
31. Shayeganrad G. Single laser-based differential absorption lidar (DIAL) for remote profiling atmospheric oxygen. Opt Lasers Eng. 2018;111:80–5.

Suggested Reading

Part of the materials presented in this chapter can be found in details in numerous quantum theories of light, optics, and laser books, as follows:

Principles of lasers, by Orazio Svelto and David C. Hanna, 5th Edition, 2010, Springer

Optics, by Eugene Hecht, 5th Edition, 2017, Pearson Addison Wesley

The Quantum Theory of Light, by Rodney Loudon 3rd Edition, 2003, Oxford University Press

Quantum Electronics, by Amnon Yariv, 3rd Edition, 1989, John Wiley & Sons

Laser and electro-optics: Fundamentals and engineering, by Christopher C. Davis, 2nd Edition, 2014, Cambridge University Press

Lasers: Fundamentals and applications, by K. Thyagarajan und A. Ghatak, 2nd dition, 2010, Springer

Semiconductor-laser fundamentals: Physics of the Gain materials, by Weng W. Chow, and Stephan W. Koch, 1999, Springer

Laser-tissue interactions: Fundamentals and applications, by Markolf H. Niemz, 3rd enlarged edition, 2007, Springer

An Open Access Encyclopedia for Photonics and Laser Technology (2012)

Laser–Tissue Interaction

3

Azhar Zam

Contents

Abstract

Since their invention, lasers have been successfully employed in many applications. The basic principle of the interaction of laser with biological tissue is explained, and how many factors may influence the results of the interaction are also discussed. The tissue optical properties, the primary factors of laser interactions, including absorption and scattering, are defined. Other factors, i.e., photochemical, photothermal, photoablation, plasma-induced ablation, and photodisruption, are also discussed.

Keywords

Lasers · Tissue optical properties · Absorption
Scattering · Photochemical · Photothermal
Photoablation · Plasma-induced ablation
Photodisruption

A. Zam (✉)
Department of Biomedical Engineering, University of Basel, Allschwil, Switzerland
e-mail: azhar.zam@unibas.ch

S. Stübinger et al. (eds.), *Lasers in Oral and Maxillofacial Surgery*,
https://doi.org/10.1007/978-3-030-29604-9_3

3.1 Introduction

Many different interactions might happen when a laser is impinging onto biological tissues. The laser parameters as well as tissue characteristics play a critical role in this diversity. In this chapter, we discuss the tissue optical properties which are essential for laser–tissue interaction. Tissue thermal properties—such as heat conduction and heat capacity—are also discussed in this chapter. On the contrary, the laser parameters, such as wavelength, exposure time, applied energy, focal spot size, energy density, and power density, are also discussed. As we will find later on in this chapter, the exposure time is a critical parameter when choosing the type of interactions. There is an unlimited number of possible combinations for the experimental parameters. However, mainly five categories of interaction types are classified today. These are photochemical interactions, thermal interactions, photoablation, plasma-induced ablation, and photodisruption. In this chapter, we thoroughly discuss each of these interaction mechanisms.

Figure 3.1 shows a double-logarithmic map with the five basic interaction types. The y-axis expresses the applied power density or irradiance in W/cm². The x-axis represents the exposure time in seconds. Two diagonals show constant energy fluences at 1 J/cm² and 1000 J/cm², respectively. According to this chart, we can roughly divide the timescale into four sections: continuous wave or exposure times >1 s for photochemical interactions, 1 min to 1 μs for thermal interactions, 1 μs to 1 ns for photoablation, and <1 ns for plasma-induced ablation and photodisruption. The difference between the latter two is attributed to different energy densities. They will be addressed separately in Sects. 3.6 and 3.7 since one of them is solely based on ionization, whereas the other is primarily associated with a mechanical effect.

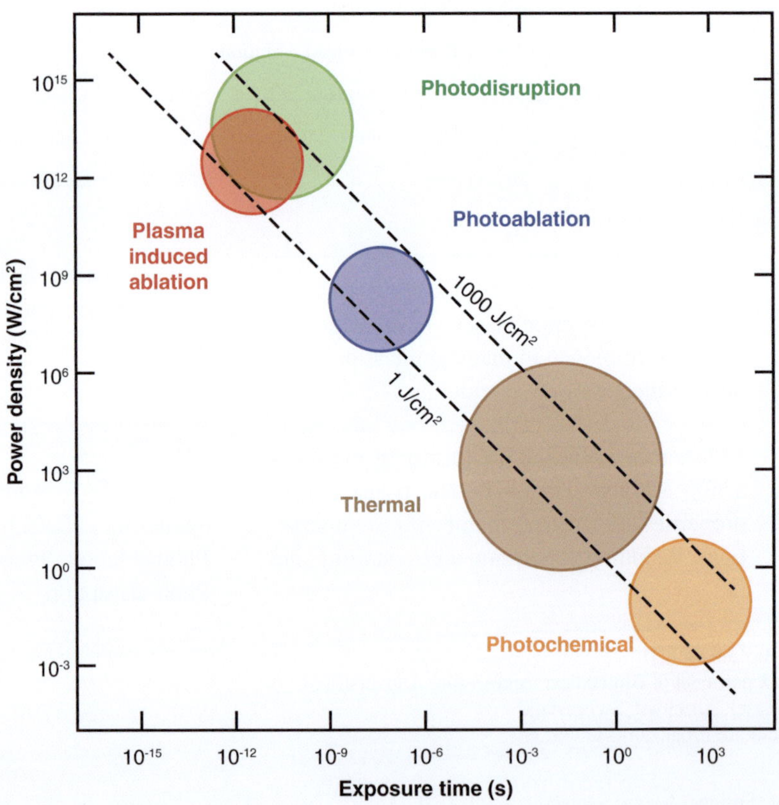

Fig. 3.1 Laser–tissue interaction map. Colored circles are rough estimation of the associated laser parameters. (Modified from [1])

3.2 Optical Properties of Tissue

In laser–tissue interaction, it is important to know about the absorbing and scattering properties of tissues. The purpose is to have better prediction of successful treatment. When we apply laser onto a highly reflecting materials, the index of refraction might be of interest. In general, we do not assume any tissue optical properties unless specified in tables or graphs. We emphasize more in the general physical interaction which mostly apply to solid and liquid. In reality, there are limitations given by the inhomogeneity of biological tissue to predict the optical properties.

3.2.1 Absorption

The intensity of light is attenuated during absorption by the biological tissue. The absorbance of tissue is defined as the ratio of absorbed and incident light intensities. A partial conversion of light energy into heat motion or certain vibrations of molecules of the absorbing material governs the process of absorption. A perfectly *transparent* medium which has no absorption will transmit the total radiant energy entering into such medium. In visible range of light, the cornea and lens can be considered as transparent media. In contrast, when the media absorb all the incident radiation, it is called *opaque*.

The terms "transparent" and "opaque" are very wavelength-dependent. This term depends on the main absorber inside the biological tissue. The cornea and lens, for instance, mainly consist of water which is highly absorbing in the infrared region, will appear *opaque* in the infrared region but *transparent* in the visible region. There is no medium known to be either transparent or opaque to all wavelengths of light.

General absorption is being considered if the substance reduces the intensity of all wavelengths by a similar fraction. If we considered the visible region, this substance would appear gray to our eyes. Colors actually originate from *selective absorption*. Basically, we can divide color as *surface* and *body colors*. Surface color is originated from surface reflection. Body color is originated from backscattering light that experiences multiple absorption and scattering inside subsurface of the substance.

The ability of a medium to absorb electromagnetic radiation depends on many factors, mainly the electronic constitution of its atoms and molecules, the wavelength of radiation, the thickness of the absorbing layer, and internal parameters such as the temperature or concentration of absorbing agents. Two laws, which describe the effect of either thickness or concentration on absorption, are commonly called Lambert's law and Beer's law and are expressed by:

$$I(z) = I_0 e^{-\mu_a z}$$

where z is the sample optical thickness, $I(z)$ is the intensity at a distance z, I_0 is the incident intensity, and μ_a is the absorption coefficient of the medium.

In biological tissues, absorption is mainly caused by either water molecules or macromolecules such as proteins and pigments, whereas absorption in the IR region of the spectrum can be primarily attributed to water molecules, proteins, and pigments mainly absorb in the UV and visible range of the spectrum. Proteins, in particular, have an absorption peak at approximately 280 nm [1].

Absorption spectra of two elementary biological absorbers—melanin and hemoglobin (HbO_2)—are shown in Fig. 3.2. Melanin is the basic pigment of the skin and is the most important epidermal chromophore. Its absorption coefficient monotonically decreases across the visible spectrum toward the infrared [2]. Hemoglobin is predominant in vascularized tissue. It has relative absorption peaks around 420, 540, and 580 nm and then exhibits a cutoff at approximately 600 nm. Most biomolecules have their complex band structure between 400 and 600 nm. Macromolecules or water is not highly absorbed in the near-infrared region. Thus, a "therapeutic window" is ranged between roughly 600 and 1200 nm. In this spectral range, biological tissues have a lower absorption, thus enabling treatment of deeper tissue structures.

As already previously stated, hemoglobin is predominant in vascularized tissue. Krypton ion

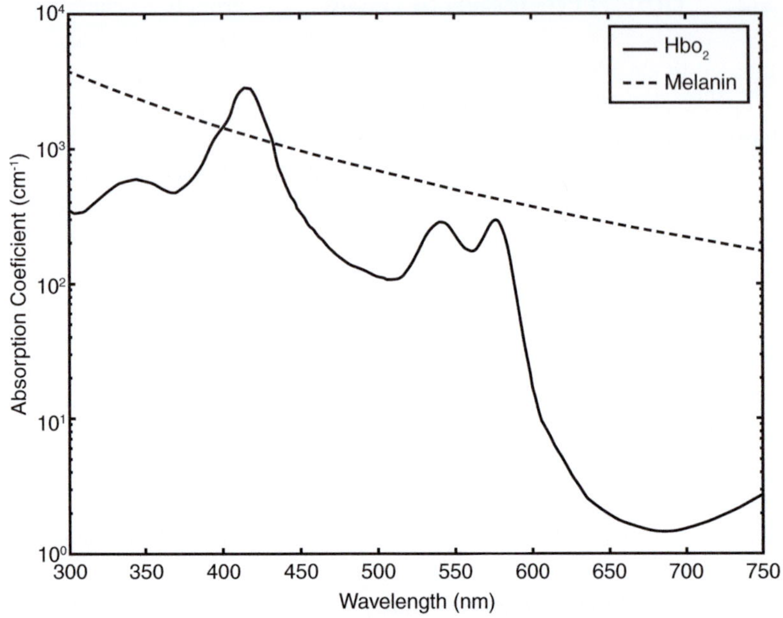

Fig. 3.2 Absorption spectra of melanin in the skin and hemoglobin (HbO_2) in blood. Relative absorption peaks of hemoglobin are at 420, 540, and 580 nm. (Data according to [2])

lasers at 531 nm and 568 nm, respectively, have almost perfectly matched wavelength with the absorption peaks of hemoglobin. Thus, these lasers can be used to coagulate blood and blood vessels. Dye lasers may also be a choice for laser treatment since their tunability can be advantageously used to match particular absorption bands of specific proteins and pigments. In some applications, special dyes and inks are used to provide enhanced absorption. Thus, we can increase specific tissue absorption which leads to better laser treatment. Moreover, we will have less damage to the adjacent tissue due to this enhanced absorption.

3.2.2 Scattering

Refractive index mismatches cause scattering of light in biological tissue at microscopic boundaries such as cell membranes and organelles. The scattering coefficient describes the scattering properties of a medium. The scattering coefficient is the product of the scattering cross section of the particles and the number density of scattering particles. The scattering cross section is an area which describes the likelihood of light being scattered by a particle. Therefore, μ_s represents the probability per unit length of a photon being scattered [3]. In the same manner as for absorption, one can define a scattering coefficient, μ_s, for a collimated source, such that [3]:

$$I(z) = I_0 e^{-\mu_s z}$$

where z is the sample optical thickness, $I(z)$ is the intensity at a distance z, I_0 is the incident intensity, and μ_s is the scattering coefficient of the medium.

The exact origins of scattering in tissue are not well known. Biological tissue is acomplex and highly heterogeneous material. There are a number of hypotheses identifying contributions to tissue scattering from various biological and biochemical microstructures, both extracellular such as collagen fibers [4, 5] and intracellular such as mitochondria [6], cell nuclei [7], and possibly a large variety of other structures such as cell membranes [8].

The angular distribution of scattering is described by the scattering phase function, $p(\theta)$, which gives us the probability of a photon to be scattered at an angle, θ, with respect to its initial direction. The phase function is normalized in such a way that $\int p(\theta)\, d\omega = 1$ (with $d\omega$ denoting integration over solid angle ω). The Henyey–

Greenstein (HG) phase function, which is originally introduced to describe scattering of light by interstellar matter [9], provides a satisfactory description of the angular patterns arising from tissue scattering [10, 11]:

$$p(\theta)=\frac{1}{4\pi}\frac{1-g^2}{\left(1-g^2+2g\cos\theta\right)^{3/2}}$$

with g being the average cosine of the scattering angle, defined as follows:

$$g=2\pi\int_0^{\pi}p(\theta)\cos\theta\sin\theta d\theta$$

The parameter g, which is also known as anisotropy factor, is very frequently used to indicate how strongly forward directed the scattering is. A typical value for tissue is in the range g = 0.7–0.95 corresponding to average scattering angles between 45° and 20°, respectively. The angular scattering pattern function for isotropic scattering has $g = 0$ and for typical biological tissue has $g = 0.9$ (see Fig. 3.3). The scattering pattern becomes more forward directed as $g \to 1$.

Another important parameter that is often used to indicate the amount of scattering present in a tissue is the reduced scattering coefficient, μ_s', which is defined as $\mu_s' = \mu_s (1 - g)$, and thus incorporates effects introduced by the anisotropic nature of scattering. The reduced scattering coefficient is the mean free path needed for the scattering to reach an isotropic scattering.

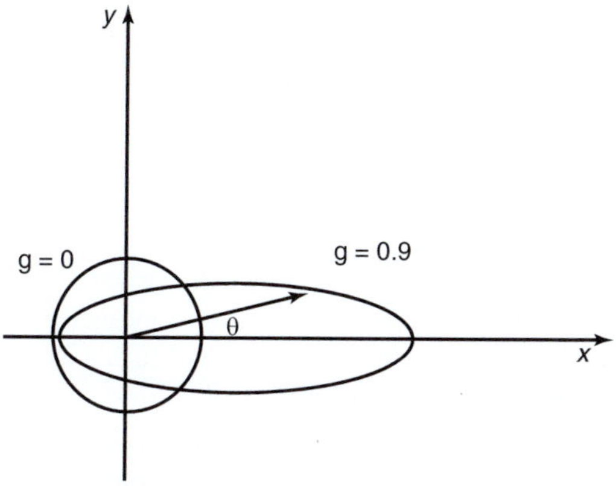

Fig. 3.3 Henyey–Greenstein scattering phase function showing the angular pattern of scattering in polar coordinates

3.3 Photochemical Interaction

Light can induce chemical effects and reactions within macromolecules or tissues. Photosynthesis is one of the most popular examples. Photochemical interaction mechanisms play a significant role during photodynamic therapy (PDT) and laser biostimulation. These two methods will be discussed in this section.

Photochemical interactions take place at very low power densities (typically 1 W/cm^2) and long exposure times ranging from seconds to continuous wave. Careful selection of laser parameters yields a radiation distribution inside the tissue that is determined by scattering. In most cases, wavelengths in the visible range (e.g., rhodamine dye lasers at 630 nm) are used because of their efficiency and their high optical penetration depths. The latter are of importance if deeper tissue structures are to be reached.

3.3.1 Photodynamic Therapy (PDT)

During PDT, spectrally adapted chromophores are injected into the body. Monochromatic irradiation may then trigger selective photochemical reactions, resulting in certain biological transformations. A chromophore compound that is capable of causing light-induced reactions in other non-absorbing molecules is called a *photosensitizer*. After resonant excitation by laser irradiation, the photosensitizer performs several simultaneous or sequential decays which result in intramolecular transfer reactions. At the end of these diverse reaction channels, highly cytotoxic reactants are released causing an irreversible oxidation of essential cell structures. Thus, the main idea of photochemical treatment is to use a chromophore receptor acting as a catalyst. Its excited states are able to store energy transferred from resonant absorption, and their deactivation leads to toxic compounds leaving the photosensitizer in its original state. Therefore, this type of

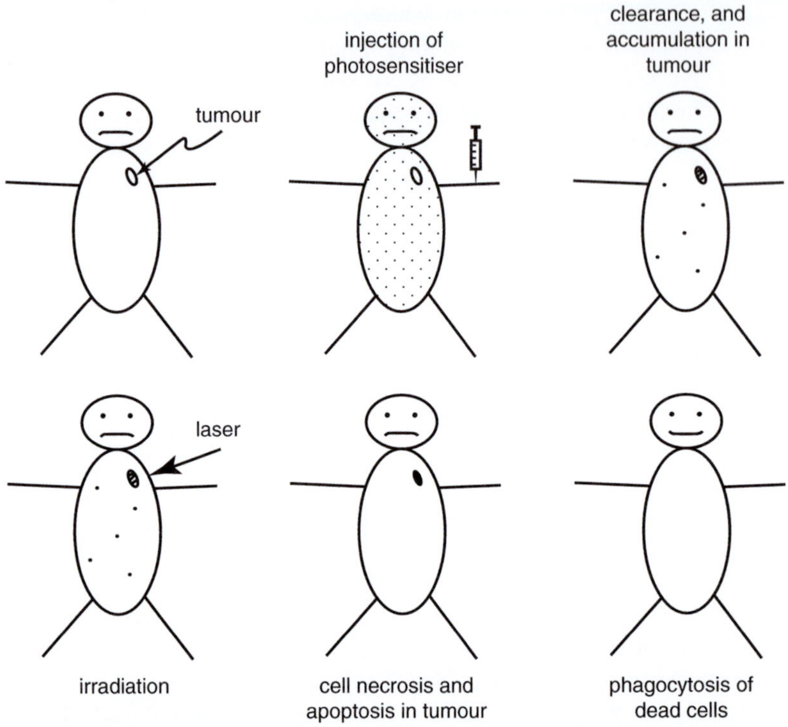

Fig. 3.4 Scheme of photodynamic therapy

interaction is also called *photosensitized oxidation*. The general procedure of photodynamic therapy is illustrated in Fig. 3.4.

At the beginning of the twentieth century, certain dyes that induce photosensitizing effects were reported [12]. In 1903, the first application of dyes in combination with light was used for treatment [13]. Later, it was observed that certain porphyrins have a long clearance period in tumor cells [14]. If by applying a laser to these dyes could change it to a toxic state, we could treat cancer cells. In 1976, the first endoscopic application of a photosensitizer in the case of human bladder carcinoma was done [15]. Today, the idea of photodynamic therapy has become one of the major pillars in the modern treatment of cancer.

3.3.2 Laser Biostimulation

Laser biostimulation also known as low-level laser therapy (LLTT) is believed to occur at very low irradiances and belongs to the group of photochemical interactions. The potential effects of extremely low laser powers (5–50 mW) on biological tissue have been found useful to stimulate the healing of wounds, skin ulcers, bed sores, pressure ulcers, and burn injuries [16]. Wound healing and anti-inflammatory properties by red or near-infrared light sources such as helium-neon lasers or diode lasers with energy fluences that lie in the range 1–4 J/cm^2 were reported [17]. In several cases, observers have noticed improvements for the patients. But in a few studies only, results could be verified by independent research groups. Moreover, contradictory results were obtained in many experiments [18].

3.4 Photothermal Interaction

Photothermal interaction happens where light energy interacts with biological tissue and increases the local temperature significantly. Either CW or pulsed laser radiation can induce thermal effects. Based on the duration and peak value of the tissue temperature achieved, we can divide the thermal interaction into *coagulation*, *vaporization*, *carbonization*, and *melting*. The summary of these thermal interactions can be found in Table 3.1.

Coagulation occurs when the final temperature of tissues is between 60 °C and 100 °C. Denaturation of proteins and collagen occurs, leading to coagulation of tissue and necrosis (death) of cells. Local temperature of tissue has to reach at least 60 °C for coagulated tissues to become necrotic. At >80 °C, membrane permeability is drastically increased, destroying the otherwise maintained equilibrium of chemical concentrations.

Vaporization occurs when tissue reaches 100 °C. Formation of gas bubbles or steam (significant increase in volume) during this phase transition results in pressure buildup and can induce mechanical ruptures and thermal decomposition of tissue fragment tissue torn open by the steam expansion, leaving behind an ablation crater with lateral tissue damage. Ablation by vaporization is purely thermomechanical, aka thermal ablation or photothermal ablation. Lateral damage can spread due to thermal diffusion from the ablation site by blood vessels. Further increase in temperature only proceeds after all water molecules have been vaporized.

Carbonization occurs when temperatures exceed 150 °C. Carbonization takes place which is observed by the blackening of adjacent tissue and the escape of smoke. Carbonization produces tissue chars where all tissue organic constituents are converted into carbon. Blackening in color reduces visibility during surgery. No benefit leads to irreparable damage of tissue. Carbonization can be avoided by cooling the tissue with either water or gas.

Melting can occur when tissue reaches temperature beyond 300 °C, depending on the target material melting point. Local temperature of tissue may reach above its melting point at sufficiently high-power density from a pulse laser.

Table 3.1 Thermal effects of laser radiation on biological tissues

Temperature (°C)	Biological effect
37	Normal
45	Hyperthermia
50	Cell immobility
60	*Coagulation*
100	*Vaporization*
>150	*Carbonization*
>300	*Melting*

3.5 Photoablation

Photoablation occurs when sufficient energy is applied into tissue to ablate it. This process should occur in a very short time before any heat can dissipate to surrounding tissue. Photoablation was first discovered in 1982 [19]. They identified it as ablative photodecomposition, meaning that material is decomposed when exposed to high-intensity laser irradiation (Fig. 3.5). The ablation process is primarily mechanical which includes thermoelastic expansion of tissue. Therefore, UV lasers generate high-energy photons mostly used for photoablation.

Photoablation typically has a threshold value of 10^7–10^8 W/cm^2 at laser pulse durations in the nanosecond range. The pulse energy determines the ablation depth up to a certain saturation limit. The beam size of the laser determines the geometry of the ablation pattern. The main advantages of this ablation technique lie in the precision of the etching process, its excellent predictability, and no thermal damage to adjacent tissue.

3.6 Plasma-Induced Ablation

Plasma-induced ablation involves exposure to optical energy concentrated in space and time with a power density of at least 10^{11} W/cm^2. High electric field of 10^7 V/cm experienced by tissue

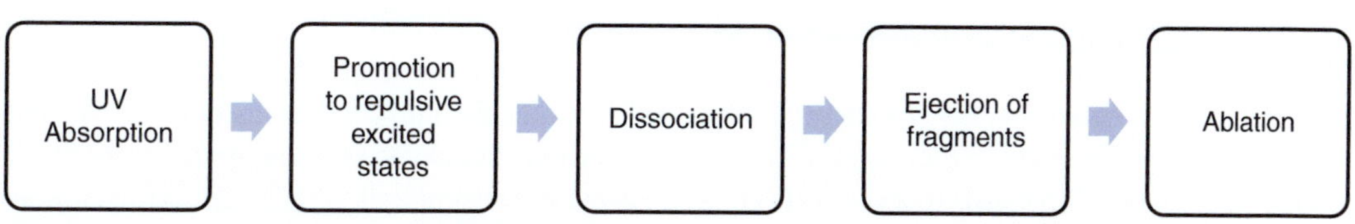

Fig. 3.5 Summary of the principle of photoablation

causes dielectric breakdown (or optical breakdown), creating a very large free electron density (plasma, or ionization of the target medium) of ~10^{18} cm^{-3} in the focal volume of the laser beam over an extremely short time period (<100's ps). High-density plasma strongly absorbs UV, visible, and IR light, leading to ablation (spatially localized to the breakdown region). Ablation is primarily caused by plasma ionization. Plasma-induced ablation can achieve very clean and well-defined removal of tissue without evidence of thermal or mechanical damage [20]. The most critical parameter of plasma-induced ablation is the local electric field strength E which determines the optical breakdown generation. If E exceeds a specific threshold value, breakdown occurs. The physical principles of breakdown have been investigated in several theoretical studies [21–24].

The initiation of plasma generation can be divided into twofold [25]. Either mode-locked laser or Q-switched laser pulses can induce a localized microplasma. In mode-locked pulses, the high electric field may induce multiphoton ionization. In Q-switched pulses, it starts with the generation of free electrons by thermionic emission which releases electrons due to thermal ionization. In general, multiphoton ionization denotes processes in which coherent absorption of several photons provides the energy needed for ionization. Multiphoton ionization is achievable only during high peak intensities as in picosecond or femtosecond laser pulses. Plasma energies and plasma temperatures, though, are usually higher in Q-switched laser pulses because of the associated increase in threshold energy of plasma formation. Thus, nonionizing side effects often accompany optical breakdown by nanosecond pulses.

The critical feature of optical breakdown is that energy deposition is possible in both pigmented tissues and nominally weakly absorbing media due to the increased absorption coefficient of the induced plasma. Furthermore, there is no restriction on the photon energy since any amount of energy can be absorbed to increase the kinetic energy of electrons. This leads to a very short rise time of the free electron plasma density of the order of ps. The irradiance must be intense enough to cause rapid ionization so that losses do not quench the electron avalanche condition for plasma growth and sustainment.

The interaction type of plasma-induced ablation can also be used for diagnostic purposes (LIBS). Laser-induced breakdown spectroscopy (LIBS) is a spectroscopic analysis of the induced plasma spark that allows evaluating the free electron density and plasma temperature in detail, and hence the information about tissue types [26] and conditions [27] can be obtained.

3.7 Photodisruption

Photodisruption is a mechanical effect resulting from high-intensity irradiation which produces plasma formation due to the ionization (optical breakdown) of biological tissue. High-energy plasma generates shock waves and other mechanical side effects which disrupt tissue structure by mechanical impact (photomechanical effect). When a laser is focused inside soft tissues or fluids, cavitation (produced by cavitation bubbles consisting of gaseous vapor and CO2) and jet formation may also take place. Unlike plasma-induced ablation, shock waves and cavitation effects spread into adjacent tissues (limited localizability of the interaction zone). Dependence of optical breakdown on laser pulse width is evident. At nanosecond pulses, shock wave formation and its effect will dominate over plasma-induced ablation. At shorter pulses, both photodisruption and plasma-induced ablation may occur (difficult to distinguish between them). In general, photodisruption can be regarded as a multi-cause mechanical effect starting with an optical breakdown. The primary mechanisms of photodisruption are *shock wave generation*, *cavitation*, and *jet formation*. Plasma formation occurs during the laser pulse and lasts for a few nanoseconds. In this time, free electrons diffuse into the surrounding medium expansion of plasma. Shock wave generation results from plasma expansion and is therefore initiated during plasma formation. After that, the shock wave propagates into adjacent tissue, leaving the focal volume, and slowed down to an ordinary acoustic wave after 30–50 ns. Cavitation starts roughly 50–150 ns after the laser pulse. The cavitation bubble usually performs several oscillations of expansion and collapses within a period of a few 100 ms. Every collapse of the bubble can also induce a jet formation if the bubble generation occurs in the vicinity of a solid boundary.

Shock wave generation occurs when there is a sudden adiabatic rise in plasma temperature to values of up to a few 10,000 K. This temperature is due to the high kinetic energy of free electrons. The energetic free electrons are not confined to the focal volume of the laser beam but diffuse into the surrounding medium instead. After a certain time delay, mass is moved and generates a shock wave. The shock wave ultimately separates from the boundary of the plasma. The shock wave initially moves at hypersonic speed but eventually slows down to the speed of sound.

Cavitation occurs if laser generates plasmas inside soft tissues or fluids. The high plasma temperature vaporizes the focal volume. Work is applied against the external pressure of the surrounding medium, and kinetic energy is being stored as potential energy in the expanded cavitation bubble. Within 1 ms, the bubble implodes as a result of the external static pressure, and the bubble content (water vapor and carbon oxides) is strongly compressed. Pressure and temperature rise again to a value achieved during optical breakdown leading to a rebound of the bubble. A second transient occurs, and the whole sequence repeats a few times until it dissipates all energy and surrounding fluids absorb all gases.

Jet formation occurs when cavitation bubbles collapse in the vicinity of a solid boundary. The impingement of the high-speed liquid on the wall can lead to severe damage and erosion of solids. If the bubble is in direct contact with the solid boundary during its collapse, the jet can cause a high impact pressure against the wall bubbles attached to solids that have the most massive damage potential. Jet velocities can be up to 156 m/s with a corresponding water hammer pressure of ~2 kbar (standard atmospheric pressure ~1 bar) [28]. A counter-jet, which points away from the solid boundary, is formed when the distance between the cavitation bubble and solid boundary is too small.

3.8 Conclusion

Laser–tissue interaction is a fundamental knowledge to have when using a laser in medical applications. This knowledge is crucial for further development of laser system in medicine. Furthermore, better knowledge of the tissue optical properties will enable accurately determined destruction of diseased tissue and its treatment in the future.

References

1. Boulnois JL. Photophysical processes in recent medical laser developments: a review. Lasers Med Sci. 1986;1(1):47–66.
2. Jacques SL. Optical properties of biological tissues: a review. Phys Med Biol. 2013;58(11):R37.
3. Tuchin VV, Tuchin V. Tissue optics: light scattering methods and instruments for medical diagnosis. Bellingham: SPIE Press; 2007.
4. Ferdman AG, Yannas IV. Scattering of light from histologic sections: a new method for the analysis of connective tissue. J Investig Dermatol. 1993;100(5):710–6.
5. Leonard DW, Meek KM. Refractive indices of the collagen fibrils and extrafibrillar material of the corneal stroma. Biophys J. 1997;72(3):1382–7.
6. Beauvoit B, Kitai T, Chance B. Contribution of the mitochondrial compartment to the optical properties of the rat liver: a theoretical and practical approach. Biophys J. 1994;67(6):2501–10.
7. Perelman LT, Backman V, Wallace M, Zonios G, Manoharan R, Nusrat A, et al. Observation of periodic fine structure in reflectance from biological tissue: a new technique for measuring nuclear size distribution. Phys Rev Lett. 1998;80(3):627.
8. Meyer RA. Light scattering from biological cells: dependence of backscatter radiation on membrane thickness and refractive index. Appl Opt. 1979;18(5):585–8.
9. Henyey LG, Greenstein JL. Diffuse radiation in the galaxy. Astrophys J. 1941;93:70–83.

10. Jacques SL, Alter CA, Prahl SA. Angular dependence of HeNe laser light scattering by human dermis. Lasers Life Sci. 1987;1(4):309–33.
11. Van Gemert MJC, Jacques SL, Sterenborg HJCM, Star WM. Skin optics. IEEE Trans Biomed Eng. 1989;36(12):1146–54.
12. Von Tappeiner H (1900) Uber die Wirkung fluoreszierender Stoffe auf Infusorien nach Versuchen von O. Raab Muench Med Wochenschr, 47(5).
13. Von Tappeiner H, Jesionek A. Therapeutische Versuche mit fluoreszierenden Stoffen. Munch Med Wochenschr. 1903;50:2042–51.
14. Auler H, Banzer G. Untersuchungen über die Rolle der Porphyrine bei geschwulstkranken Menschen und Tieren. Z Krebsforsch. 1942;53(2):65–8.
15. Kelly JF, Snell ME. Hematoporphyrin derivative: a possible aid in the diagnosis and therapy of carcinoma of the bladder. J Urol. 1976;115(2):150–1.
16. Bihari I, Mester AR. The biostimulative effect of low level laser therapy of long-standing crural ulcers using helium neon laser, helium neon plus infrared lasers, and noncoherent light: preliminary report of a randomized double blind comparative study. Laser Therapy. 1989;1(2):97–8.
17. Berki T, Nemeth P, Hegedüs J. Biological effect of low-power helium-neon (HeNe) laser irradiation. Lasers Med Sci. 1988;3(1–4):35–9.
18. Moore KC, Hira N, Broome IJ, Cruikshank JA. The effect of infra-red diode laser irradiation on the duration and severity of postoperative pain: a double blind trial. Laser Therapy. 1992;4(4):145–9.
19. Srinivasan R, Mayne-Banton V. Self-developing photoetching of poly (ethylene terephthalate) films by far-ultraviolet excimer laser radiation. Appl Phys Lett. 1982;41(6):576–8.
20. Huang H, Yang L-M, Bai S, Liu J. Smart surgical tool. J Biomed Opt. 2015;20(2):028001.
21. Seitz F. On the theory of electron multiplication in crystals. Phys Rev. 1949;76(9):1376.
22. Yablonovitch E, Bloembergen N. Avalanche ionization and the limiting diameter of filaments induced by light pulses in transparent media. Phys Rev Lett. 1972;29(14):907.
23. Bloembergen N. Laser-induced electric breakdown in solids. IEEE J Quantum Electron. 1974;10(3):375–86.
24. Sacchi CA. Laser-induced electric breakdown in water. J Opt Soc Am B. 1991;8(2):337–45.
25. Puliafito C, Steinert R. Short-pulsed Nd:YAG laser microsurgery of the eye: biophysical considerations. IEEE J Quantum Electron. 1984;20(12):1442–8.
26. Abbasi H, Rauter G, Guzman R, Cattin PC, Zam A. Differentiation of femur bone from surrounding soft tissue using laser induced breakdown spectroscopy as a feedback system for smart laserosteotomy. In biophotonics: photonic solutions for better health care VI. Int Soc Opt Photon. 2018;10685:1068519.
27. Abbasi H, Rauter G, Guzman R, Cattin PC, Zam A. Laser-induced breakdown spectroscopy as a potential tool for autocarbonization detection in laserosteotomy. J Biomed Opt. 2018;23(7):071206.
28. Vogel A, Lauterborn W, Timm R. Optical and acoustic investigations of the dynamics of laser-produced cavitation bubbles near a solid boundary. J Fluid Mech. 1989;206:299–338.

Part II

Clinical and Technical Applications

Prevention and Treatment of Oral Mucositis in Cancer Patients Using Photobiomodulation (Low-Level Laser Therapy and Light-Emitting Diodes)

4

Cesar Augusto Migliorati

Contents

Abstract

Oral mucositis (OM) is one of the most impacting oral complications negatively affecting the quality of life of cancer patients being treated with high-dose chemotherapy and radiation of the head and neck. It is an acute adverse effect that can be devastating and could affect cancer prognosis. Prevention and management strategies have not been successful. Photobiomodulation is a form of light therapy delivered to human tissues by lasers, light-emitting diodes, and even broadband light. It interferes in the way human cells repair tissues in a nonthermal and nonionizing fashion. There is mounting evidence that photobiomodulation (PBM or low-level laser therapy) can be effective in preventing OM and/or reducing the severity of this important complication. This chapter describes current modeling of the pathobiology and clinical characteristics of OM, the burden on the cancer patient, and the use of PBM as a preventative and/or therapeutic management of this oral complication.

Keywords

Oral mucositis · Photobiomodulation · Laser therapy · Low-level laser therapy · Oral complications of cancer therapy

C. A. Migliorati (✉)
Department of Oral and Maxillofacial Diagnostic Sciences, University of Florida College of Dentistry, Gainesville, FL, USA
e-mail: cmigliorati@dental.ufl.edu

4.1 Introduction

Advances in cancer therapy have changed the way cancer patients are treated. In many instances, depending on the staging a malignancy is detected, oncologists aim to cure. Clinically, this means the use of aggressive and multiple chemotherapeutic agents and/or radiation therapy. To achieve cure, cytotoxic regimens are

S. Stübinger et al. (eds.), *Lasers in Oral and Maxillofacial Surgery*,
https://doi.org/10.1007/978-3-030-29604-9_4

being used at the price of severe adverse events for the cancer patient. These adverse side effects can develop in clusters making quality of life miserable. The burden to the patient can be so severe that oncologists must alter therapy protocols to levels that can be tolerated by the patient. The negative result can be a change in the prognosis. One of the most severe adverse event of cancer therapies is **oral mucositis (OM)**.

Photobiomodulation (PBM) is defined as the use of various forms of light delivery to help accelerate tissue healing. This can be achieved by using low-level lasers, light-emitting diodes, and broadband light. Shining light in tissues that need repair leads to changes in the absorption of light by tissue chromophores, a process that is nonthermal and nonionizing and that elicits photochemical and photophysical effects that stimulate tissue repair [1, 2].

In this chapter, we briefly discuss how researchers and clinicians combine the use of PBM to prevent, manage, and treat oral mucositis. We explain what OM is, the current pathobiological modeling that explains the molecular basis of this process, and then how PBM can alter the mechanisms that lead to OM formation. Furthermore, we discuss the current science that supports the use of PBM to prevent and treat this important complication of cancer therapies. In addition, we address a recent concern that the use of PBM in cancer patients could stimulate cancer cells and promote cancer resistance.

4.2 Oral Mucositis

Alimentary mucositis is a general term that describes this complication affecting the entire gastrointestinal system. Oral mucositis (OM) refers to this adverse event occurring solely in the oral mucosa. It is one of the most important and damaging oral complications of cancer therapies [3, 4]. Risk factors are associated with patient characteristics such as genetic polymorphisms, age, oral health, and smoking [5]. The severity of OM varies depending on the type of therapy being used, including radiation of the head and neck and high-dose chemotherapy, associated or not with radiation. The complication can start insidiously presenting clinically as erythema but progressing to become ulcerated. OM affects more often nonkeratinized areas of the oral mucosa and can develop in several anatomic sites depending on the severity. The ulcerative form can bleed easily and can be covered by a layer of necrotic cells and fibrin characterized clinically as a white pseudomembrane [6]. Common signs and symptoms include pain and discomfort at rest, when eating, and when swallowing; burning sensation; difficulty swallowing or talking; and bleeding from the ulcerated areas. These signs and symptoms can significantly alter patient quality of life [7].

There are several scoring criteria for oral mucositis. The scale proposed by the World Health Organization (WHO) is one of the most used. It goes from grades 0 to 4 and is based on both clinical and functional features (Table 4.1, Fig. 4.1).

The prevention and management of OM is an unresolved issue. With the development of cytotoxic cancer treatment protocols that usually combine different agents such as high-dose chemotherapy and radiation of the head and neck, the risk of OM grades 3 and 4 has increased, altering the patient's quality of life and the tumor prognosis. Several remedies have been suggested over the years without observed efficacy and scientific support. So far, the only approved intervention for OM is palifermin (Kepivance®) [8]. This therapy is expensive, and its use is aimed at only a small number of patients in the cancer populations at risk.

Clinicians have relied on clinical experience and observations about the development of OM depending on the type of therapy. One hundred

Table 4.1 WHO oral mucositis scoring criteria

0 = Normal
1 = Soreness with or without erythema; no ulceration
2 = Ulceration and erythema; patient can swallow a solid diet
3 = Ulceration and erythema; patient cannot swallow a solid diet
4 = Severe ulceration and erythema; alimentation not possible

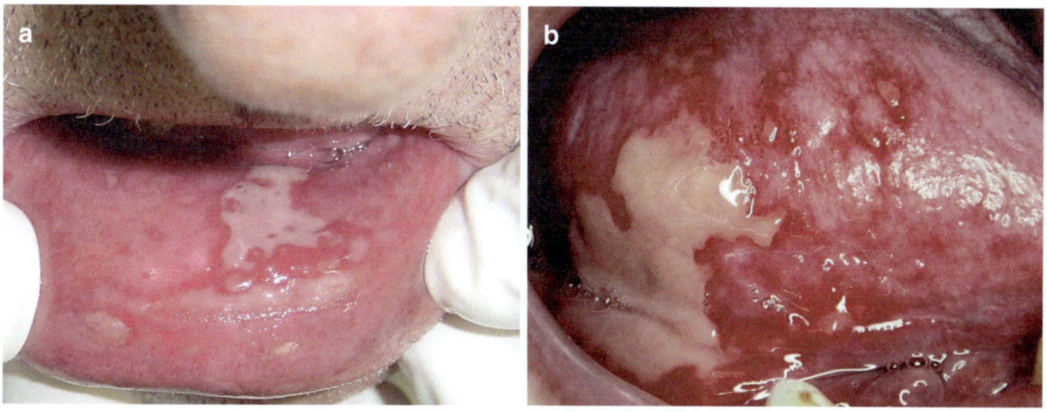

Fig. 4.1 Oral mucositis. (**a**) A patient being treated with high-dose chemotherapy developed oral mucositis on the labial mucosa. (**b**) A patient with head and neck cancer treated with radiation developed oral mucositis on the lateral and ventral tongue

percent of patients treated with ionizing radiation of the head and neck will develop some degree of OM. The ulcers may prevent eating and affect swallowing and speech [9].

The current pathobiology modeling of OM and the discovery of various molecular pathways involved on the formation of this adverse reaction have opened the opportunity for the exploration of new ways to prevent and treat this important complication of cancer therapy [3, 10, 11]. The pathobiology of mucositis has been described to occur in five distinct stages. The initial stage starts with a direct injury to DNA by radiation and chemotherapy resulting in clonogenic basal epithelial cell death. Of importance is the formation of reactive oxygen species (ROS). This process in combination with the toxicity of chemotherapy and radiation trigger biological events such as the activation of NF-ƙB, Wnt, p53, and their associated pathways. The next stage of the process is the signaling and amplification in which the activation of NF-ƙB and sphingomyelinases by ROS and radiation leads to the production of pro-inflammatory cytokines such as TNF-α that will activate more NF-ƙB and sphingomyelinases leading to tissue injury and cell death. NF-ƙB can stimulate the upregulation of genes that can cause a second phase of tissue damage. Pro-inflammatory cytokines TBF-α and interleukins can lead to the amplification of the tissue injury and cell apoptosis. At this stage, tissue damage overcomes epithelial healing resulting in tissue ulceration. Ulcers become colonized by oral cavity bacteria. The breakdown of bacterial cell wall allows for cytotoxic products to penetrate into the submucosa. This process will stimulate macrophages to produce even more pro-inflammatory cytokines and further augment tissue damage [6, 12–15].

In patients being treated with chemotherapy, the OM process is acute. It develops in the first few days of therapy and will start healing in about 2–3 weeks when the toxic effects of chemotherapy start to ware off. In patients treated with radiation therapy, the damage is cumulative. The treatment is delivered daily, 5 days a week, and can last for up to 7 weeks. This causes the oral mucosal damage to prolong up to the end of therapy and longer. These variations in the type of therapy have to be considered by clinicians when talking about prevention and treatment of OM. There are several suggestions in the literature on how to manage OM. However, they are not supported by solid evidence. In 1994, the mucositis study group of the Multinational Association of Supportive Care in Cancer and the International Society of Oral Oncology developed the first evidence-based guidelines [4]. These guidelines reported measures that were recommended and those that were only suggestions, due to the lack of solid scientific evidence. One of the recommendations for the prevention and management of OM included patient education, basic oral care, and palliative care [4, 16, 17]. Whereas initially the use of lasers only received a suggestion level of evidence, a large body of publications became available in the literature, suggesting that lasers and LED could have a positive impact on both the prevention and management of the complication. A systematic review confirmed that the use of lasers and other forms of light in oral mucositis confirmed that there was sufficient evidence to support the use of the technology in the prevention and treatment of oral mucositis [18]. The MASCC/ISOO mucositis guidelines were recently updated and included the use of lasers as one recommendation at a level II evidence [19, 20].

There are still a number of unanswered questions regarding the science behind the effect of light over tissues. In spite of the large number of studies in the literature, the variety of devices, parameters of light delivery, and protocols used in the treatment of patients, additional evidence is needed in order to determine ideal protocols [2]. One must also consider that available studies are from individual centers and that multicenter controlled studies are not yet available.

4.2.1 Photobiomodulation (PBM) and Oral Mucositis

Photobiomodulation can be achieved with the use of different forms of light: low-level laser therapy (LLLT), light-emitting diodes (LED), and white light. In the following, we address two basic and important questions related to the use of PBM in OM in cancer patients:

1. **What are the ideal parameters used in PBM and by what mechanisms can it influence the complex pathobiological mechanism of OM preventing its appearance or decreasing its severity?**

   As discussed above, OM is a complex process that starts within tissues following the use of high-dose chemotherapy and/or radiation therapy of the head and neck. It is an early process that initiates when cancer treatment commences and is already in development before changes can be seen on the oral mucosal tissues by clinical examination. Thus, preventative measures must start earlier in the process, most likely when tissue aggression also starts.

   PBM involves the use of red and near-infrared light with the goal of stimulating healing, relieving pain, and reducing inflammation [21]. It also triggers an immune response. The interaction of tissues and light is dependent on the light absorption by tissue chromophores. The primary chromophores in this process have been identified as cytochrome c oxidase in mitochondria, and calcium ion channels [22]. PBM is the result of this process [22]. This change in cell metabolism has been recently confirmed [23]. The current hypothesis explaining how light increases cytochrome c oxidase activity is that nitric oxide can be photodissociated by the absorption of a photon of red light, leading to increased rates of respiration inside of cells and ATP production, improving healing conditions [24]. This mechanism is activated by PBM resulting in anti-inflammatory effects, justifying the use of light to treat OM [21].

   Considering that PBM can stimulate healing and the fact that the type of light, the amount of energy density, the wavelength used, and the time of light are applied to the tissues, one must determine what the ideal protocol to deliver PBM is. The number of publications in this field continues to grow. However, a variety of devices, parameters, and protocols of light delivery are being reported. Studies are done in individual institutions, are not controlled, and, therefore, are passive of flaws. Currently, there is a lack of multicenter studies [18, 25].

   The current protocol recommended in the MASCC/ISOO mucositis guidelines was published recently, and it was based on a randomized controlled study done in Seattle at the Seattle Cancer Care Alliance (Fred Hutchinson Cancer Research Center) [19, 20].

> The recommendation by the panel of experts is for the use of low-level laser therapy (wavelength 650 nm, power at 40 mW, and each square centimeter of tissue treated with the required time to reach the energy dose of 2 J/cm^2), to prevent OM in patients receiving hematopoietic stem cell transplant (HSCT) conditioned with high-dose chemotherapy with or without total body irradiation.

In preventive protocols, the technique to apply the light is by lightly touching the tip of the probe on the areas were OM develops with more frequency. The probe covers point by point during the time determined to be ideal for the case, until the entire desired area has been illuminated. When mucositis has developed, the technique is the same, but now only the ulcerated areas and the surrounding tissues are illuminated (Fig. 4.2).

In addition, based on weaker evidence supporting effectiveness in the treatment setting listed above, the panel of experts suggests:

> The use of low-level laser therapy (wavelength around 632.8 nm) to prevent OM in patients undergoing radiation therapy without concomitant chemotherapy, for head and neck cancer patients.

It is important to keep in mind that the mucositis guidelines of MASCC/ISOO are evidence-based and that recommendation for use of a therapy for either prevention or treatment of OM is based on studies that are flawless and have a high level of evidence [19].

Since these guidelines became available, a large number of studies have been published supporting the evidence that light therapy can be beneficial in the prevention and treatment of OM in cancer patients receiving a variety of therapies in different populations both in adults and in pediatric patients [20, 25–34]. However, determining the ideal parameters is still a key question. It appears that both laser light and light-emitting diodes (LEDs) have similar effects on tissues and OM. However, using the correct parameters will improve the efficacy of the technology and the outcomes of therapy.

In view of the variety of parameters reported in various studies in the literature, a comprehensive list of parameters and their explanation have been suggested to help researchers when they design studies and report their results [35, 36]. This will allow for a better standardization of protocols and replication of results.

2. **If PBM is so robust to alter the complex inflammatory process involved in the formation of OM and stimulate healing of cells and tissues, could it also stimulate cancer cells present in areas where PBM is applied and promote tumor protection?**

PBM use to prevent and treat OM has been widely used in countries around the world. The only protective requirement when using PBM is eye protection. This barrier is provided by the manufacturers of PBM units by means of special eyewear that filters the specific wavelength being used. No other adverse

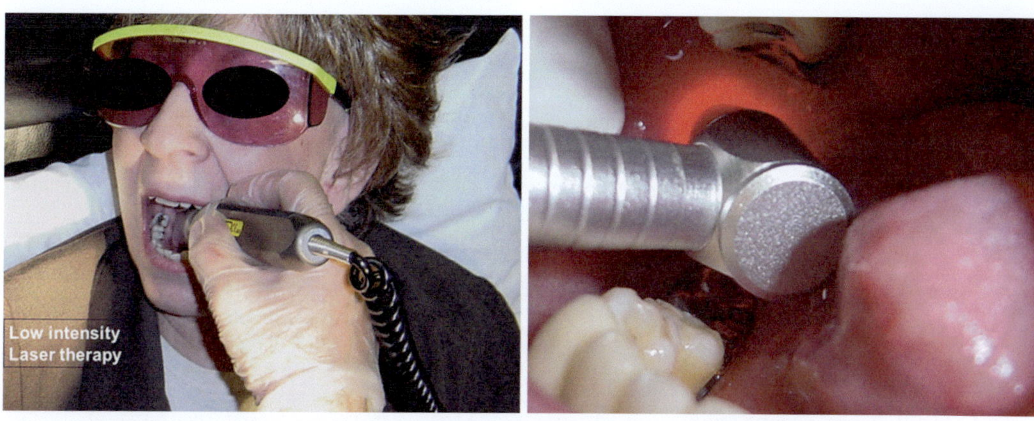

Fig. 4.2 A breast cancer patient receiving preventive application of laser

effects have been reported in years of use of this technology. PBM is not ionizing and, therefore, does not have the capacity to cause DNA damage. It also does not produce heat [2]. A recent concern was raised based on the protective effects this technology has on oral tissue and its capacity to stimulate cells. It has been asked whether the robust effect of PBM on tissues and cell could promote tumor protection or stimulate malignant cells to form a new tumor [37].

PBM technology has been used for several decades, and still there have been no reports that the technology has affected malignancy. The prevention and treatment of OM have been extensively discussed in the literature as demonstrated in this chapter. Medical oncologists work together with oral oncologists and support the use of PBM in their patients. In recent years, the side effect of medications has been growing to alarming rates, and antibiotic resistance is a current problem. In addition to the use of PBM in the oral cavity, oncologists are also using this technology in cancer patients. For example, PBM is used in breast cancer patients to manage secondary lymphedema [38].

Nevertheless, no matter how the question about potential activation of malignant cell by PBM is evaluated, a strong scientific support has yet to be produced. Clinicians are advised not to use PBM in areas where visible malignancy can be seen. With the objective of providing evidence in this area, researchers have looked into existing literature. A retrospective study of head and neck cancer patients treated with radiation therapy and also with PBM to prevent oral mucositis evaluated the safety of the use of this technology in 152 patients with stages III and IV squamous cell carcinomas (OSCC). Clinicopathological features and survival outcomes were similar to previously published data. There was no evidence that PBM negatively impacted outcome of treatment of the primary cancer, recurrence, second cancers, or survival of the primary index OSCC [39]. A prospective study is underway.

4.2.2 New Beneficial Evidence

- A recent study suggested that PBM can positively impact on the long-term survival of cancer patient receiving concurrent chemoradiation. This is the first evidence of this benefit that will need to be further evaluated when additional long-term studies are conducted [39].
- The cost-effectiveness of associating the use of PBM with specialized oral care in patients treated with hematopoietic stem cell transplantation (HSCT) has been evaluated. The use of this protocol in the study group demonstrated a decreased in OM severity. Less severity was associated with the less need for parenteral nutrition, prescription of opioids, pain in the oral cavity, and fever. On the contrary, the non-PBM group had an increase in the hospitalization costs of about 30% higher. Thus, it appears that when OM is less severe, it also helps to minimize hospitalization costs associated with HSCT [40].
- The use of PBM associated with specialized oral care before, during, and after HSCT has also been shown to improve quality of life of HSCT patients [41].

The increase in research in the field of PBM and its applications in the prevention and treatment of OM requires a close monitoring of the literature for new advances. Building a stronger scientific support for the use of this technology in cancer patients is of great importance.

References

1. Arany PR. Photobiomodulation therapy: communicating with stem cells for regeneration? Photomed Laser Surg. 2016;34(11):497–9.
2. Arany PR. Craniofacial wound healing with photobiomodulation therapy: new insights and current challenges. J Dent Res. 2016;95(9):977–84.
3. Sonis ST. Mucositis: the impact, biology and therapeutic opportunities of oral mucositis. Oral Oncol. 2009;45(12):1015–20.
4. Rubenstein EB, Peterson DE, Schubert M, Keefe D, McGuire D, Epstein J, et al. Clinical practice guide-

lines for the prevention and treatment of cancer therapy-induced oral and gastrointestinal mucositis. Cancer. 2004;100(9 Suppl):2026–46.
5. Eduardo FP, Bezinelli L, Luiz AC, Correa L, Vogel C, Eduardo CP. Severity of oral mucositis in patients undergoing hematopoietic cell transplantation and an oral laser phototherapy protocol: a survey of 30 patients. Photomed Laser Surg. 2009;27(1):137–44.
6. Sonis ST. Pathobiology of oral mucositis: novel insights and opportunities. J Support Oncol. 2007;5(9 Suppl 4):3–11.
7. Elting LS, Keefe DM, Sonis ST, Garden AS, Spijkervet FK, Barasch A, et al. Patient-reported measurements of oral mucositis in head and neck cancer patients treated with radiotherapy with or without chemotherapy: demonstration of increased frequency, severity, resistance to palliation, and impact on quality of life. Cancer. 2008;113(10):2704–13.
8. Sonis ST. Efficacy of palifermin (keratinocyte growth factor-1) in the amelioration of oral mucositis. Core Evid. 2010;4:199–205.
9. Lalla RV, Sonis ST, Peterson DE. Management of oral mucositis in patients who have cancer. Dent Clin N Am. 2008;52(1):61–77, viii
10. Sonis ST, Elting LS, Keefe D, Peterson DE, Schubert M, Hauer-Jensen M, et al. Perspectives on cancer therapy-induced mucosal injury: pathogenesis, measurement, epidemiology, and consequences for patients. Cancer. 2004;100(9 Suppl):1995–2025.
11. Sonis ST. Pathobiology of mucositis. Semin Oncol Nurs. 2004;20(1):11–5.
12. Fox BS, Sonis S. TNF and oral mucositis: response to effect of selective inhibitors of inflammation on oral mucositis: preclinical studies. Radiother Oncol 2009; 92:472–6. Radiother Oncol. 2010;94(1):123; author reply -4
13. Logan RM, Gibson RJ, Sonis ST, Keefe DM. Nuclear factor-kappaB (NF-kappaB) and cyclooxygenase-2 (COX-2) expression in the oral mucosa following cancer chemotherapy. Oral Oncol. 2007;43(4):395–401.
14. Logan RM, Stringer AM, Bowen JM, Yeoh AS, Gibson RJ, Sonis ST, et al. The role of pro-inflammatory cytokines in cancer treatment-induced alimentary tract mucositis: pathobiology, animal models and cytotoxic drugs. Cancer Treat Rev. 2007;33(5):448–60.
15. Sonis ST. New thoughts on the initiation of mucositis. Oral Dis. 2010;16(7):597–600.
16. McGuire DB, Correa ME, Johnson J, Wienandts P. The role of basic oral care and good clinical practice principles in the management of oral mucositis. Support Care Cancer. 2006;14(6):541–7.
17. McGuire DB, Johnson J, Migliorati C. Promulgation of guidelines for mucositis management: educating health care professionals and patients. Support Care Cancer. 2006;14(6):548–57.
18. Migliorati C, Hewson I, Lalla RV, Antunes HS, Estilo CL, Hodgson B, et al. Systematic review of laser and other light therapy for the management of oral mucositis in cancer patients. Support Care Cancer. 2013;21(1):333–41.
19. Lalla RV, Bowen J, Barasch A, Elting L, Epstein J, Keefe DM, et al. MASCC/ISOO clinical practice guidelines for the management of mucositis secondary to cancer therapy. Cancer. 2014;120(10):1453–61.
20. Schubert MM, Eduardo FP, Guthrie KA, Franquin JC, Bensadoun RJ, Migliorati CA, et al. A phase III randomized double-blind placebo-controlled clinical trial to determine the efficacy of low level laser therapy for the prevention of oral mucositis in patients undergoing hematopoietic cell transplantation. Support Care Cancer. 2007;15(10):1145–54.
21. Hamblin MR. Mechanisms and applications of the anti-inflammatory effects of photobiomodulation. AIMS Biophys. 2017;4(3):337–61.
22. Passarella S, Karu T. Absorption of monochromatic and narrow band radiation in the visible and near IR by both mitochondrial and non-mitochondrial photoacceptors results in photobiomodulation. J Photochem Photobiol B. 2014;140:344–58.
23. Hamblin MR. Mechanisms and mitochondrial redox signaling in photobiomodulation. Photochem Photobiol. 2018;94(2):199–212.
24. Lane N. Cell biology: power games. Nature. 2006;443(7114):901–3.
25. Bjordal JM, Bensadoun RJ, Tuner J, Frigo L, Gjerde K, Lopes-Martins RA. A systematic review with meta-analysis of the effect of low-level laser therapy (LLLT) in cancer therapy-induced oral mucositis. Support Care Cancer. 2011;19(8):1069–77.
26. Zecha JA, Raber-Durlacher JE, Nair RG, Epstein JB, Elad S, Hamblin MR, et al. Low-level laser therapy/photobiomodulation in the management of side effects of chemoradiation therapy in head and neck cancer: part 2: proposed applications and treatment protocols. Support Care Cancer. 2016;24(6):2793–805.
27. Bjordal JM. Low level laser therapy (LLLT) and World Association for Laser Therapy (WALT) dosage recommendations. Photomed Laser Surg. 2012;30(2):61–2.
28. Antunes HS, de Azevedo AM, da Silva Bouzas LF, Adao CA, Pinheiro CT, Mayhe R, et al. Low-power laser in the prevention of induced oral mucositis in bone marrow transplantation patients: a randomized trial. Blood. 2007;109(5):2250–5.
29. Antunes HS, Herchenhorn D, Small IA, Araujo CM, Viegas CM, Cabral E, et al. Phase III trial of low-level laser therapy to prevent oral mucositis in head and neck cancer patients treated with concurrent chemoradiation. Radiother Oncol. 2013;109(2):297–302.
30. Silva GB, Mendonca EF, Bariani C, Antunes HS, Silva MA. The prevention of induced oral mucositis with low-level laser therapy in bone marrow transplantation patients: a randomized clinical trial. Photomed Laser Surg. 2011;29(1):27–31.
31. Freire Mdo R, Freitas R, Colombo F, Valenca A, Marques AM, Sarmento VA. LED and laser photobiomodulation in the prevention and treatment of oral mucositis: experimental study in hamsters. Clin Oral Investig. 2014;18(3):1005–13.

32. Weissheimer C, Curra M, Gregianin LJ, Daudt LE, Wagner VP, Martins MAT, et al. New photobiomodulation protocol prevents oral mucositis in hematopoietic stem cell transplantation recipients-a retrospective study. Lasers Med Sci. 2017;32(9):2013–21.
33. Whelan HT, Connelly JF, Hodgson BD, Barbeau L, Post AC, Bullard G, et al. NASA light-emitting diodes for the prevention of oral mucositis in pediatric bone marrow transplant patients. J Clin Laser Med Surg. 2002;20(6):319–24.
34. Hodgson BD, Margolis DM, Salzman DE, Eastwood D, Tarima S, Williams LD, et al. Amelioration of oral mucositis pain by NASA near-infrared light-emitting diodes in bone marrow transplant patients. Support Care Cancer. 2012;20(7):1405–15.
35. Zecha JA, Raber-Durlacher JE, Nair RG, Epstein JB, Sonis ST, Elad S, et al. Low level laser therapy/photobiomodulation in the management of side effects of chemoradiation therapy in head and neck cancer: part 1: mechanisms of action, dosimetric, and safety considerations. Support Care Cancer. 2016;24(6):2781–92.
36. Tuner J, Jenkins PA. Parameter reproducibility in photobiomodulation. Photomed Laser Surg. 2016;34(3):91–2.
37. Sonis ST, Hashemi S, Epstein JB, Nair RG, Raber-Durlacher JE. Could the biological robustness of low level laser therapy (Photobiomodulation) impact its use in the management of mucositis in head and neck cancer patients. Oral Oncol. 2016;54:7–14.
38. MT EL, JG EL, de Andrade MF, Bergmann A. Low-level laser therapy in secondary lymphedema after breast cancer: systematic review. Lasers Med Sci. 2014;29(3):1289–95.
39. Antunes HS, Herchenhorn D, Small IA, Araujo CMM, Viegas CMP, de Assis Ramos G, et al. Long-term survival of a randomized phase III trial of head and neck cancer patients receiving concurrent chemoradiation therapy with or without low-level laser therapy (LLLT) to prevent oral mucositis. Oral Oncol. 2017;71:11–5.
40. Bezinelli LM, de Paula Eduardo F, da Graca Lopes RM, Biazevic MG, de Paula Eduardo C, Correa L, et al. Cost-effectiveness of the introduction of specialized oral care with laser therapy in hematopoietic stem cell transplantation. Hematol Oncol. 2014;32(1):31–9.
41. Bezinelli LM, Eduardo FP, Neves VD, Correa L, Lopes RM, Michel-Crosato E, et al. Quality of life related to oral mucositis of patients undergoing haematopoietic stem cell transplantation and receiving specialised oral care with low-level laser therapy: a prospective observational study. Eur J Cancer Care. 2016;25(4):668–74.

5 Photodynamic Reactions for the Treatment of Oral-Facial Lesions and Microbiological Control

Mariana Carreira Geralde, Michelle Barreto. Requena, Clara Maria Gonçalves de Faria, Cristina Kurachi, Sebastião Pratavieira, and Vanderlei Salvador Bagnato

Contents

Abstract

In this chapter, we introduce the fundamentals of photodynamic reactions and applications for the treatment of oral-facial lesions, and microbiological control are presented.

Keywords

Photodynamic therapy · Photosensitizer
Light · Cancer · Oral infections

Mariana Carreira Geralde, Michelle B. Requena, and Clara Maria Gonçalves de Faria are contributed equally to this work.

M. C. Geralde · M. B. Requena · C. M. G. de Faria
C. Kurachi · S. Pratavieira (✉)
São Carlos Institute of Physics, University of São Paulo, São Carlos, SP, Brazil
e-mail: cristina@ifsc.usp.br; prata@ifsc.usp.br

V. S. Bagnato
São Carlos Institute of Physics, University of São Paulo, São Carlos, SP, Brazil

Faculty Fellow at the Hagler Institute for Advanced Study and Visiting Professor at the Department of Biomedical Engineering - Texas A&M University, College Station, TX, USA
e-mail: vander@ifsc.usp.br

S. Stübinger et al. (eds.), *Lasers in Oral and Maxillofacial Surgery*,
https://doi.org/10.1007/978-3-030-29604-9_5

5.1 Introduction

Photodynamic reaction is a process that involves the interaction between light and a photosensitizer (PS) in a biological environment. Currently, this modality has been applied as a local treatment for cancer and also for infections caused by bacteria, fungi, or virus [1]. The first biological photodynamic action was reported by Oscar Raab in 1900, when he observed that the toxicity of acridine hydrochloride against *Paramecium caudatum* was dependent on the amount of light, thus publishing the first article on photodynamic effects of chemical compounds [2].

Later, the first clinical applications of the technique with the use of eosin as PS and light were applied for the treatment of lupus vulgaris, syphilis, psoriasis, and superficial skin cancer [3]. Although in all these potential findings, around 1928 with the emergence of antibiotics age, the further development and investigation of the inactivation photodynamic effect were significantly decreased [4].

The photodynamic action occurs when the PS in its fundamental state (S_0) is excited by light with a well-suited wavelength to an electronic excited state and, later, through an intercrossing system process, to a triplet excited state (T_1). After that, there are two possible reactions, type I reaction (via free radical formation) and type II (via singlet oxygen formation), depending on the PS characteristics. The photodynamic reactions and the biological targets are summarized in Fig. 5.1.

In the type I reaction, the PS excited can interact with the biological substrate (BS) transferring electrons or deducting a hydrogen atom, as the Eqs. (5.1) and (5.2), while, in the type II reaction, the PS excited can react with molecular oxygen ($^3O_2$) producing the singlet oxygen ($^1O_2$) that is a reactive oxygen species, according to the Eq. (5.3):

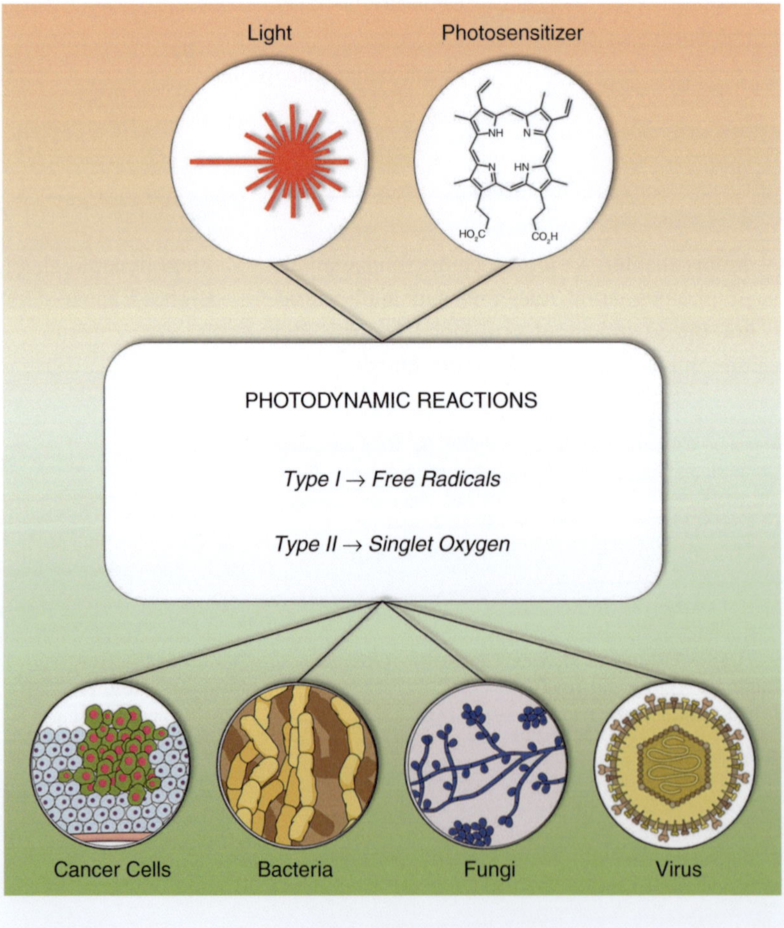

Fig. 5.1 Photodynamic reactions promoted by the interaction of the light and the photosensitizer. The main application targets are cancer cells, bacteria, fungi, and virus. The death mechanisms can be activated by free radicals (type I reaction) or singlet oxygen formation (type II reaction)

$$T_1 + SBH_2 \rightarrow HS_0 + SBH \quad (5.1)$$

$$T_1 + SB \rightarrow S_0 + SB^- \quad (5.2)$$

$$T_1 + {}^3O_2 \rightarrow S_0 + {}^1O_2 \quad (5.3)$$

These reactions result in toxic products responsible for the biological target's damage, and it is highly unlikely that microorganisms and cells acquire resistance to the treatment, which is a significant advantage when compared to the antibiotics mechanisms.

When the photodynamic reactions are used to treat cancer, the technique is known as photodynamic therapy (PDT). PDT is also used in non-oncological lesions as in wet age-related macular degeneration, acne, psoriasis, and atherosclerosis [5–7]. Depending on the PS localization, the cell death in PDT can be caused by necrosis when the PS is mainly located in the plasma membrane, by apoptosis if it is localized in the mitochondria or lysosomes, and by autophagia if it is held in the endoplasmic reticulum [8].

PDT allows a localized treatment since the PSs accumulate preferentially in the target cells, and it is possible to perform local irradiation [9, 10]. This selectivity is another significant advantage when PDT is compared to the other cancer treatments, once it can preserve healthy cells and tissues. The main disadvantage of PDT is the limited light penetration, which results in a limited tumor necrosis. This technique can only be used for superficial tumors; in bulky tumors, as of head and neck cancers (HNC), the combination of PDT with surgery and radiation therapy, or multiple sessions, is usually needed. Other related disadvantages are pain during the irradiation procedure mainly only using the topical PDT, and with the systemic PDT, the skin photosensitivity can last for weeks or months. Nevertheless, analgesics and anti-inflammatory can be prescribed by the physician based on patient needs; there is no reported evidence of adverse effects of PDT in combination with these drugs.

The light source for the irradiation is chosen depending on the region to be treated. For internal organs, the irradiation is mainly applied by a laser with optical fiber to achieve the desired location. In contrast, to perform an external treatment is possible to irradiate using laser or light-emitting diode (LED) systems [11, 12]. The typical light parameters range from 80 to 200 mW/cm^2 with total delivered dose from 80 to 150 J/cm^2. Hence the irradiation takes from 10 to 30 min to be completed. Figure 5.2 shows examples of light sources for treatment by photodynamic reactions. For superficial basal cell carcinoma (BCC) lesions, some groups have pre-

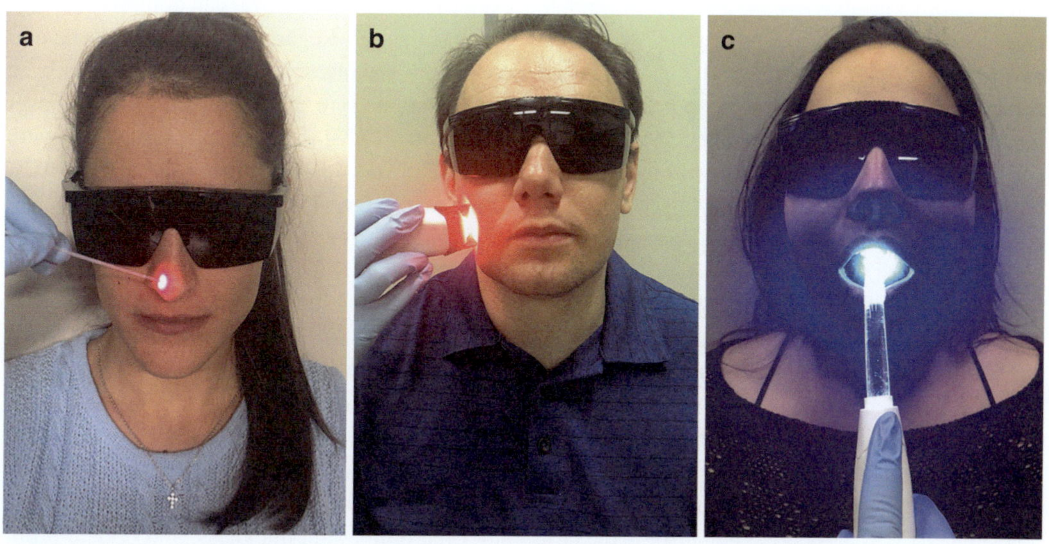

Fig. 5.2 Examples of light sources application for PS activation: (**a**) diode laser coupled to an optical fiber for cancer treatment; (**b**) red LED device for cancer treatment; (**c**) blue LED device for oral cavity decontamination

sented sunlight as an alternative PDT light source. The procedure using the sun as a light source is known as daylight PDT and has been used in numerous studies [13–16]. But here, consideration must be performed, since the dosimetry cannot be well-controlled, due to high variability associated with the meteorological conditions.

As PDT is based on simple concepts, it could be used in any type of well-oxygenated lesion for which it is possible to deliver PS and light. However, in practice, it is not that simple. Due to the limitation imposed by light penetration, dark lesions, such as melanoma or pigmented basal cell carcinoma, are not adequate for PDT. Also, bulky or internal tumors are challenges for sufficient and uniform irradiation. For a useful treatment with PDT, it is essential to afford enough amounts of light and drug, ensuring precise dosimetry for each application [17].

5.2 Photodynamic Therapy in Facial Lesions

The main malignant lesions in the facial skin are superficial and nodular basal cell carcinoma (BCC) and squamous cell carcinoma (SCC), whereas the primary nonmalignant lesions are actinic cheilitis, psoriasis, actinic and seborrheic keratosis, Bowen's disease (squamous cell carcinoma in situ), and sebaceous hyperplasia. PDT can be applied as an alternative to the traditional treatments to all these facial lesions, with the advantages of having better cosmetic results in comparison with surgery, for example. The photosensitizer can be applied intravenously or topically. The systemic delivery of the PS is recommended for more aggressive types of cancer or internal diseases. Beil et al. reviewed relevant results of PDT using systemic PS delivery to PDT treatment of head and neck cancers (HNC), though there is a significant side effect of the systemic application, the prolonged photosensitivity, during weeks depending on the PS.

When the PS is topically applied, we call it topical PDT. The most used prodrugs for topical PDT are 5-aminolevulinic acid (ALA) and methyl aminolevulinate (MAL). ALA is a precursor in the biosynthesis of the endogenous protoporphyrin IX (PpIX). Due to metabolic changes in altered cells, they present the behavior to produce more PpIX and have a different pharmacokinetics time of its elimination. The steps of PpIX formation after topical cream application are summarized in Fig. 5.3. After the cream application, the prodrug molecule (e.g., ALA) reaches the mitochondria, where the PpIX is synthesized and thus converted into heme to produce hemoglobin molecules. To avoid exceeding heme molecules to be converted back to ALA by negative feedback autoregulation, the ALA vehicle cream contains ferrochelatase inhibitors (such as ethylenediaminetetraacetic acid, EDTA) to interrupt heme formation at PpIX step and allow PpIX accumulation in cells. Abnormal cells show characteristics that interfere with the clearance of the accumulated PpIX. Thus, although the mechanisms are not clearly elucidated, it is observed that those cells usually take much longer time to completely clear the extra PpIX molecules when compared to normal cells [18].

Topical PDT is a simple procedure, it can be performed in an ambulatory setting, and after the treatment, the patient receives instructions related to pain control and post-procedure care.

The BCC is considered a nonmetastatic type of cancer. It is the most incident non-melanoma skin cancer, affecting mainly the head and neck regions [19, 20]. The surgical procedure is the standard protocol applied, though there are elder patients with comorbidities that prevent the surgery or even cases that the removal can compromise anatomic structures. Regarding a better cosmetic outcome and less invasive treatment, PDT has been widely applied in non-melanoma skin cancer treatment [21, 22], including BCC [23, 24] with similar success to the surgery. When the BCC lesion is less than 2 mm in thickness, the topical PDT is preferred. Figure 5.4 presents a BCC lesion treated with systemic PS (Photogem—hematoporphyrin derivative) administration; also its follow-up is 30 and 180 days after PDT.

For squamous cell carcinoma, PDT can be indicated but only using the systemic photosensitizer administration. This is a more invasive cancer and requires a higher PDT dose to be treated. The planning of the PDT irradiation must consider the tumor site, thickness, and optical properties, mainly absorbance.

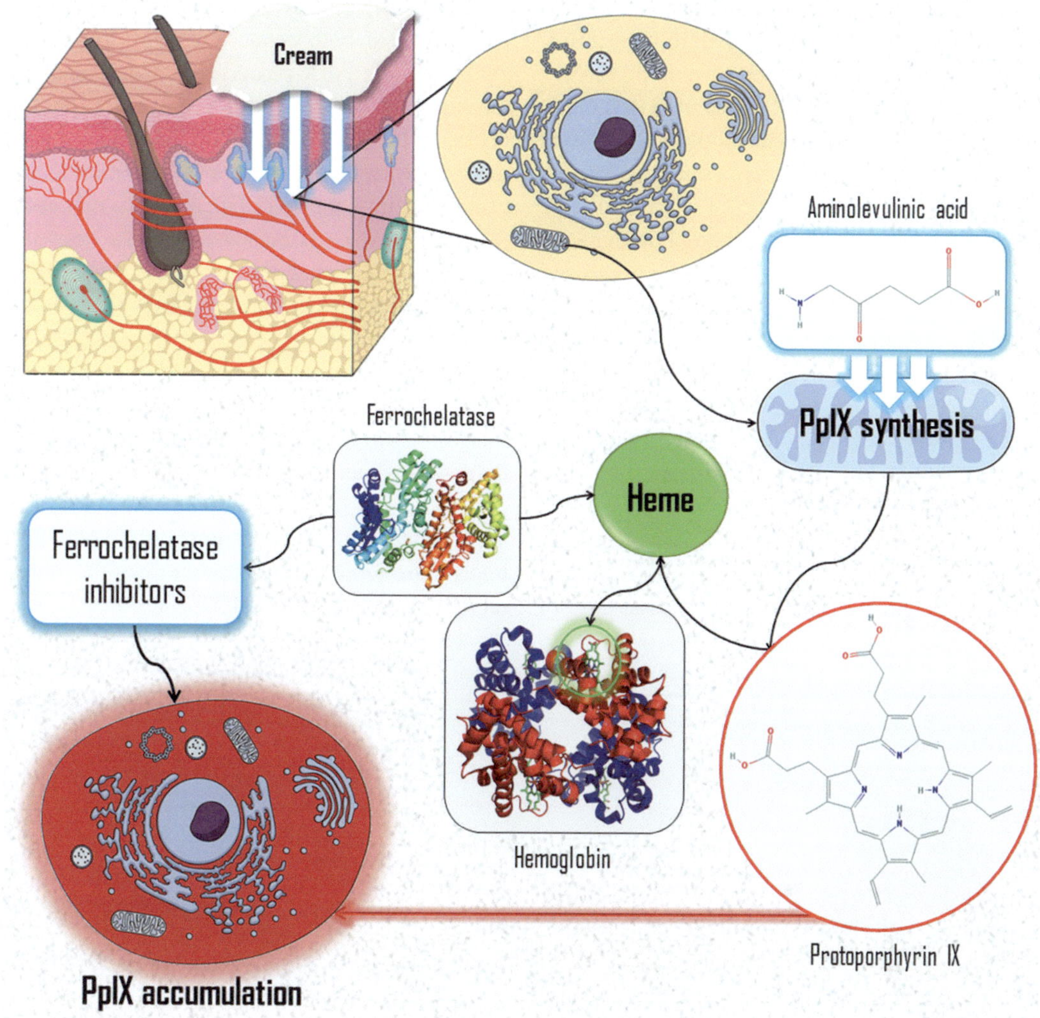

Fig. 5.3 PpIX accumulation after ALA cream topical application

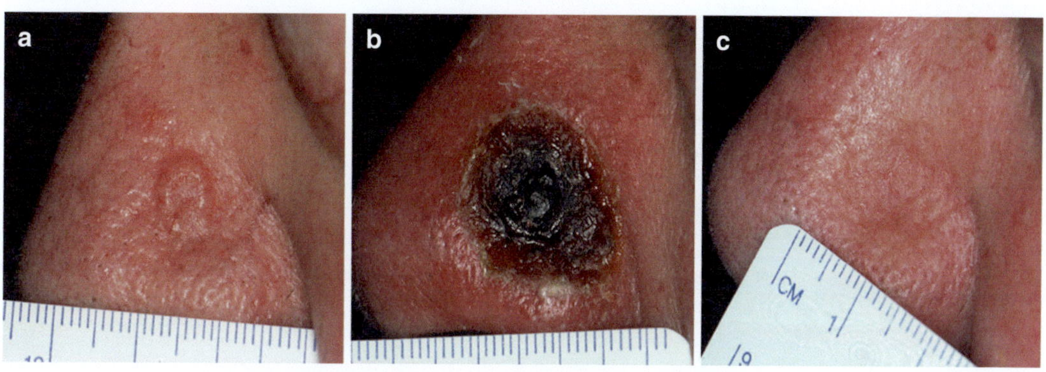

Fig. 5.4 BCC lesion: (**a**) before the PDT treatment; (**b**) 30 days after the treatment with the presence of necrotic tissue; (**c**) 180 days after the treatment

Cutaneous melanoma is not a current indication for PDT, due to its high visible light absorbance. The PDT is inefficient to this pigmented lesion since the light will be absorbed in the first cell layers, resulting in reduced light penetration and no PDT response in depth. Another issue is because melanoma is highly invasive, and PDT has no effect at a distance, i.e., no photodynamic response will occur away from the irradiated tissue.

In the literature, several studies can be found showing the success of PDT in the treatment of nonmalignant lesions as actinic cheilitis [14, 25–28], psoriasis [6, 29], actinic and seborrheic keratosis [13, 30, 31], Bowen's disease [32–34], sebaceous hyperplasia [35, 36].

When a patient with facial lesion is referred to be treated with topical PDT, the lesion is usually scarified, to remove crusts and a particular layer of stratum corneum, allowing a better permeation and penetration of both cream and light. The cream containing the PpIX precursor is then applied on the lesion as a layer about 1 mm thick, and an occlusive bandage is placed on the lesion to keep the cream in place and to avoid undesired light exposure during the drug-light interval. After about 3 h, the bandage is removed, and the lesion is cleaned with gauze and is ready to receive irradiation. Figure 5.5 shows the steps of a typical clinical PDT procedure for skin cancer using topical medication. The lesion morphology with the white light image, followed by the widefield fluorescence images before the cream application (endogenous fluorescence), after 3 h of incubation (the red color corresponds to the PpIX fluorescence), and after the irradiation (PpIX consumption). White light images also represent the appearance of the treated region 7 and 30 h after PDT.

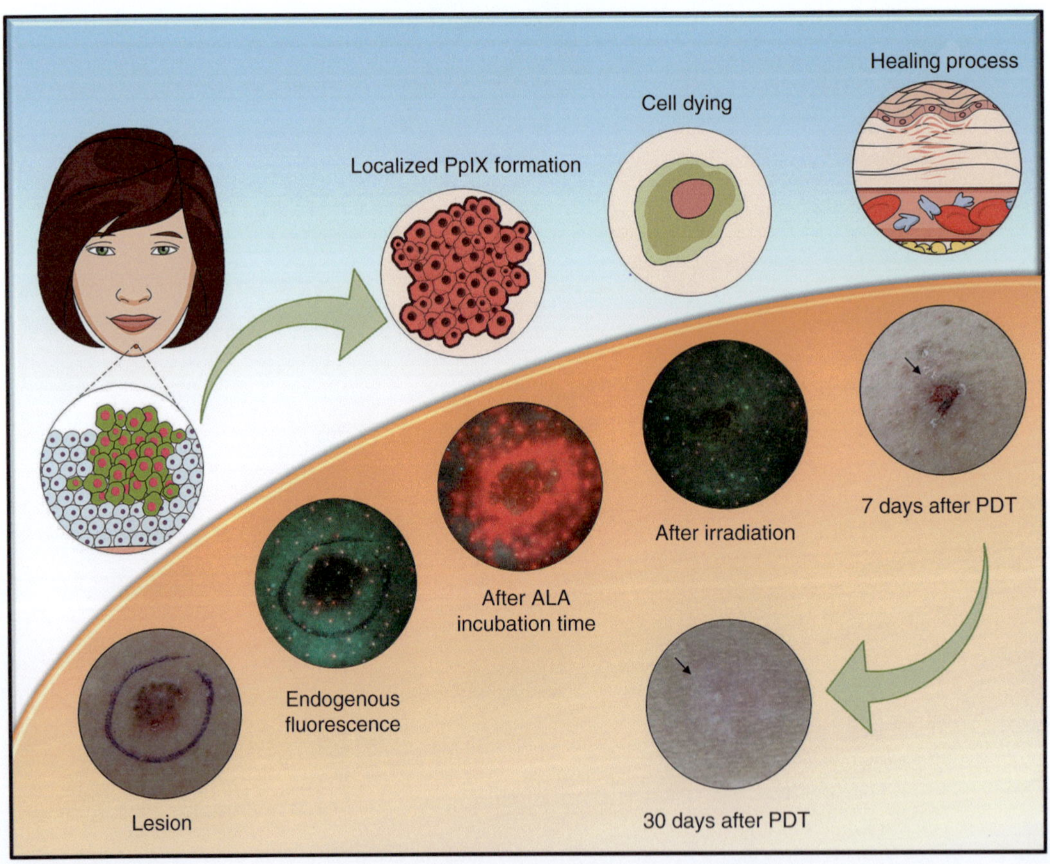

Fig. 5.5 Summary of a facial lesion treated with topical PS application

5.3 Photodynamic Therapy of Head and Neck Cancers

HNC consists in an anatomically and histopathologically diverse group of malignancies located in about 35 different sites of the region but mainly in the lips, mouth, pharynx, larynx, salivary glands, paranasal sinuses, and skin of the head and neck [37]. Their treatment is a clinical challenge since it affects important structures, such as vital nerves, vessels and tracks, and the ones essential for basic sensations. Additionally, the overall survival rates have remained unchanged for many decades, and significant increases in it have been achieved only recently. In the United States, 5-year survival increased from 54.7% in 1992–1996 to 65.9% in 2002–2006 [38, 39].

Standard treatments include surgery and chemoradiotherapy. Surgical resection is still controversial, with opinions divided between a conservative and observative approach and a traditional one, in which large margins are employed to try to prevent recurrences [40, 41]. On the contrary, radiation exposure in the tissues surrounding the tumor due to radiotherapy results in short- and long-term consequences such as xerostomia, mucositis, taste loss, radiation caries, trismus, dental decay, dysphagia, and, occasionally, osteoradionecrosis and the formation of scar tissue. However, even in cases that present excellent cure rates, their long-term sequelae substantially and negatively impact the quality of life [41]. Additionally, there are cases of recurrence after surgery and chemoradiotherapy in which the tumor site is not easily accessible [42].

In that context, PDT has emerged as an alternative treatment that could improve the quality of life of patients, as it protects surrounding tissues and results in excellent cosmetic outcomes, as well as provides a way to treat inaccessible tumors via interstitial PDT with local fibers [42, 43]. In the mid-1980s, there were initial clinical trials in head and neck tumors restricted to advanced disease patients with poor prognosis. Still, good results in a small number of patients were reported [44–49]. Since then, several types of tumors have been treated with PDT [50]. PDT for HNC can be indicated as a curative treatment, when the lesion volume can be entirely irradiated, or as a palliative technique; in this case, aiming to control or decrease the tumor size is indicated in combination with the radiotherapy and surgery.

There are good reviews on the topic, Civantos et al. reported an overall view focusing on clinical application of the past 30 years of PDT experience in HNC treatment regarding mechanisms of action, available data, and historical development [50]. Gondivkar et al. also presented a recent review on the subject, focused on protocols, details, and results obtained in 1985–2015, covering 26 studies and a total of 988 patients [51]. They reported complete response following PDT of oral potentially malignant lesions in 27% of these studies and 16–100% in HNC patients.

5.3.1 Protocols and Determining Factors in the Outcome

Diverse protocols have been used in preclinical and clinical trials, comprising wavelengths from 585 to 660 nm, fluence rates, photosensitizers, and incubation times. Light sources reported include light-emitting diodes (LEDs), dye lasers, and diode lasers, with power densities in the interval of 50–500 mW/cm^2. Photosensitizers (PSs) used in clinical trials varied from hematoporphyrin derivatives, Photofrin, aminolevulinic acid (ALA), meta-tetra(hydroxyphenyl)chlorin, choline e6, Photosan, and Foscan. It could be employed in a gel, cream, or emulsion form when applied topically, or intralesionally and intravenously. The PS choice is mostly based on regulatory agencies approval, cancer type, and site and tumor volume, which correlates to light penetration required. The PS doses employed and the time between application and irradiation vary widely, the last one ranging from 24 to 96 h for intravenous administrations and 1–5 h for topical application [51]. Many parameters in PDT, combined with the intrinsic heterogeneity of tumors, limit the comparison and advances in the modality since it becomes difficult to isolate the dependence of successful outcomes with a variable. Some factors that are known to impact the treatment are briefly described next.

5.3.2 Lesion Size and Appearance

Tumor volume and appearance are crucial factors for determining PDT results. However, most of the studies fail to correlate them with treatment outcome. As pointed out by Gondivkar et al., the recurrence differences between the results from Selvam et al., Grant et al., and Jerjes et al. (0%, 36%, and 19%, respectively) suggest that dysplasia, type, volume, and surface of the lesion could impact the effectiveness of the therapy [47, 52, 53]. Future investigations are needed to determine the influence of these factors in PDT.

5.3.3 Dosimetry

As mentioned before, light dose, or fluence rate, is one of the leading protocol parameters, and it has a significant role in determining the success or failure of PDT. Light distribution is hugely affected by spatial and temporal diversity in the optical properties of the tissue, which impacts the light dose delivered in the tumor volume. Therefore, it is known that advances in dosimetry lead to better clinical outcomes [50]. The total delivered dose is dependent on the number of PDT employed. However, its effectiveness also depends on the number of PDT sessions. Hosokawa et al. reported no additional effect of the second or third PDT compared to a single one, in the treatment of 33 patients with head and neck squamous cell carcinoma [43].

5.3.4 Site

The success of PDT is highly dependent on the anatomical tumor site and type. For example, subgroup analysis from the study of Karakullukcu identified that lesions from the oral tongue and floor of mouth have more favorable outcomes relative to other oral cavity sites, the oropharynx, or the nasal cavity [54]. In 2015, Cerrati et al. reviewed the PDT literature for oral cavity cancer comparing it with surgical treatment. They found no statistical difference between the groups concerning local control and recurrences [55]. For lip squamous cell carcinomas, PDT is also very efficient, especially for field cancerization cases, in which leukoplakia and erythroplakia compromise large areas of the lip surface [56]. However, PDT should not be the single therapeutic modality of tumors with more than 3 mm of invasion depth, as additional treatment of the neck would be essential [50].

There is proper evidence that suggests that PDT would be an alternative to endoscopic resection for treating superficial lesions of early-stage larynx cancer. A study of Shafirstein et al. reported complete response in 68% of the 29 patients treated with PDT using HPPH as a PS [57]. As mentioned before, it presents the advantage of minimal normal tissue destruction. Nevertheless, there are no available data on the quality of life of PDT patients compared to conventional approaches [50].

Interstitial PDT (iPDT) is performed for bulky tumors or cancer sites thicker than 5 mm. PS is given via intravenous or intralesional administration, and light is delivered using fibers. The main advantage of iPDT is the possibility of protecting and sparing nerves and essential structures that often surround the tumor, preventing severe functional deficiencies caused by surgery and chemoradiotherapy. PDT also helps in the preservation of elastin and collagen fibers, when compared to other treatment modalities, which may reduce the risks of thrombosis or rupture of normal arteries [38]. It is also a useful option for a palliative measure and treatment of recurrent tumors [38, 58, 59]. The main groups investigating iPDT uses are from the University College London, who uses ultrasound to guide the laser fibers, and a group from the Netherlands Cancer Institute, who uses computer tomography and magnetic resonance imaging-guided catheters and cylindrical diffusers [50].

A summary of the main advantages and disadvantages of PDT is presented in Table 5.1.

Table 5.1 Summary of the main advantages and disadvantages of PDT

Advantages	Disadvantages
Negligible effect on underlying functional structures	Limited penetration depth
Excellent cosmetic outcomes	Nonspecific tissue uptake
Does not have the cumulative toxicity	Phototoxicity
Cost-effective	Local pain
Increased quality of life after treatment	Swelling and edema

5.4 Photodynamic Inactivation

There are many terms in the literature to describe photodynamic reactions for microorganism inactivation, such as photodynamic inactivation (PDI), antimicrobial photodynamic therapy (aPDT), photodynamic antimicrobial chemotherapy (PACT), photoactivated disinfection (PAD), and photodynamic disinfection (PDD) [60–64].

Microorganisms, especially bacteria, have a high multiplication rate, and if a mutation occurs that assists a single microbe to survive in the presence of an antibiotic, it will become predominant in the microbial population creating a drug-resistant strain. With the increase of bacteria resistant to antibiotics stress, there is a need for the development of different antimicrobial therapies; this is one of the reasons why the Raab idea was again a topic of investigation on this area [63].

PDI is an alternative for the treatment of diseases caused by antibiotic-resistant pathogens and has shown a promising outcome for multidrug-resistant infections. There are still no reports of the development of microorganism resistance to PDI, even after numerous attempts at induction by repetition of cycles of this technique [63]. Further, antibiotics administration may cause side effects, commonly gastrointestinal disturbances, in addition to allergies caused by penicillins, uptake of tetracyclines into the bones and teeth, arthropathies induced by quinolones, headache, dizziness, metallic taste, or alcohol intolerance with metronidazole [65]. In this context, PDI is considered a potential tool to renew the treatment of infectious diseases.

The PDI for microorganisms is based on the accumulation of photosensitizer (PS) preferentially in the therapeutic target such as bacteria, not on the surrounding cells or tissues, and also on lower resistance to PDT damage when compared to the mammalian host cells. Such condition is essential for the subsequent activation of low-light fluences (often called "light doses," which is a correlation with the amount of energy delivered to the target cells); a toxic effect does not occur in host cells [2]. The technique is already used clinically as a treatment for various infectious diseases, such as skin ulcers, oral candidiasis, periodontal diseases, and acne vulgaris [66–70].

One important disease that can be treated by PDI and affects oral cavity is denture stomatitis, which is erythematous candidiasis associated with the continuous denture use and/or its poor hygiene, as well as immunosuppression, mucosal trauma, smoking, and others. Commonly denture stomatitis is asymptomatic; however, it can be painful even and may cause taste changes and swallowing difficulty. PDI mediated by Photodithazine® and Photogem® as PS is already applied to treat denture stomatitis in patients [71–73]. Alves et al. (2018) inactivated *Candida* spp. using Photodithazine® gel and red light irradiation; the protocol was applied three times a week for 15 days (six sessions). Forty-five days after the last PDI session, the colony-forming units per milliliter (CFU/mL) values were lower than found before the treatment [73].

For periodontal diseases, another relevant infection that has been already related to bacterial endocarditis, PDI is used with different synthetic dyes, such as methylene blue, toluidine blue, porphyrins, chlorines, Photodithazine®, and, more recently, curcumin, which is a natural PS, and has been applied to avoid collateral effects and drug interactions [4, 65]. PDI application has a relative advantage on antibiotics administration for periodontal diseases, whereas the high rate of bacterial resistance to most antibiotics used in periodontology, the increased number of immunosuppressed patients, and also the periodontal infections are frequently caused by many diverse pathogens which require different antibiotics administration enhancing the risks of adverse reactions [65].

Photodynamic reactions are also an alternative procedure to inactivate pathogenic microbes in the oral mucosa and periodontal tissue. The current antimicrobial mouthwash for oral hygiene has several drawbacks [74]. Further, numerous infectious diseases may affect the oral cavity, motivating the use of PDI in dentistry. Several studies using photosensitizers as mouthwash followed by the irradiation of the oral cavity were performed, and the inactivation is compared with the traditional mouthwash [75–77].

In addition to diseases of the oral cavity, many studies applied PDI to treat acne vulgaris and other skin infections. Most studies conclude that PDI is considered as an effective treatment for acne or an auxiliary treatment, especially in patients who do not respond to topical therapy and oral antibacterials. The most commonly used PS to treat acne vulgaris is the aminolevulinic acid (ALA) excited by red or blue light, although it is possible to use other PS such as indocyanine green [68, 78–82].

Still, on head and neck infections, Blanco et al. (2017) proposed PDI with curcumin and blue light as an innovative treatment for pharyngotonsillitis, which shares the same challenge as other infectious diseases concerning the fight against antibiotic-resistant microorganisms. In 2050, the number of deaths caused by these pathogens is expected to reach ten million people per year [83].

The approaches here presented play a relevant role in offering alternatives for the use of PDI as a treatment for head and neck infectious diseases. The advantages provided concerning the aesthetic results for skin applications are a positive aspect and frequently decisive for the patient acceptance of the treatment. The ability to provide therapy with little-to-none side effects is also relevant, particularly concerning drug-resistant microorganisms. Thus, these therapies may be offered either as the first choice or as supportive therapy, or even as a last resource when other techniques have failed in providing results.

Acknowledgments The authors acknowledge the support provided by Brazilian funding agencies Coordenação de Aperfeiçoamento de Pessoal de Nível Superior - Brasil (Capes) - Finance Code 001, CNPq (465360/2014-9), and São Paulo Research Foundation (FAPESP) with grants 2013/07276-1 (CEPOF) and 2014/50857-8 (INCT).

References

1. Wilson BC, Patterson MS. The physics, biophysics and technology of photodynamic therapy. Phys Med Biol. 2008;53(9):R61–109.
2. Maisch T. Anti-microbial photodynamic therapy: useful in the future? Lasers Med Sci. 2007;22(2):83–91.
3. Dougherty TJ, Kaufman JE, Goldfarb A, Weishaupt KR, Boyle D, Mittleman A. Photoradiation therapy for the treatment of malignant tumors. Cancer Res. 1978;38:2628–35.
4. Santezi C, Reina BD, Dovigo LN. Curcumin-mediated photodynamic therapy for the treatment of oral infections-a review. Photodiagn Photodyn Ther. 2018;21:409–15.
5. Amemiya T, Nakajima H, Katoh T, et al. Photodynamic therapy of atherosclerosis using YAG-OPO laser and Porfimer sodium, and comparison with using argon-dye laser. Jpn Circ J. 1999;63(4):288–95.
6. Choi YM, Adelzadeh L, Wu JJ. Photodynamic therapy for psoriasis. J Dermatolog Treat. 2014;6634:1–6.
7. Sessler JL, Miller RA. Texaphyrins: new drugs with diverse clinical applications in radiation and photodynamic therapy. Biochem Pharmacol. 2000;59(7):733–9.
8. Abrahamse H, Hamblin MR. New photosensitizers for photodynamic therapy. Biochem J. 2016;473(4):347–64. https://doi.org/10.1042/BJ20150942.
9. Wachowska M, Muchowicz A, Firczuk M, Gabrysiak M, Winiarska M, Wańczyk M, et al. Aminolevulinic acid (ALA) as a prodrug in photodynamic therapy of cancer. Molecules. 2011;16(12):4140–64.
10. de Paula Campos C, de Paula D'Almeida C, Nogueira MS, Moriyama LT, Pratavieira S, Kurachi C, et al. Fluorescence spectroscopy in the visible range for the assessment of UVB radiation effects in hairless mice skin. Photodiagn Photodyn Ther. 2017;20:21–7.
11. Mang TS. Lasers and light sources for PDT: past, present and future. Photodiagn Photodyn Ther. 2004;1:43–8.
12. Grecco C, Buzzá HH, Stringasci MD, Andrade CT, Vollet-Filho JD, Pratavieira S, et al. Single LED-based device to perform widefield fluorescence imaging and photodynamic therapy. SPIE Proc. 2015;9531:953121. https://doi.org/10.1117/12.2185925.
13. Wiegell SR, Wulf HC, Szeimies RM, Basset-Seguin N, Bissonnette R, Gerritsen MJP, et al. Daylight photodynamic therapy for actinic keratosis: an international consensus: International Society for

Photodynamic Therapy in Dermatology. J Eur Acad Dermatol Venereol. 2012;26:673–9.
14. Levi A, Wulf HC, Enk CD. Two cases of actinic cheilitis responsive to daylight-activated photodynamic therapy (DA-PDT). Photodermatol Photoimmunol Photomed. 2013;29:268–71.
15. Vicentini C, Tylcz JB, Betrouni N, Mortier L, Mordon S. Is daylight-PDT a good treatment option during solar eclipse? Photodiagn Photodyn Therap. 2015;12:376–7.
16. Shumack S, et al. Daylight PDT: a convenient, similarly effective, and nearly painless alternative to conventional PDT. J Dtsch Dermatol Ges. 2013;11:87.
17. de Faria CMG, Inada NM, Kurachi C, Bagnato VS. Determination of the threshold dose distribution in photodynamic action from in vitro experiments. J Photochem Photobiol B Biol. 2016;162:168–75.
18. Uehlinger P, Zellweger M, Wagnières G, Juillerat-Jeanneret L, van den Bergh H, Lange N. 5-Aminolevulinic acid and its derivatives: physical chemical properties and protoporphyrin IX formation in cultured cells. J Photochem Photobiol B. 2000;54(1):72–80.
19. Scrivener Y, Grosshans E, Cribier B. Variations of basal cell carcinomas according to gender, age, location and histopathological subtype. Br J Dermatol. 2002;147(1):41–7.
20. Bastiaens MT, Hoefnagel JJ, Bruijn JA, Westendorp RGJ, Vermeer BJ, Bavinck JNB. Differences in age, site distribution, and sex between nodular and superficial basal cell carcinomas indicate different types of tumors. J Invest Dermatol. 1998;110(6):880–4.
21. Cabete J, Rafael M, Cravo M, Moura C, Sachse F, Pecegueiro M. Long-term recurrence of nonmelanoma skin cancer after topical methyl aminolevulinate photodynamic therapy in a dermato-oncology department. An Bras Dermatol. 2015;90(6):846–50.
22. Griffin L, Lear J. Photodynamic therapy and nonmelanoma skin cancer. Cancers (Basel). 2016;8(10):98. http://www.mdpi.com/2072-6694/8/10/98
23. Horn M, Wolf P, Wulf HC, Warloe T, Fritsch C, Rhodes LE, et al. Topical methyl aminolaevulinate photodynamic therapy in patients with basal cell carcinoma prone to complications and poor cosmetic outcome with conventional treatment. Br J Dermatol. 2003;149:1242–9.
24. Ramirez DP, Kurachi C, Inada NM, Moriyama LT, Salvio AG, Vollet Filho JD, et al. Experience and BCC subtypes as determinants of MAL-PDT response: preliminary results of a national Brazilian project. Photodiagn Photodyn Ther. 2014;11(1):22–6.
25. Sotiriou E, Apalla Z, Koussidou-Erremonti T, Ioannides D. Actinic cheilitis treated with one cycle of 5-aminolaevulinic acid-based photodynamic therapy: report of 10 cases. Br J Dermatol. 2008;159:261–2.
26. Alexiades-Armenakas M. Commentary on photodynamic therapy of actinic cheilitis. Dermatol Surg. 2015;41:199–200.
27. Yazdani Abyaneh MA, Falto-Aizpurua L, Griffith RD, Nouri K. Photodynamic therapy for actinic cheilitis: a systematic review. Dermatol Surg. 2015;41(2):189–98.
28. Ribeiro CF, Souza FHDM, De Jordão JM, Haendchen LC, Mesquita L, Schmitt JV, et al. Photodynamic therapy in actinic cheilitis: clinical and anatomopathological evaluation of 19 patients. An Bras Dermatol. 2012;87(3):418–23.
29. Almutawa F, Thalib L, Hekman D, Sun Q, Hamzavi I, Lim HW. Efficacy of localized phototherapy and photodynamic therapy for psoriasis: a systematic review and meta-analysis. Photodermatol Photoimmunol Photomed. 2015;31:5–14.
30. Ericson MB, Wennberg A-M, Larkö O. Review of photodynamic therapy in actinic keratosis and basal cell carcinoma. Ther Clin Risk Manag. 2008;4(1):1–9.
31. Nolan M. EMA approved new drugs: photodynamic therapy for actinic keratosis. Eur J Hosp Pharm. 2013;20:60.
32. Suarez-Perez JA, Herrera E, Herrera-Acosta E, Lopez-Navarro N, Martin-Cuevas P, Bosch R. Photodynamic therapy in the treatment of extensive Bowen disease. J Am Acad Dermatol. 2013;68(4):AB164.
33. Morton CA, Whitehurst C, McColl JH, Moore JV, MacKie RM. Photodynamic therapy for large or multiple patches of Bowen disease and basal cell carcinoma. Arch Dermatol. 2001;137(3):319–24.
34. Han J, Kim JE, Park GH, Won CH, Chang SE, Lee MW, et al. Photodynamic therapy of the Bowen disease. J Dermatol. 2012;39:252.
35. Richey DF. Aminolevulinic acid photodynamic therapy for sebaceous gland hyperplasia. Dermatol Clin. 2007;25:59–65.
36. Alster TS, Tanzi EL. Photodynamic therapy with topical aminolevulinic acid and pulsed dye laser irradiation for sebaceous hyperplasia. J Drugs Dermatol. 2003;2:501–4.
37. Staffieri A, Sebastian P, Kapre M, Kazi R, Varghese BT. Essentials of head and neck cancer. Delhi: Byword Books Private Limited; 2011. 280 p.
38. Lou P-J, Jäger HR, Jones L, Theodossy T, Bown SG, Hopper C. Interstitial photodynamic therapy as salvage treatment for recurrent head and neck cancer. Br J Cancer. 2004;91(3):441–6.
39. Rettig EM, D'Souza G. Epidemiology of head and neck cancer. Surg Oncol Clin N Am. 2015;24(3):379–96.
40. Rigual NR, Thankappan K, Cooper M, Sullivan MA, Dougherty T, Popat SR, et al. Photodynamic therapy for head and neck dysplasia and cancer. Arch Otolaryngol Neck Surg. 2009;135(8):784.
41. Vissink A, Jansma J, Spijkervet FKL, Burlage FR, Coppes RP. Oral sequelae of head and neck radiotherapy. Crit Rev Oral Biol Med. 2003;14(3):199–212.
42. Nelke KH, Pawlak W, Leszczyszyn J, Gerber H. Photodynamic therapy in head and neck cancer. Postepy Hig Med Dosw. 2014;68:119–28.
43. Hosokawa S, Takebayashi S, Takahashi G, Okamura J, Mineta H. Photodynamic therapy in patients with head and neck squamous cell carcinoma. Lasers Surg Med. 2018;50(5):420–6.
44. Harris DM, Hill JH, Werkhaven JA, Applebaum EL, Lobraico RV, Waldow SM. Porphyrin fluorescence

and photosensitization in head and neck cancer. Arch Otolaryngol Head Neck Surg. 1986;112(11):1194–9.
45. Wenig BL, Kurtzman DM, Grossweiner LI, Mafee MF, Harris DM, Lobraico RV, et al. Photodynamic therapy in the treatment of squamous cell carcinoma of the head and neck. Arch Otolaryngol Head Neck Surg. 1990;116(11):1267–70.
46. Feyh J, Goetz A, Müller W, Königsberger R, Kastenbauer E. Photodynamic therapy in head and neck surgery. J Photochem Photobiol B. 1990;7(2–4):353–8.
47. Grant WE, Hopper C, Speight PM, Macrobert AJ, Bown SG. Photodynamic therapy of malignant and premalignant lesions in patients with "field cancerization" of the oral cavity. J Laryngol Otol. 1993;107(12):1140–5.
48. Biel MA. Photodynamic therapy of head and neck cancers. Semin Surg Oncol. 2010;11(5):355–9.
49. Biel M. Advances in photodynamic therapy for the treatment of head and neck cancers. Lasers Surg Med. 2006;38(5):349–55.
50. Civantos FJ, Karakullukcu B, Biel M, Silver CE, Rinaldo A, Saba NF, et al. A review of photodynamic therapy for neoplasms of the head and neck. Adv Ther. 2018;35(3):324–40.
51. Gondivkar SM, Gadbail AR, Choudhary MG, Vedpathak PR, Likhitkar MS. Photodynamic treatment outcomes of potentially-malignant lesions and malignancies of the head and neck region: a systematic review. J Investig Clin Dent. 2017;2017:e12270.
52. Selvam N, Sadaksharam J, Singaravelu G, Ramu R. Treatment of oral leukoplakia with photodynamic therapy: a pilot study. J Cancer Res Ther. 2015;11(2):464.
53. Jerjes W, Upile T, Hamdoon Z, Mosse CA, Akram S, Hopper C. Photodynamic therapy outcome for oral dysplasia. Lasers Surg Med. 2011;43(3):192–9.
54. Karakullukcu B, van Oudenaarde K, Copper MP, Klop WM, van Veen R, Wildeman M, et al. Photodynamic therapy of early stage oral cavity and oropharynx neoplasms: an outcome analysis of 170 patients. Eur Arch Otorhinolaryngol. 2011;268(2):281–8.
55. Cerrati EW, Nguyen SA, Farrar JD, Lentsch EJ. The efficacy of photodynamic therapy in the treatment of oral squamous cell carcinoma: a meta-analysis. Ear Nose Throat J. 2015;94(2):72–9.
56. Kübler AC, de Carpentier J, Hopper C, Leonard AG, Putnam G. Treatment of squamous cell carcinoma of the lip using Foscan-mediated photodynamic therapy. Int J Oral Maxillofac Surg. 2001;30(6):504–9.
57. Shafirstein G, Rigual NR, Arshad H, Cooper MT, Bellnier DA, Wilding G, et al. Photodynamic therapy with 3-(1′-hexyloxyethyl) pyropheophorbide-a for early-stage cancer of the larynx: phase Ib study. Head Neck. 2016;38(S1):E377–83.
58. Jerjes W, Upile T, Hamdoon Z, Nhembe F, Bhandari R, Mackay S, et al. Ultrasound-guided photodynamic therapy for deep seated pathologies: prospective study. Lasers Surg Med. 2009;41(9):612–21.
59. Jerjes W, Upile T, Hamdoon Z, Mosse CA, Akram S, Morley S, et al. Interstitial PDT for vascular anomalies. Lasers Surg Med. 2011;43(5):357–65.
60. Cassidy CM, Tunney MM, McCarron PA, Donnelly RF. Drug delivery strategies for photodynamic antimicrobial chemotherapy: from benchtop to clinical practice. J Photochem Photobiol B Biol. 2009;95(2):71–80.
61. Haukvik T, Bruzell E, Kristensen S, Tønnesen HH. Photokilling of bacteria by curcumin in different aqueous preparations. Studies on curcumin and curcuminoids XXXVII. Pharmazie. 2009;64(10):666–73.
62. Street CN, Gibbs A, Pedigo L, Andersen D, Loebel NG. In vitro photodynamic eradication of Pseudomonas aeruginosa in planktonic and biofilm culture. Photochem Photobiol. 2009;85(1):137–43.
63. Kharkwal GB, Sharma SK, Huang YY, Hamblin MR. Photodynamic therapy for infections: clinical applications. Lasers Surg Med. 2011;43(7):755–67.
64. Romano RA, Pratavieira S, Silva APD, da Kurachi C, Guimarães FEG. Light-driven photosensitizer uptake increases Candida albicans photodynamic inactivation. J Biophotonics. 2017;10(11):1538–46.
65. Meisel P, Kocher T. Photodynamic therapy for periodontal diseases: state of the art. J Photochem Photobiol B Biol. 2005;79(2):159–70.
66. Christodoulides N, Nikolidakis D, Chondros P, Becker J, Schwarz F, Rössler R, et al. Photodynamic therapy as an adjunct to non-surgical periodontal treatment: a randomized, controlled clinical trial. J Periodontol. 2008;79(9):1638–44.
67. Lei X, Liu B, Huang Z, Wu J. A clinical study of photodynamic therapy for chronic skin ulcers in lower limbs infected with Pseudomonas aeruginosa. Arch Dermatol Res. 2015;307(1):49–55.
68. Moftah NH, Ibrahim SM, Wahba NH. Intense pulsed light versus photodynamic therapy using liposomal methylene blue gel for the treatment of truncal acne vulgaris: a comparative randomized split body study. Arch Dermatol Res. 2016;308(4):263–8.
69. Scwingel AR, Barcessat ARP, Núñez SC, Ribeiro MS. Antimicrobial photodynamic therapy in the treatment of oral candidiasis in HIV-infected patients. Photomed Laser Surg. 2012;30(8):429–32.
70. Yang Y, Sang J, Liao N, Wei F, Liao W, Chen J. Off-label photodynamic therapy for recalcitrant facial flat warts using topical 5-aminolevulinic acid. Lasers Med Sci. 2016;31(5):929–36.
71. Mima EG, Vergani CE, Machado L, Massucato EMS, Colombo L, Bagnato VS, et al. Comparison of photodynamic therapy versus conventional antifungal therapy for the treatment of denture stomatitis: a randomized clinical trial. Clin Microbiol Infect. 2012;18(10):E380–8.
72. Ribeiro DG, Pavarina AC, Dovigo LN, De Oliveira Mima EG, MacHado AL, Bagnato VS, et al. Photodynamic inactivation of microorganisms present on complete dentures. A clinical investigation Photodynamic disinfection of complete dentures. Lasers Med Sci. 2012;27(1):161–8.

73. Alves F, Alonso GC, Carmello JC, Mima EG de O, Bagnato VS, Pavarina AC. Antimicrobial photodynamic therapy mediated by photodithazine® in the treatment of denture stomatitis: a case report. Photodiagn Photodyn Ther. 2018;21:168–71.
74. Adad Donato R, Pratavieira S, Grecco C, Brugnera-Jú A, Bagnato VS, et al. Clinical comparison of two photosensitizers for oral cavity decontamination. Photomed Laser Surg. 2017;35(2):105–10.
75. Santezi C, Tanomaru JMGG, Bagnato VS, Júnior OBO, Dovigo LN. Potential of curcumin-mediated photodynamic inactivation to reduce oral colonization. Photodiagn Photodyn Ther. 2016;15:46–52.
76. Araújo NC, Fontana CR, Gerbi MEM, Bagnato VS. Overall-mouth disinfection by photodynamic therapy using curcumin. Photomed Laser Surg. 2012;30(2):96–101.
77. Leite DPV, Paolillo FR, Parmesano TN, Fontana CR, Bagnato VS. Effects of photodynamic therapy with blue light and curcumin as mouth rinse for oral disinfection: a randomized controlled trial. Photomed Laser Surg. 2014;32(11):627–32.
78. Pinto MCDC, Fujita AKL, De Menezes PFC, Bagnato VS. Photodynamic therapy with 5-aminolevulinic acid (ALA) in the treatment of acne: a case study. Clin Dermatol. 2017;1(1):114.
79. Genina EA, Bashkatov AN, Simonenko GV, Odoevskaya OD, Tuchin VV, Altshuler GB. Low-intensity indocyanine-green laser phototherapy of acne vulgaris: pilot study. J Biomed Opt. 2004;9(4):828–34.
80. Zhang L, Wu Y, Zhang Y, Liu X, Wang B. Topical 5-aminolevulinic photodynamic therapy with red light vs intense pulsed light for the treatment of acne vulgaris: a split face, randomized, prospective study. Dermatoendocrinol. 2018;9(1):1–9.
81. Posadzki P, Car J. Light therapies for acne. JAMA Dermatol. 2018;154(5):597–8.
82. Hongcharu W, Taylor CR, Chang Y, Aghassi D, Suthamjariya K, Anderson RR. Topical ALA-photodynamic therapy for the treatment of acne vulgaris. J Invest Dermatol. 2000;115(2):183–92.
83. Blanco KC, Inada NM, Carbinatto FM, Giusti AL, Bagnato VS. Treatment of recurrent pharyngotonsillitis by photodynamic therapy. Photodiagn Photodyn Ther. 2017;18:138–9.

Biophotonic Based Orofacial Rehabilitation and Harmonization

6

Rosane de Fatima Zanirato Lizarelli
and Vanderlei Salvador Bagnato

Contents

Abstract

Dentistry is a field that has been evaluated to act beyond the teeth. Treatment of diseases such as gingivitis, neuralgia, and others is common nowadays. The constant demand created by the highest life expectations of men and women requires constantly changing procedures. Geriatric dentistry is, today, a specialty among the general dental activities. This constant evolution is directing dentistry to offer patients much more than the conventional curative procedures, also migrating to rehabilitation and to aesthetic restoration to promote full harmonization. Based on modern technologies, with special attention to those promoted by biophotonics, orofacial rehabilitation and harmonization is becoming a reality. In this chapter, we describe a collection of procedures and technologies that has allowed orofacial biophotonics-based rehabilitation and harmonization to become a new specialty for modern dentistry.

Keywords

Laser · LED · Dentistry · Rehabilitation Orofacial · Biophotonics

6.1 Introduction

Biophotonics is the use of light in the areas of health, for the purposes of the diagnosis, treatment, and maintenance of biological systems. Within dentistry, the competence of the dental

R. de Fatima Zanirato Lizarelli (✉) · V. S. Bagnato
Biophotonics Laboratory - Physics Institute of Sao Carlos, University of São Paulo, São Carlos, Brazil

S. Stübinger et al. (eds.), *Lasers in Oral and Maxillofacial Surgery*,
https://doi.org/10.1007/978-3-030-29604-9_6

surgeon is required to prevent, diagnose, treat, and preserve patients' orofacial health. It is part of this profession to be up to date with all the innovative, scientifically established procedures.

Biophotonics, using different light sources, associated or not with other therapies (dermocosmetics, peelings, kinesiotherapies, etc.) came to add and contribute at different levels e.g., from the diagnosis of tissues to the treatment and treatment plan itself; the microbiological control of infections (e.g., caries, periodontitis, acnes, herpes), loss of sensation (paresthesias), loss of motor activity (paralyses), acute and chronic pain (photodynamic therapy); photoactivation of biomaterials (resin restorative materials and bleaching agents); selective ablation of hard and soft tissues and of biomaterials; preservation of healthy structures, and also in the management of dysfunctions, which may or may not be established in the orofacial region.

In this way, lasers and LEDs, intense pulsed light (IPL) and radiofrequency (RF), high-intensity focused ultrasound (HIFU) and high-intensity laser therapy, ablative or non-ablative, fractional or non-fractional, will also aid us in tissue and muscular toning, integumentary whitening/decontamination, and aesthetic orofacial corrections.

Considering non-invasive procedures, photobiomodulation is the area of biophotonics where light sources operating at low or medium intensity are used.

6.2 Photonic Therapies for Orofacial Rehabilitation and Harmonization

Considering the use of laser and LED light, it is possible to work from real-time optical diagnosis, with violet LEDs, performing dental lightening, with photodynamic therapy and photoactivation, laser surgery for ultra-conservative plastics and removal of carious tissue. But without doubt, the most frequently explored area that has a much broader field of action has been photobiomodulation and its combination with other therapies, such as chemical and mechanical treatments, both for the integumentary system and for the orofacial neuromuscular system.

In this way, we will review the indications of the most commonly used spectral bands and their associations with kinesiotherapies (photokinesiotherapy) and with chemical–physical treatments (photopeelings).

The intention of these therapies is to minimize the effects of aging using all the knowledge of anatomy, reconstituting the joviality without giving a plasticized, artificial aspect, with rhytidoplasty considered the gold standard.

Face squaring most often starts from the age of 30, and, depending on genetic standards and the neutralizing ability of each person's free radicals, wrinkles may or may not arise early.

Prophylaxis for patients with high muscular strength and very expressive people prevents the early appearance of static wrinkles. For this purpose, it is possible to use photobiomodulation with light-emitting red (600–700 nm) and low total energy per application point (1 J) or infrared laser with high total energy per application point (around 5 J), associating with the functional elastic bandages (Phototaping) or even using botulinum toxin.

Orofacial rehabilitation/harmonization is, at the moment, a field of dentistry rather than a specialization. It brings together various very specific areas that intersect with each other and that seek the same goal of managing senescence and preventing the senility of the stomatognathic system.

6.2.1 Photobiomodulation

Photobiomodulation has become established as an intelligent "instrument" in managing the cellular, tissue and systemic physiological responses, in different directions, but all with the same objective: to return the synesthetic and holistic homeostasis, resulting in systemic functionality.

Phototherapy, called photobiomodulation since 2015 [1], a term that encompasses all light sources that modulate systemic physiological responses without ablating (removing) tissues, has been shown to be a very efficient option within dentistry. Relief of acute and chronic pain, drainage of inflammatory processes and tissue repair can be performed or supplemented with light at low intensity. Using higher and controlled doses and protocols, it is also able to improve the quality of the tissues under repair, avoiding keloids and apparent scars, lightened patches of skin, mucous and dental surfaces, promoting the microbiological and tumor control of regions affected by infections or uncontrolled mitoses, recovering cellular functions damaged by time.

Currently, we consider the visible spectral range and the near infrared as the lights whose chromophores in the biological tissue absorb them and, therefore, result in the promotion of a photobiomodulatory effect; however, a recently published article by Hamblin [2], also cites the possibility of light emitting in the medium infrared, where there is a considerable temperature rise, also to be absorbed, but by the water molecules and, as a consequence, increases the influx of calcium ions into the intracellular environment.

Here, we highlight some interesting photobiomodulatory characteristics of each spectral range, from violet to near infrared. According to Daghastanli [3], the lights in the visible portion have the following spectral bands: violet from 390 to 455 nm, blue from 455 to 492 nm, green from 492 to 577 nm, yellow from 577 to 597 nm, amber from 597 to 622 nm, red from 622 to 780 nm. Above 780 nm, the infrared spectrum begins, the next one considered to be 780 to 1500 nm, an average of 1500 to 5600 nm and distance of 5600 to 10,600 nm.

6.2.1.1 Red Light (622–780 nm)

Red light is absorbed by the cytochrome c-oxidase, then causing oxidation of nicotinamide adenine dinucleotide (NAD) and consequently changing the state of mitochondrial and cytoplasmic oxy-reduction. This change in the electron transport velocity of the respiratory chain generates an increase in the proton-motor force, in the electrical potential of the mitochondrial membrane, in the acidity of the cytoplasm, and in the amount of endocellular adenosine tri-phosphate (ATP).

The increase in intracellular H + ion concentration results in changes in the sodium (Na^+) and potassium (K^+) pump in the cell membrane, increasing the permeability to calcium ions (Ca^{2+}) to the intracellular medium. The increased amount of this cation affects the level of the cyclic nucleotides that modulate the synthesis of RNA and DNA [4]. It changes the oxy-red state of the cell, promoting chemical and enzymatic reactions for the dissociation of internal components, immediately releasing the nitric oxide molecules previously attached to the cytochrome c-oxidase, and then accelerating the metabolism; this reflects vasodilation at the tissue level [5].

It is a spectral band that can be used in protocols for nutrition, oxygenation, and tissue repair, facilitating all other steps provided in the protocols, so that it can be associated in several treatments.

In addition, we know that for the light to be absorbed by cytochrome c-oxidase, phototoxication of nitric oxide occurs, which is responsible for the immediate increase in vasodilation and improvement in tissue oxygenation.

In addition, in an editorial of *Photomedicine and Laser Surgery*, Sommer and Trelles [6] developed the following idea: the near infrared light (670 nm—red) at low intensities for biostimulation is fundamental to regulating the ATP content in cells, and when applied in a pulsed mode, to the activation of cellular metabolism.

Thus, red light can promote the treatment of vitiligo—in very low doses 3 J/cm^2 – reorganization of fibroblasts, melanocytes, keratinocytes, and melanoblasts ([7, 8]; be antioxidant [9, 10]; decrease the expression of metalloproteinases; and promote an "FPS 15-like" effect by preventing post-inflammatory hyperpigmentation by increasing nerve growth factor (NGF), protecting melanocytes from UVB [11].

Moshkovska and Mayberry [9] and Huang et al. [12] already mentioned the benefits of intravascular therapy with red laser, also being an antioxidant and systemically treating some diseases.

Red laser is low intensity, because it penetrates less, mainly by the mechanism of absorption through which it interacts with the biological tissue is indicated for superficial lesions such as tissue repair (healing and local drainage), muscle relaxation, or to photoactivate biomaterials/dermocosmetics for topical application.

Red light (laser or LED) at low intensity also promotes mitochondrial biogenesis, that is, it restores the conditions for the cells to rebalance their metabolism. Recent work shows that 630 nm (37 mW/cm^2, 75 mW) LED irradiation with 16 J/cm^2 radiant exposure was able to induce a proliferative response in stem cells of the pulp tissue of deciduous teeth without affecting mitochondrial function or inducing senescence [13].

A recent study by Oh et al. [14] showed that the LED, emitting in the range of 660 nm, under an energy density of 10–20 J/cm^2, was able to inhibit tyrosinase activity, reducing UVB-induced melanogenesis in the skin (in vitro and in vivo). They concluded that the red LED ± 660 nm is a potential integumentary depigmentation.

6.2.1.2 Near Infrared Light (780–1500 nm)

Light emitting in the spectral range of the near infrared can be absorbed by the cytochrome c-oxidase in the mitochondrial respiratory chain, too. However, it can also be absorbed in the biomembranes, the photophysical polarity of the membranes that results in the alteration of the conduction of neural stimuli and the permeability of these biomembranes.

Cytoplasmic membrane permeability increases in relation to the Ca^{2+}, Na^+ and K^+ ions, determining an increase in cell membrane receptor activity. As a result, endorphin synthesis and the action potential of neural cells increase, whereas the amount of bradykinin as well as the activity of C-fibers leading to painful stimuli diminishes. This sequence of events results in relief of pain symptoms [4]. Infrared laser/LED are wavelengths that act in the relief of acute and chronic pain, lymphatic drainage, and bone and neural repair, being considered, in aesthetic treatment, essential when the cause is the accumulation of free radicals in the system. Considering the integumentary system, it is hypothesized that, once this spectral band is absorbed by the membrane proteins, it can then be absorbed by the aquaporins, for example, thus stimulating its action, which is the transport of transmembrane water molecules (from the dermis to the epidermis). This could promote active epidermal hydration.

The infrared laser in low intensity is more penetrating, but because it interacts through changes in the polarity of the biomembranes, it has been the wavelength of choice for neural and bone repair, and also to promote immediate and temporary analgesia, as it works by altering the potential of these biomembranes.

As with red light, it can also be delivered in the target tissue at the dental clinic, both in a timely manner and in a larger area, when the idea of concentrating the delivered light penetrates a little more and the diffusion in the cluster generates the opposite effect, keeping the greater percentage of the energy absorbed in the more superficial layers.

Several studies with infrared, laser, and/or LED light, associated with exercises and other kinesiotherapies, have demonstrated a great ability to accelerate neuro-muscular rehabilitation, both facially and in the body. This possibility opens a very important window for orofacial rehabilitation procedures, as it would not only be suitable for reconditioning the system to perform its functions, but also to prevent the loss of efficiency that is physiologically occurring with the aging of the stomatognathic system. This approach will be discussed in Sect. 6.2.2 on photokinesiotherapy.

6.2.1.3 Blue Light (455–492 nm)

Blue light is able to accelerate chemical reactions, including cell metabolism. Absorbed by the flavoproteins [15], in the mitochondrial respiratory chain, hemoglobin, porphyrins, and cytochrome c were reduced [16], but also absorbed by cryptochromes [2], in biological tissues, and by most biomaterials because of their spectral range.

Upon absorption by flavoproteins and cryptochromes, the blue light promotes an increase in the influx of some ions, such as calcium, magnesium, and zinc, improving the cellular metabolism.

It can be used as a photoactivator and photoaccelerates polymerization of monomers in restorative materials and to induce the production of singlet oxygen in photodynamic therapies, when the photosensitizer and/or the target bacterium (as for example, the bacterium of acne, *Propionibacterium acnes* [17] and the bacteria of periodontal disease) absorb blue wavelengths [18, 19].

However, even within photobiomodulation, it can decompose hydrogen peroxide present in cells (metabolism products) [18] and/or biomaterial (dental bleaching agents). The action, when absorbed by the peroxides, results in the breaking of large light-absorbing molecules and of these peroxides, transforming double bonds into simple ones, reducing the absorption of light, and then there will be whitening of the skin and dental tissue (enamel and dentin) and hydration of the tissues [20, 21].

In addition to this mechanism, through controlled thermotherapy, when the source emits with medium intensity, a facilitation occurs in the decomposition of the peroxides and diffusion of the products to the interstitial space, in the soft tissues, inducing swelling and acting as a hydrating agent by wetting, promoting the change in the superficial tension of the skin, with the aesthetic effect of expansion of the tissues.

In addition, once absorbed, blue light may induce the production of collagen and elastin, being able to accelerate cellular metabolism as much as or more than the red wavelength [22].

Another hypothesis on tegument hydration (skin = epidermis, dermis, and cutaneous attachments) is that the blue spectrum accelerates the function of keratin in making the stratum corneum more resistant and impermeable, acting as an occlusion agent for the epidermis, reducing loss (reducing transepidermal water loss).

A more recently discovered function: low doses (3–16 J/cm^2) are able to modulate immature and mature Langerhans cells (dendritic cells), modulating proinflammatory cytokines locally and in lymph nodes [23].

6.2.1.4 Amber Light (577–622 nm)

Amber light emits into a spectral range of 577–622 nm. It has the best peak of absorption by cytochrome c oxidase, according to Poyton and Ball [24]. Thus, as well as wavelengths emitting red (600–700 nm), it interferes with mitochondrial respiration by accelerating the rate of endocellular ATP production and promotes a large release of nitric oxide (NO), which is responsible for vasodilation and neurotransmission.

It is therefore recommended to accelerate the repair of soft tissues of the tegument (gingiva, epidermis, and dermis) and the conjunctiva, such as assisting the return of muscle toning in a case of facial paralysis during the neuromuscular rehabilitation process.

Regarding its penetrability into the biological tissue, it is already known that amber light reaches the connective tissue, i.e., in the skin, it reaches the papillary dermis. Figure shows a measure where this situation is very clear. However, orofacial tissues, because they are very thin, may have the benefit of this light in deeper layers, reaching muscle tissue.

WEISS et al. [25, 26] presented an experience of more than 2 years treating 900 patients with dermatological diseases, using amber LED (±590 nm) as the only instrument or associated with other therapies (Light Intense Pulsed (LIP), RF, ablative lasers, for example). They observed the following clinical effects of this amber light: an anti-inflammatory effect, acceleration in tissue repair, decreased gene expression of collagenase in photodark skins, and thus a suitable light for skin aging management treatments as well as post-treatment of more aggressive surgical procedures [27, 28].

Another study by the same group [25, 26] confirmed with standardized experiments that the photomodulation treatment has the potential to modulate the production of matrix metalloproteinases (MMPs) after thermal lesions. Therefore, combined amber LED treatments with non-ablative thermal techniques, such as ILP or dye laser, may be beneficial.

To McDaniel (2005), the patent was granted to manufacture all the equipment with amber LED, whether alone or associated with the infrared laser, in the continuous (CW), periodic (keyed) or pulsed modes. He presented the methods and how to use them to regulate cell proliferation and gene expression in the production of collagen.

A recently published article by Chen et al. [29] demonstrated that amber light at 585 nm with fluences of 10–20 J/cm^2 was able to induce autophagy of melanocytes and decrease melanogenesis, confining their indication to tissue whitening.

6.2.1.5 Violet Light (390–455 nm)

In this emission range, the photons have more energy; therefore, being highly absorbed, the penetrability of this light into the biological tissues is quite superficial, remaining in the epithelial band of the mucous membranes and in the epidermis of the skin. In this way, fluorescence can also be easily observed and seen with the naked eye or with filters; thus, it is a welcome spectral range for both optical diagnostics and surface treatments.

Absorption chromophores consist of derivatives of porphyrins, flavoproteins, and terminal oxidases; oxyhemoglobin and melanin; and long chain molecules with delocalized electrons [30].

In addition, it is important to note that the effects of nitric oxide (NO) and NO molecules on the surface of the lungs have been shown to be associated with the effects of vasoconstriction and decontamination [31], and with the use of a high-performance tooth-whitening agent (Lever et al., 2010).

Some studies have shown that violet light is more efficient than blue light for decontamination of skin, mucosa, and even osseo-integrated implants [32–34], and is very well indicated as a photonic agent for facial peelings [35], promoting excellent clinical results by softening facial expression marks and wrinkles.

However, it is a spectral band that can generate many free radicals that are deleterious to important molecules, such as carotenoids (natural skin antioxidants) and fibroblasts present in the dermis [36]; the dose and frequency of application should be monitored. It is worth remembering here the importance of dosimetry in the clinical success of photobiomodulation.

6.2.1.6 Green Light (492–577 nm)

There are still few studies on green light. According to HAMBLIN [2], green light is absorbed by the opsins. One of the best defined signaling events that occurs after opiate light activation is the opening of light ion channels, such as members of the calcium channel family of transient receptor potential (TRP). TRP channels are now known as pleiotropic cellular sensors that measure the response to a wide range of external stimuli (heat, cold, pressure, taste, smell) and are involved in various cellular processes.

The light emitted in this spectral range is able to reach the dermo-epidermal junction in the skin, as well as the dentinal tissue of the dental organ, and is therefore an interesting tool for the mechanisms of maintenance of skin metabolism and protection of the pulp. However, this is just a suggestion; studies need to check these potentialities, because only a few studies on green light have been published so far:

- Antioxidant effect on photoaged skin [37].
- Increased angiogenesis [38].
- Acceleration in the process of repair in burned skin [39].
- Anti-inflammatory effect on burned skin [40].
- Acceleration in the cellular metabolism (increase in the concentration of calcium ions) and an increase in the gene expression for osteogenesis, from the stem cells [41].
- Excessive increase in the entry of calcium ions (oxidation), greatly increasing free radicals and inhibiting the proliferation of adipocytes (from the stem cells) [42].

We performed clinical research, with laboratorial measurements of electromyography and ultrasound of the dermis, to evaluate the effect of photobiomodulation with purple light (blue LED + red laser) and yellow light (amber LED + infrared laser) in women aged 35–55 years (Fig. 6.1).

Figures 6.2 and 6.3 present digital photographs and comparative measurements of the initial and final (after 30 days) situation of one of the participants in the light research group. It is a simple, easy-to-perform orofacial biophotonics session, which can be used not only as a single treatment but also as an operative sequence of the mid and late postoperative periods of other more invasive procedures (peelings, HIFU, LIP, etc.). The session lasts around 60 to 90 min.

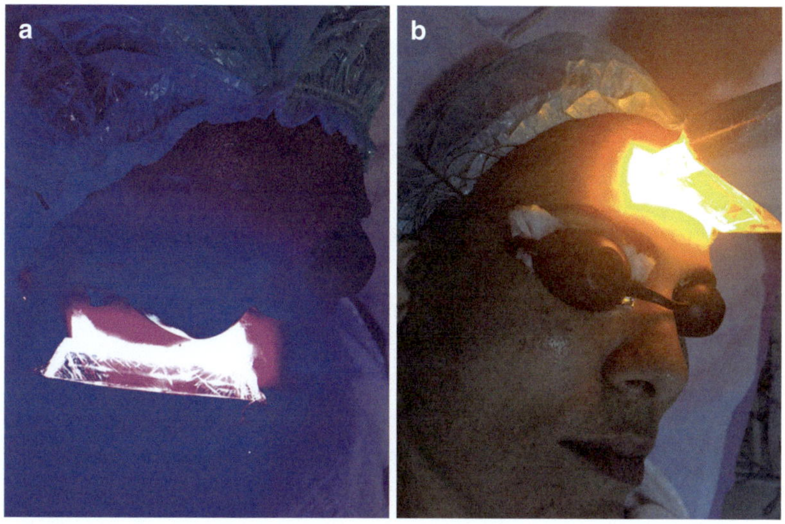

Fig. 6.1 Photobiomodulation with (**a**) purple light (blue LED + red laser) and (**b**) yellow light (amber LED + infrared laser; Venus, MMOptics, São Carlos, SP, Brazil)

In Fig. 6.1, facial photographs are presented without the eye covering, because it is very important to look closely at the region of the periocular muscles. It is very interesting to see how much the photobiomodulation has changed in the clinical orofacial aspect of the patient (Fig. 6.2). Of course, owing to the instructions on the correct method of hygiene, hydration, and protection that she received, in the first session, when she received the dermocosmetics and started using them, her home care could already contribute to the improvement in integumentary health. However, very different from the cases studied in the control group, where the participants did not receive irradiation or any other stimuli (kinesiotherapies), the patient in the present case leaves very easily observed evidence that photobiomodulation can cause homeostasis to return, not only to the skin, but also to the orofacial neuromuscular system. This is because the clinical aspect presented after the eight sessions of laser/LED irradiation appears to be calm with diminished expression marks, which could be understood as the balance of the orofacial muscle force vectors or, simply, neuromuscular reprogramming.

Figure 6.3 shows results from the same patient as shown in Fig. 6.1, where this reprogramming seems to be more evident. In Fig. 6.2a, the electromyography of the frontal bundles of the right and left occipital–frontal muscles (left side, above), before and after the treatment, as well as the right and left orbicularis muscles (left side, below), both in isometry (elevation of the eyebrows and forced closure respectively), showed an improvement in the electromyographic signal, which can be translated as an improvement of muscle toning. In Fig. 6.2b, it was the integumentary system covering the orbicularis muscle of the right eye (above) and the frontal bundle of the right occipital frontal muscle (below) that were evaluated under dermal ultrasound (Dermascan, FCFRP/USP Cosmetology Lab), comparing the initial (left) and final (right) situations, when there was a significant improvement in echogenicity, which can be translated as an improvement in tegumentary (skin) toning.

6.2.2 Photokinesiotherapies

Photokinesiotherapy is a program of active, passive, and/or active isometric muscle movements, associated with photobiomodulation, lasers, and LEDs, in the pre- and post-time, i.e., preparing and preserving the tissues to be worked on, providing an efficient metabolism, and then draining the free radicals resulting from this work. The main goal is muscular toning and the consequent improvement of health

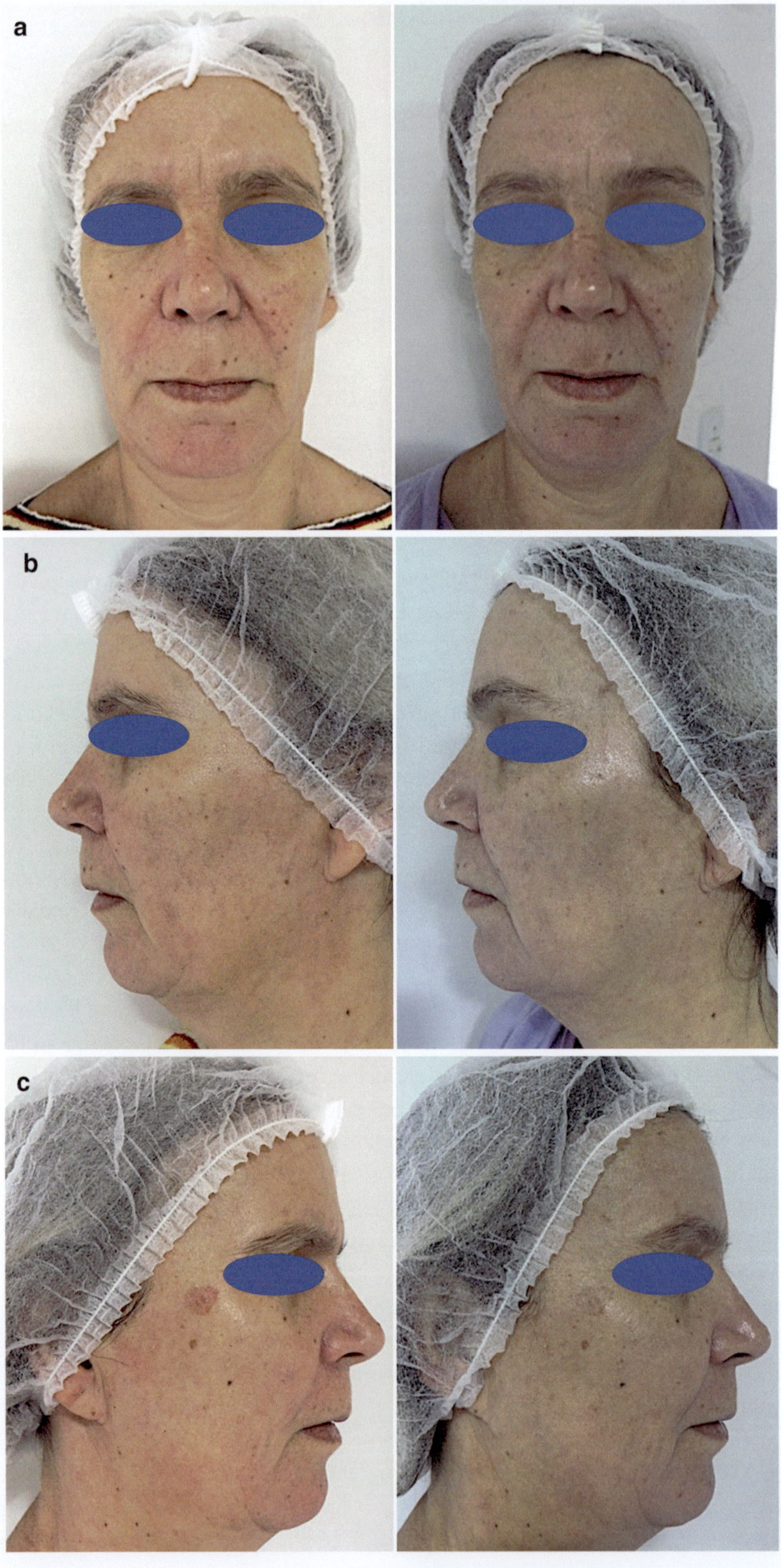

Fig. 6.2 Management of senescence with photobiomodulation: patient G.P.M., 48 years old, female, single, administrative assistant. She sought treatment to improve facial tone. Initial (left) and final (right) clinical appearance in (**a**) frontal, (**b**) left lateral and (**c**) right lateral positions. The clinical sequence, in all the sessions, was: hygiene/exfoliation; irradiation with "purple" light (blue LED + red laser) for 30 s, stopped and in contact throughout the face; irradiation with "yellow" light (amber LED + infrared laser) for 5 min in each facial quadrant (Venus, MMO, São Carlos, SP, Brazil); application of moisturizer with filter (Neofarma/Lizarelli) (personal archive)

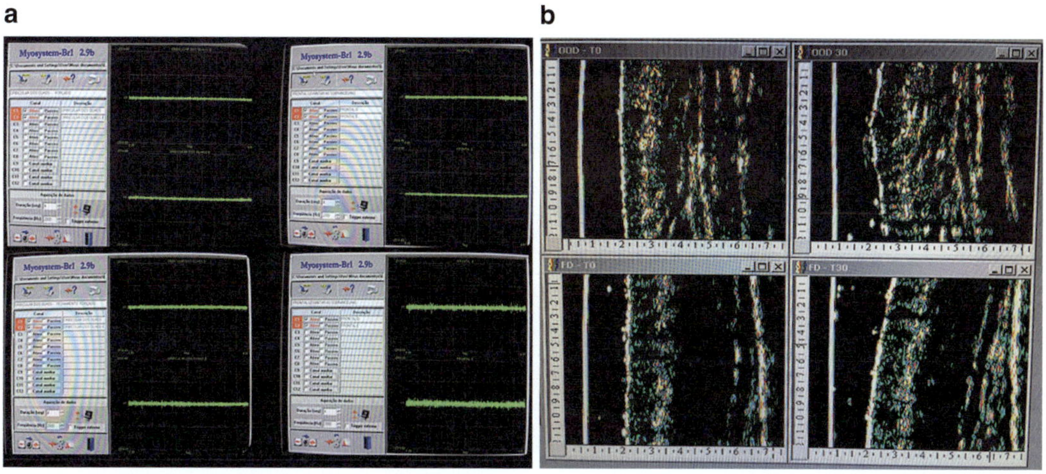

Fig. 6.3 Data on (**a**) electromyography (**b**) ultrasound of the dermis (Dermascan, Lab. Cosmetology of FCFRP / USP) of the orbicularis oculi muscles (Fig. 6.2a, b, below) and frontal view of the occipital–frontal muscles (Fig. 6.2a, b, above), participant of the light group (personal archive)

(improved toning, hydration, and elasticity) of the integumentary system, i.e., the skin.

As the name describes, it is the symbiotic combination of photobiomodulation and kinesiotherapy.

The idea of this new approach, within the rehabilitation of the stomatognathic system, came about with orofacial neuromuscular behavior in the face of senescence (natural physiological aging), senility (senescence associated with traumas or other pathological conditions) and also due to disuse or "misuse" of orofacial muscles.

If the neuromuscular system is dysfunctional, one of the aesthetic and functional consequences presented is orofacial disharmony, through an imbalance of facial proportions, asymmetries, and wrinkles or dynamic and/or static rhytids. Physical orofacial pain may or may not be associated, but in the vast majority of cases, psychological pain and personal dissatisfaction may be present, requiring rehabilitative therapy.

Light sources could be associated with this treatment proposal, in addition to the kinesiotherapies themselves (which will be described below), as well as the therapies capable of managing or reprogramming the entire orofacial neuromuscular system, that is, the orthopedic function of the jaws and the application of botulinum toxin, therapeutic procedures already established within dentistry.

We understand kinesiotherapies to be all the therapeutic modalities with which we can promote muscular movement to cure an illness.

Kinesiotherapies could be classified, in a more didactic way, into:

1. Passive kinesiotherapies: when the patient receives therapy without exerting a physical effort of his own, e.g., mechanical stimuli with massage (stretching, drainage, among others), with equipment such as ultrasound and also with functional elastic bandages, electrical stimuli with equipment (Farádica, Australian, Russian chains).
2. Active kinesiotherapies: mechanical stimuli with self-massage, mechanical stimuli with isometric and isotonic exercises.

We have noticed that a loss of efficiency of the neuromuscular responses occurs over the years. It is sometimes a disabling situation that facilitates the instigation of orofacial dysfunctions, resulting in discomfort, pain and functional loss, and aesthetic disharmony.

For the dental surgeon to offer efficient treatments, it must be understood that, given the cellular nature of these neural and muscular tissues, the quest to maintain physiological homeostasis demands care in the mitochondrial functions. Damaged mitochondria are not only less bioenergy efficient, they can also lead to sarcopenia (loss of skeletal muscle mass and strength due to aging) and loss of muscle function. But they also generate larger amounts of free radicals (reactive oxygen species, ROS) by interfering with and compromising mechanisms of control in cell quality and, finally, showing a greater tendency toward apoptosis.

A large body of evidence indicates that mitochondria are the main source of ROS during chronic muscle inactivity. The experimental evidence also suggests that chronic muscle inactivity causes large disturbances in intracellular calcium homeostasis [43–45], which may lead to the modification of the management of mitochondrial calcium and increased oxidant production [46].

The metabolic plasticity of skeletal myofibers depends to a large extent on the dynamic nature of mitochondria and the ability of these organelles to alter their organization (i.e., shape and size) and position within a cell in response to intracellular and extracellular signals [47]. The mitochondrial morphology is regulated by continuous fusion and fission events that are not only crucial for the determination of the organelle form but also for the transmission of sensitive signals to the oxidation–reduction reactions, maintenance of mitochondrial DNA integrity, and regulation of the pathways of cell death [48]. The equilibrium between fusion and fission depends on a complex machine of mitochondrial dynamics.

Mitochondrial dynamics is centrally involved in the maintenance of cellular homeostasis. In fact, the fusion of isolated mitochondria results in the formation of a mitochondrial network, which allows the mitochondria to mix their content, redistribute metabolites, proteins, and mitochondrial DNA, and avoid the local accumulation of abnormal mitochondria [49]. The fission secretes the components of the mitochondrial network that are irreversibly damaged or unnecessary, allowing its autophagic removal [50]. There is, therefore, a functional link between mitochondrial dynamics and autophagy, which is essential for mitochondrial quality control [51]. An imbalance in mitochondrial fusion–fission events, associated with altered mitochondrial degradation, contributes to the mitochondrial imbalance observed in atrophied muscles.

Thus, it seems very clear that the prevention, treatment, and maintenance of orofacial muscular health, that is, the toning of the orofacial muscles, depends directly on mitochondrial functionality. So how could photobiomodulation accomplish this "mitochondrial management"?

XU et al. presented a very interesting study in rats. They induced oxidative mitochondrial stress by electrical stimuli, subsequently treating with laser therapy, and concluded that photobiomodulation significantly reduced ROS production and restored mitochondrial function, which may form a basis for the use of photobiomodulation to treat mitochondrial dysfunction induced by exercise or skeletal muscle fatigue.

Also, degenerative diseases, such as Parkinson's and Alzheimer's, have been studied to promote not only their treatment with associated light, but also to prevent those diseases that result in orofacial senility. According to Tegowska and Wosinska [52], although mitochondria constantly generate free radicals, from which they are protected by their own defensive systems, in some situations these systems become deregulated, which leads to mitochondrial defects based on free radicals. This causes an energy deficit in the neurons and an additional increase in the association of free radicals. The nature of these processes is initially protective because of their antioxidant action, but as the amount of formations increases, the beneficial effect decreases. They become a storage site for substances that improve the processes of free radicals, which makes them toxic. This is approach of the primary causal factor for Alzheimer's, suggesting the use of methylene-based drugs, laser, or insulin applied intranasally.

In 2014, Agrawal et al. showed evidence that photobiomodulation may also be effective if delivered to normal cells or tissue prior to the actual trauma in a preconditioning mode. The muscles are protected, the nerves feel less pain and there is even protection against a subsequent heart attack. These examples point the way to the wider use of photobiomodulation as a preconditioning modality to prevent pain and increase healing after surgical/medical procedures, and possibly to increase athletic performance.

Nguyen et al. [53] evaluated mitochondria of muscle cells irradiated with near infrared light (800–950 nm) under low intensity (22.8 J/cm^2) and suggested that exposure to this light source repeated for 4 consecutive days seemed to increase oxidative stress and mitochondrial regulatory proteins upstream AMPK (3.1-fold), p38 (2.8-fold), PGC-1α (19.7%), Sirt1 (26.8%), and reduced RIP140 (23.2%), but the regulation of mitochondrial content (Tfam, NRF-1, Sirt3, cytochrome c, ETC subunits) was not altered. The data indicated that light in the near infrared spectrum alters mitochondrial biogenesis signaling and may represent a mechanistic link to the clinical benefits.

Albuquerque-Pontes et al. [54] performed a study to evaluate photobiomodulation (laser and LED) in mice with Duchenne muscular dystrophy. They compared controls with experimental groups irradiated with a cluster probe with nine diodes (1 × 905-nm super-pulsed laser diode, 4 × 875-nm infrared LEDs, and 4 × 640-nm red LEDs, manufactured by Multi Radiance Medical®, Solon-OH, USA), three times a week for 14 weeks, using low doses (1 or 3 J) and high doses (10 J) applied at a single point (anterior tibial muscle, bilaterally). We analyzed the functional performance, muscular morphology, and the gene and protein expression of dystrophin. Photobiomodulation at a dose of 10 J significantly improved ($p < 0.001$) functional performance compared with all other experimental groups. Muscular morphology was improved by all doses, with better results at doses of 3 and 10 J. The genetic expression of dystrophy was significantly increased, with doses of 3 J ($p < 0.01$) and 10 J ($p < 0.01$), compared with the control group. Regarding the protein expression of dystrophy, doses of 3 J ($p < 0.001$) and 10 J ($p < 0.05$) also showed a significant increase in relation to the control group. They concluded that photobiomodulation can preserve mainly the muscular morphology and improve the muscular function of the mice through the modulation of gene expression for dystrophy. In addition, as it is a non-pharmacological treatment with no side effects and easy to perform, it can be seen as a promising tool for the treatment of Duchenne muscular dystrophy.

Considering aging, Brito et al. [55] conducted a study on infrared laser photobiomodulation 780 nm, 40 mW, 3.2 J to each point, remodeling of connective tissue, and skeletal muscle regeneration in elderly rats. Eight points were irradiated on the skin referring to the anterior tibial muscle, 2 h after the injury with cryotherapy. In the histomorphological analysis, the treated group showed a significant decrease in the inflammatory infiltrate ($p < 0.001$), as well as increasing the immature fibers and the new blood vessels at 7 days compared with the untreated group ($p < 0.05$). In addition, the treatment induced a better distribution of collagen at 7 days compared with the untreated group ($p < 0.05$). In conclusion, low-energy level laser therapy demonstrated a modulating effect on the muscle repair process in elderly animals with regard to collagen remodeling and morphological aspects of muscle tissue.

This work by Brito et al. [55] makes it clear that low-dose irradiation (up to 3 J) in the infrared spectrum modulates trauma without "destroying" the opportunity that this controlled trauma allows the aged tissues to at least partially recover their tone.

We have developed a logical sequence of orofacial exercises (active kinesiotherapy). This sequence or spreadsheet is shown in Fig. 6.4. The patients perform this sequence daily in their homes, which takes, on average, 45 min. As part of the treatment, these patients attend the clinic twice a week and receive the photobiomodulation with purple light (blue LED + red laser) followed by yellow light (amber LED + infrared laser). This photobiomodulation seeks to tone the stomatognathic system, stimulating not only the neural and muscular connections but also its relationship with the integumentary system. Therefore, it is possible to optimize nutritional changes, to drain metabolites, but to guarantee, by preparing exfoliation (prior to irradiation) and with the isometric movements of the exercises, the microleaves necessary to stimulate neocollagenesis (Fig. 6.5).

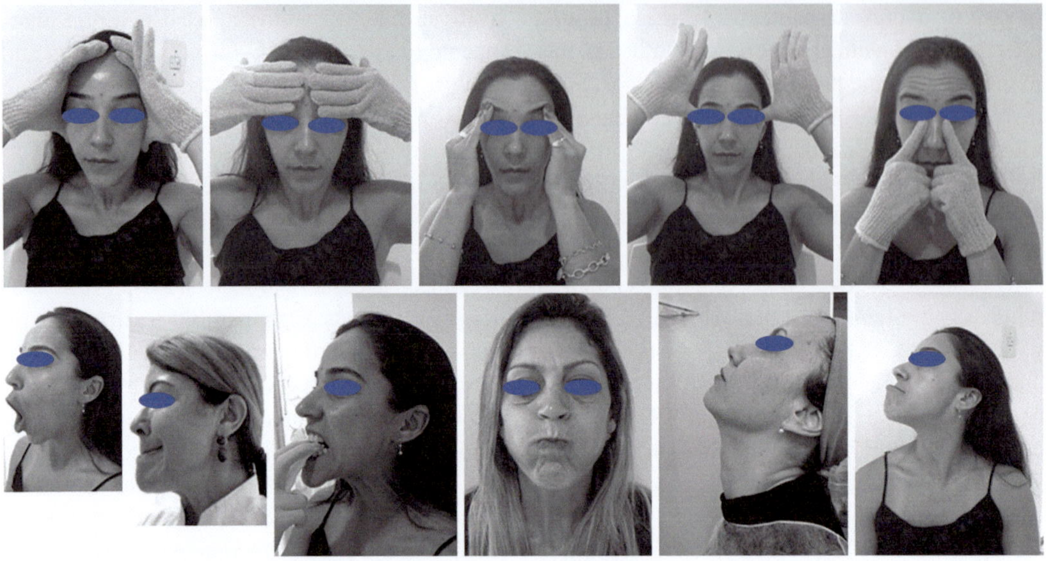

Fig. 6.4 Orofacial exercise sequence using isometric movements addressing the three parts of face: superior third (forehead, eyes, and nose root)—the five exercises on top; the middle third (cheeks, face-lift muscles, buccinator muscles, and masseters)—the first four exercises bottom; and lower third of the face (contour of the face, suprahyoid muscles, and responsible for the protrusion of the mandible)—the last two exercises bottom. It is possible to observe one participant (Fig. 6.5) before and after treatment using photobiomodulation and orofacial exercises

There is a gap to be filled with legitimate dental actions that can reduce the discomfort of our patients caused by trauma, dysfunction, and orofacial aging. Association with therapies that promote different physiological stimuli, optical (lasers and LEDs), mechanical (functional elastic bandages and facial exercises) and electrical (Australian current), has presented very fast results for orofacial neuromuscular rebalancing as well as in the nutritional stimulus and metabolic characteristics of the facial integumentary system, a fact that decelerates natural senescence [56].

6.3 Photopeelings

Peeling consists in a very common procedure aimed at "peeling" the integumentary system. Different layers can be removed, in a controlled manner, at different depths. It means that different goals can be pursued: from the improvement in the permeation of cosmetic assets to the pro-inflammatory stimulus in the dermis, as a stimulus for the neo-formation of proteins (collagen, elastin, reticulin), as well as glycosaminoglycans (e.g., hyaluronic acid).

It is believed that this modality of treatment is one of the oldest forms of rejuvenation. It is effective, flexible, and has a histological, chemical, toxicological, and clinical base. The interesting thing about this procedure is that it can be adapted to most circumstances within the limits of its indications.

Historically, the use of this philosophy of "controlled destruction" to "rejuvenate" the skin, presents very interesting reports. Cleopatra and many women of ancient Egypt bathed in fermented milk to soften and invigorate the skin; and even though they lacked the scientific knowledge about what they were doing, they were actually performing superficial peeling with an alpha-hydroxy acid called lactic acid, which is derived from milk. There are also indications that Turkish women used fire to scorch the skin, and

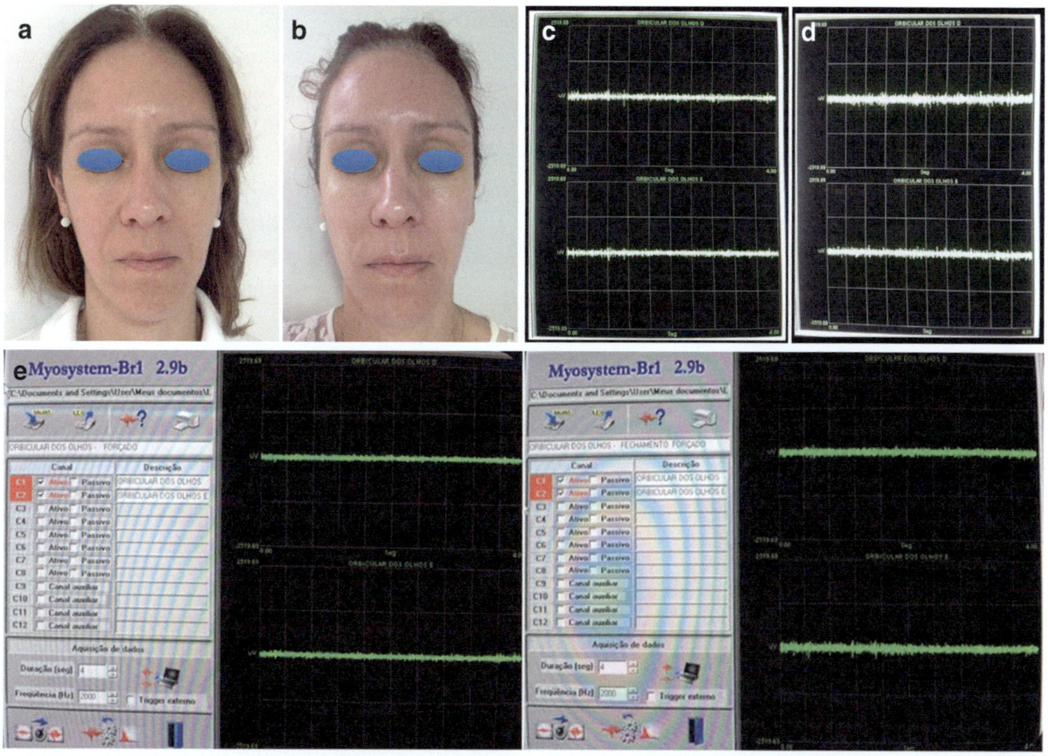

Fig. 6.5 Digital photographs of face (**a**) initially and after (**b**) eight sessions of photobiomodulation in association with orofacial exercises; electromyography of the orbicularis oculis (**c**—top, right side, and, **d**—below, left side); and echogenicity (skin ultrasound) of the right masseter before (**e**—top) and after treatment (**c**—bottom)

then promoted a light exfoliation, whereas Indian women were given a mixture of urine and pumice on the skin to stimulate epidermal desquamation [57]. Also, the Greeks and Romans used some procedures, such as cataplasms containing mustard, sulfur, and corrosive limestone sublimate [58].

Peels can be classified as mechanical, physical, chemical, enzymatic or biological, cryogenic, photomodulated, or photoactivated.

At the end of the nineteenth century, the Norwegian doctor Niels Finsen was already considering preparing his patients' skin with pyrogallic acid ointment to allow better absorption of UV light in the treatment of lupus vulgaris. This could be considered a light photomodulated peeling.

When using a chemical, physical or enzymatic peeling associated with light sources for photobiomodulation, before and after, we considered a photomodulated peeling. This ensures the preparation of the tissue to receive the aggressive procedure and the control of the inflammation generated (and desired) for better healing and tissue neoformation.

Photomodulated or photoactivated peelings are characterized by the presence of acids (alpha hydroxy acids and beta hydroxy acids) with the function of promoting a peeling, which, in association with a light source, becomes more efficient, either by accelerating their reactions or by interacting with its target tissue making it more reactive. Therefore, we consider photoactivated peeling when at least one of the components of this chemical formulation has the ability to absorb light at a specific wavelength (color) with a high quantum yield of ROS formation capable of generating damage of the target tissue stimulating the tissue repair.

Photoactivated peeling is an effective, safe, reproducible, non-melanogenic procedure, and always results in tegmental "whitening," as, minimally, it improves the tissue metabolism and the drainage of the metabolites.

According to Manoel et al. [59] and Menezes [60], photoactivated peels using active chemicals such as methylene blue (Photoskin; Dr. Peel, SP, Brazil), curcumin (Photopeel and Photoskin; Dr. Peel), and glycosides, and procyanidins (Photomelan Peel; Dr. Peel) act by promoting the structuring of the epidermis (thickening) and dermis (stimulation of collagen and other biomolecules), which is very well indicated for aged and dehydrated skin.

An example of a very interesting commercial product with antioxidant, whitening, and skin resurfacing function is Photopeel (Dr Peel). It is a blend of acids combined with curcumin, derived from saffron, and has an absorption band in blue–violet and blue (400–490 nm). Interestingly, depending on the conditions presented by the patient's skin and the timing of the treatment plan, the peeling session with Photopeel can act by preparing, treating or maintaining the health (aesthetics and function) of the skin. It is very well indicated for treatment of acneic skin (Fig. 6.6) and also as an antioxidant and whitening treatment (Fig. 6.7).

Another interesting option is the combination of a physical (electric) peeling with photobiomodulation, resulting in photoelectroabrasion. New Skin (MMO) equipment is a dual technology for multiple treatment purposes. It acts as an electric peeling, promoting the superficial removal of stains through electrodermabrasion, but also as an electro-stimulator, inducing a punctual inflammatory response, that will lead to tissue repair through the activation of the cicatricial process of the treated tissue. The red light type LED, which accompanies the equipment, can be used prior to the procedure, preparing the repair metabolism, and also the post-procedure of this electric peeling, aimed at a more homogeneous and efficient repair and a well-directed control of post-inflammatory staining, being well indicated in the immediate postoperative period of 7 and 14 days respectively. Figure 6.8 shows a clinical case.

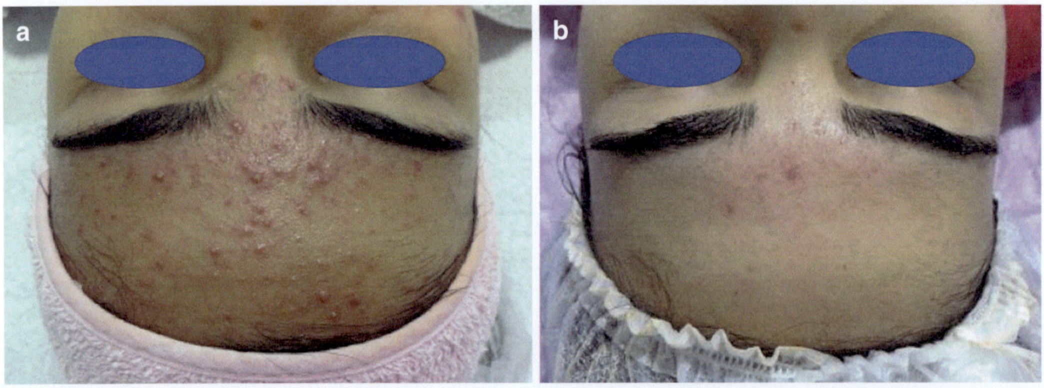

Fig. 6.6 (**a**) Teen patient J.C.L., 15 years old, female, student, phototype III, sought care, accompanied by parents. In the anamnesis, it was observed that the patient had harmful habits, such as excessive junk food and a low daily consumption of water, besides not being well oriented as regards the minimal and necessary home care for her type of face, acne grade 3. The patient received photobiomodulation and photoactivated peeling based on acids and curcumin (Photopeel; Neofarma–Dr. Peel, SP, Brazil) photoactivated with blue LED (Elite, DMC, São Carlos, SP, Brazil) for 3 months, and 2 weekly sessions, to control the acne disease. (**b**) After treatment, the patient presented a significant improvement, including self-esteem and social coexistence (personal file)

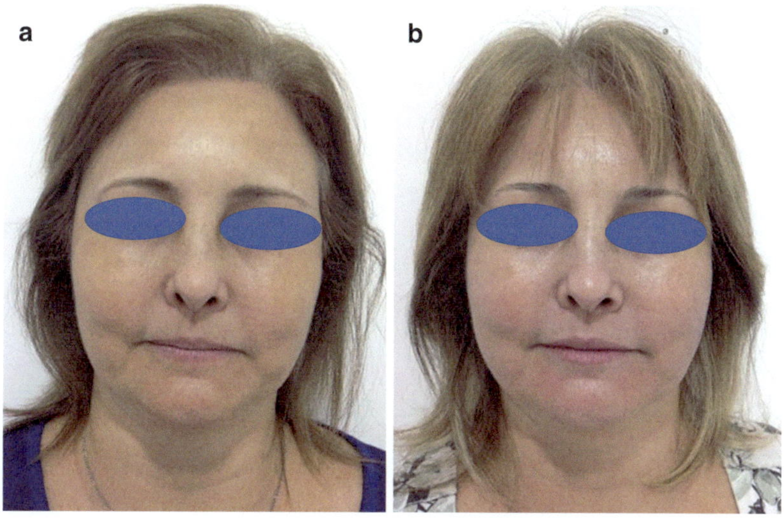

Fig. 6.7 (**a**) Patient R.C.F., 50 years old, married, presented a clinical appearance of decreased tissue toning and lack of vitality. The patient received six sessions with photo-activated peeling (Photopeel; Dr. Peel) photoactivated with blue LED (Elite; DMC), weekly, and intercalated sessions of photokinesiotherapy (orofacial exercises and light), totaling 2 months of treatment for rehabilitative orofacial biophotonics, (**b**) resulting in a healthier, youthful, and toned appearance, as well as lighter skin. The patient's eyes were not covered because of the importance of observing the improvement in upper palpebral tissue flaccidity and her ptosis (tissue and muscular toning; personal archive)

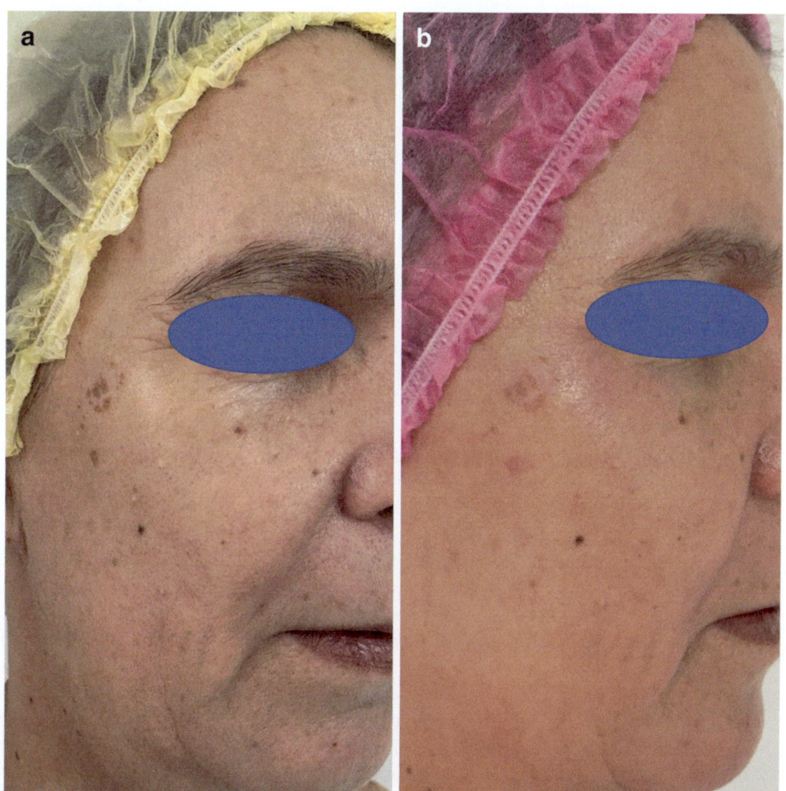

Fig. 6.8 Patient G.P.M., 48 years old, female, single, administrative assistant. She sought treatment to improve facial tone. (**a**) Initial and (**b**) 7 days after the procedure using photomodulated (red LED) electrodermabrasion (New Skin; MMOptics, São Carlos, SP, Brazil) clinical appearance in the right lateral position

6.4 Conclusion

The use of different light sources as a unique tool or in combination with other therapies could facilitate orofacial rehabilitation, preventing senescence and dental dysfunction. These proposed functional treatments allow a great aesthetic result, promoting orofacial harmonization. In fact, having knowledge about how to use biophotonics to prevent orofacial sarcopenia is mandatory for all general dentists or specialists in the rehabilitation of the stomatognathic system. We think in this way because the possibilities presented here, photobiomodulation, phototherapies, and photopeelings not only allow to treat dysfunctions caused by sarcopenia and uncontrolled senescence, they can also prevent unbalanced aging of the stomatognathic system.

References

1. Anders JJ, Lanzafame RJ, Arany PR. Low-level light/laser therapy versus photobiomodulation therapy. Photomed Laser Surg. 2015;33:183–4.
2. Hamblin MR. Mechanisms and applications of the anti-inflammatory effect of photobiomodulation. Aims Biophys. 2017;4(3):337–61.
3. Daghastanli NA (2017). http://ebm.ufabc.edu.br/wp-content/uploads/2011/10/aula-01-a-04_Laser_2012.pdf. Accessed 24 December 2017.
4. Lizarelli RFZ. Protocolos clínicos odontológicos—uso do laser de baixa intensidade. 4 ed. São Carlos: Return Propaganda e Publicidade, Maio; 2010. 88p. Il
5. Karu TI. Mechanisms of low power laser light action on cellular level. In: Simunovic Z, editor. Lasers in medicine and dentistry: basic science and upt-to-date clinical applications of low-energy level laser therapy—Lllt, Cap. 4. Vitagraf: Rijeka-Croácia; 2000. p. 99–125.
6. Sommer AP, Trelles A. Light pumping energy into blood mitochondria: a new trend against depression? Photomed Laser Surg. 2014;32(2):59–60.
7. Lan CC, Wu CS, Chiou MH, Hsieh PC, Yu HS. Low-energy helium-neon laser induces locomotion of the immature melanoblasts and promotes melanogenesis of the more differentiated melanoblasts: recapitulation of vitiligo repigmentation in vitro. J Invest Dermatol. 2006;126(9):2119–26.
8. Lan CC, Wu CS, Chiou MH, Chiang TY, Yu HS. Low-energy helium-neon laser induces melanocyte proliferation via interaction with type IV collagen: visible light as a therapeutic option for vitiligo. Br J Dermatol. 2009;161(2):273–80.
9. Moshkovska T, Mayberry J. It is time to test low level laser therapy in Great Britain. Postgrad Med J. 2005;81:436–41.
10. Lim W, et al. Effect of 635nm light-emitting diode irradiation on intracellular superoxide anion scavenging independent of the cellular enzymatic antioxidant system. Photomed Laser Surg. 2012;30(8):451–9.
11. Yu HS, et al. Helium-neon laser irradiation stimulates migration and proliferation in melanocytes and induces repigmentation in segmental-type vitiligo. J Invest Dermatol. 2003;120(1):56–64.
12. Huang SF, et al. Effects of intravascular laser irradiation of blood in mitochondria dysfunction and oxidative stress in adults with chronic spinal cord injury. Photomed. Laser Surg. 2012;30(10):579–86.
13. Vale KLD, et al. The effects of photobiomodulation delivered by light emitting diode on stem cells from human exfoliated deciduous teeth: a study on the relevance to pluripotent stem cell viability and proliferation. Photomed Laser Surg. 2017;35(2):659–65.
14. Oh CT, Kwon TR, Choi EJ, et al. Inhibitory effect of 660nm Led on melanin synthesis in in vitro and in vivo. Photodermatol Photoimmunol Photomed. 2017;33:49–57.
15. Karu TI. Ten lectures on basic science of laser phototherapy. Roseville: Prima Books; 2008. 400p. il
16. Nelson DL, Cox MM. Principios de bioquímica de Lehninger. 6th ed. New York: W. H. Freeman; 2014.
17. Wheeland RG, Koreck A. Safety and effectiveness of a new blue light device for the self-treatment of mild-to-moderate acne. J Clin Aesthetic Dermatol. 2012;5(5):25–31.
18. Oyamada A, Ikai H, Nakamura K, Hayashi E, Kanno T, Sasaki K, Niwano Y. In vitro bactericidal activity of photo-irradiated oxydol products via hydroxyl radical generation. Biocontrol Sci. 2013;18(2):83–8.
19. Fontana CR, Song X, Polymeri A, Goodson JM, Wang X, Soukos NS. The effect of blue light on periodontal biofilm growth in vitro. Lasers Med Sci. 2015;30(8):2077–86.
20. Lizarelli RFZ, Grandi NDP, Florez FLE, Grecco C, Almeida-Lopes L. Clinical study on orofacial photonic hydration using phototherapy and biomaterials. Biophotonics South America. Proc SPIE. 2015;9531:95311W. https://doi.org/10.1117/12.2181132.
21. Menezes RFC, Requena MB, Lizarelli RFZ, Bagnato VS. Blue led irradiation to hydration of skin. Biophotonics South America. Proc SPIE. 2015;9531:95311W. https://doi.org/10.1117/12.2181196.
22. Lavi R, Ankri R, Sinyakov M, et al. The plasma membrane is involved in the visible light-tissue interaction. Photomed Laser Surg. 2012;30(1):14–9.
23. Carvalho-Costa TM, Mendes MT, Silva MC, Rodrigues V, et al. Light emitting diode at 460 ± 20 nm increases the production of IL-12 and IL-6 in murine dendritic cells. Photomed Laser Surg. 2017;35(10):560–6. https://doi.org/10.1089/pho.2016.4244.
24. Poyton RO, Ball KA. Therapeutic photobiomodulation nitric oxide and a novel function of mito-

chondrial cytochrome C oxidase. Discov Med. 2011;11(57):154–9.
25. Weiss RA, et al. Clinical experience with light-emitting diode (Led) photomodulation. Dermatol Surg. 2005a;31:1199–205.
26. Weiss RA, McDaniel DH, Geronemus RG, Weiss MA. Clinical trial of a novel non-thermal Led array for reversal of photoaging: clinical, histologic and surface profilometric results. Lasers Surg Med. 2005b;36:85–91.
27. Alster TS, Wanitphakdeedecha R. Improvement of postfractional laser erythema with light-emitting diode photomodulation. Dermatol Surg. 2009;35:813–5.
28. Sauder DN. Light-emitting diodes: their role in skin rejuvenation. Int J Dermatol. 2010;49:12–6.
29. Chen L, Xu Z, Jiang M, et al. Light emitting diode 585nm photobiomodulation inhibiting melanin synthesis and inducing autophagy in human melanocytes. J Dermatol Sci. 2018;89:11–8.
30. Bashkatov AN, Genina EA, Kochubey VI, Tuchin VV. Optical properties of human skin, subcutaneous and mucous tissues in the wavelength range from 400 to 2000 nm. J Phys D Appl Phys. 2005;38:2543–55.
31. Dijkstra AT, Majoie IML, Van Dongen JWF, Van Weelden H, Van Vloten WA. Photodynamic therapy with violet light and topical aminolaevulinic acid in the treatment of actinic keratosis, Bowen's disease and basal cell carcinoma. J Eur Acad Dermatol Venereol. 2001;15:550–4.
32. Lipovsky A, Nitzan Y, Gedanken A, Lubart R. Visible light-induced killing of bacteria as a function of wavelength: implication for wound healing. Lasers Surg Med. 2010;42:467–72.
33. Bumah VV, Masson-Meyers DS, Cashing S, Enwemeka CS. Wavelength and bacterial density influence the bactericidal effect of blue light on methicillin-resistant Staphylococcus aureus (Mrsa). Photomed Laser Surg. 2013;31(11):547–53. https://doi.org/10.1089/pho.2012.3461.
34. Giannelli M, Landini G, Materassi F, Chellini F, Antonelli A, Tani A, Nosi D, Zecchi-Orlandini S, Rossolini GM, Bani D. Effects of photodynamic laser and violet-blue led irradiation on Staphylococcus aureus biofilm and Escherichia coli lipopolysaccharide attached to moderately rough titanium surface: in vitro study. Lasers Med Sci. 2017;32(4):857–64. https://doi.org/10.1007/s10103-017-2185-y.
35. Fournier N, Fritz K, Mordon S. Use of nonthermal blue (405 to 420 nm) and near-infrared light (850 to 900 nm) dual-wavelength system in combination with glycolic acid peels and topical vitamin C for skin photorejuvenation. Dermatol Surg. 2006;32:1140–6.
36. Mahmoud BH, Hexsel CL, Hamzavi IH, Lim UW. Effects of visible light on the skin. Photochem Photobiol. 2008;84:450–62.
37. Comorosan S, Polosan S, Jipa S, Popescu I, Marton G, Ionescu E, Cristache L, Badila D, Mitrica R. Green light radiation effects on free radicals inhibition in cellular and chemical systems. J Photochem Photobiol B. 2011;102:39–44.
38. Sousa AP, Paraguassu GM, Silveira NT, Souza J, Cangussú MC, Santos JN, Pinheiro AL. Laser and Led phototherapies on angiogenesis. Lasers Med Sci. 2013;28(3):981–7.
39. Catao MHCV, Nonaka CFW, Albuquerque RLC Jr, Bento PM, Costa RO. Effects of red laser, infrared, photodynamic therapy, and green Led on the healing process of third-degree burns: clinical and histological study in rats. Lasers Med Sci. 2015;30(1):421–8.
40. Catao MHCV, Costa RO, Nonaka CFW, Albuquerque RLC Jr, Costa IRRS. Green Led light has anti-inflammatory effects on burns in rats. Burns. 2016; 42(2):392–6.
41. Wang Y, Huang YY, Wang Y, Lyu P, Hamblin MR. Photobiomodulation (blue and green light) encourages osteoblastic-differentiation of human adipose-derived stem cells: role of intracellular calcium and light-gated ion channels. Sci Rep. 2016; 6:33719.
42. Wang Y, Huang YY, Lyu P, Hamblin MR. Red (660nm) or near-infrared (810nm) photobiomodulation stimulates, while blue (415nm), green (540nm) light inhibits proliferation in human adipose-derived stem cells. Sci Rep. 2017;7(1):7781.
43. Soares JM, Duarte JA, Carvalho J, Appell HJ. The possible role of intracellular Ca2+ accumulation for the development of immobilization atrophy. Int J Sports Med. 1993;14:437–9.
44. Ingalls CP, Warren GL, Armstrong RB. Intracellular Ca^{2+} transients in mouse soleus muscle after hindlimb unloading and reloading. J Appl Physiol. 1999;87:386–90.
45. Weiss N, et al. Altered myoplasmic Ca(2+) handling in rat fast-twitch skeletal muscle fibres during disuse atrophy. Pflugers Arch. 2010;459:631–44.
46. Brookes PS, et al. Calcium, Atp, and Ros: a mitochondrial love-hate triangle. Am J Phys Cell Phys. 2004;287:C817–33.
47. Liesa M, Palacín M, Zorzano A. Mitochondrial dynamics in mammalian health and disease. Physiol Rev. 2009;89:799–845.
48. Schafer A, Reichert AS. Emerging roles of mitochondrial membrane dynamics in health and disease. Biol Chem. 2009;390:707–15.
49. Ono T, Isobe K, Nakada K, Hayashi JI. Human cells are protected from mitochondrial dysfunction by complementation of Dna products in fused mitochondria. Nat Genet. 2001;28:272–5.
50. Twig G, Elorza A, Molina AJ, et al. Fission and selective fusion govern mitochondrial segregation and elimination by autophagy. EMBO J. 2008a;27:433–46.
51. Twig G, et al. Mitochondrial fusion, fission and autophagy as a quality control axis: the bioenergetic view. Biochim Biophys Acta. 2008b;1777:1092–7.
52. Tegowska E, Wosinska A. The role of biological sciences in understanding the genesis and a new therapeutic approach to Alzheimer's disease. Postepy Hig Med Dosw. 2011;65:73–92.
53. Nguyen LM, Malamo AG, Larkin-Kaiser KA, Borsa PA, Adhihetty PJ. Effect of near-infrared light

exposure on mitochondrial signaling in C2C12 muscle cells. Mitochondrion. 2014;14(1):42–8.
54. Albuquerque-Pontes GM, et al. Photobiomodulation therapy protects skeletal muscle and improves muscular function of mdx mice in a dose-dependent manner through modulation of dystrophin. Lasers Med Sci. 2018;33(4):755–64. https://doi.org/10.1007/s10103-017-2405-5.
55. Brito A, et al. Effect of photobiomodulation on connective tissue remodeling and regeneration of skeletal muscle in elderly rats. Lasers Med Sci. 2017;33(3):513–21. https://doi.org/10.1007/s10103-017-2392-6.
56. Lizarelli RFZ. Reabilitação biofotônica orofacial. São Carlos: Compact; 2018. 400p. il
57. Peelings faciais. Programa de Educação Continuada a Distância—Portal da Educação, 2015.
58. Brody HJ, Monheit GD, Resnik SS, Alt TH. A history of chemical peelings. Dermatol Surg. 2000;26:405–9.
59. Manoel CA, Paolillo FR, Menezes PFC. Conceitos fundamentais e práticos da fotoestética. São Carlos: Compacta; 2014.
60. Menezes PFC. Aplicação da luz na dermatologia e estética. São Carlos: Compacta; 2017. 283p. il

Use of Er:YAG Laser in Conservative Dentistry and Adhesion Process

7

Gianfranco Semez and Carlo Francesco Sambri

Contents

Abstract

This chapter deals with the use of Er:YAG laser in conservative laser dentistry as well as its part in the interaction with the adhesion process. Er:YAG laser is helpful in conservative dentistry. Its property to be absorbed by water and apatite can help clinicians in selective and microinvasive decay removal from tooth structure. The importance of using repeatable clinical protocol, to obtain a very strong adhesion effect with materials, brings medium- and long-term results of efficacy in conservative rehabilitations. The precision of the laser beam and its selectivity give the possibility to create new shapes for conservative cavity preparation.

Keywords

Er:YAG laser · Conservative dentistry · Micro leakage · Adhesion · Threshold ablation

G. Semez (✉) · C. F. Sambri
Semez srl, Trieste, Italy

7.1 Er:YAG Laser Interaction with Enamel and Dentine

Up until today, preservative dentistry has been defined as that branch of dental practice that concerns all clinical procedures carried out with a view to preserving natural teeth and ensuring their functioning within a framework of preserving both oral health and the overall health of the patient (definition: School of Dental Medicine at the University of Geneva). Within that framework, we can define what are the real aims of preservative dentistry thanks to the current expertise and technology in the field of the treatment of hard dental tissue that we have set out to achieve:

1. *Prevention and the safeguarding of the integrity of the tooth:* the techniques and procedures carried out on the patient with a view to reducing the amount of cariogenic bacteria in the mouth in order to reduce the incidence of disturbances to the enamel and dentine tissue.
2. *Curative treatment and restoration:* microinvasive techniques for the removal of infected

S. Stübinger et al. (eds.), *Lasers in Oral and Maxillofacial Surgery*,
https://doi.org/10.1007/978-3-030-29604-9_7

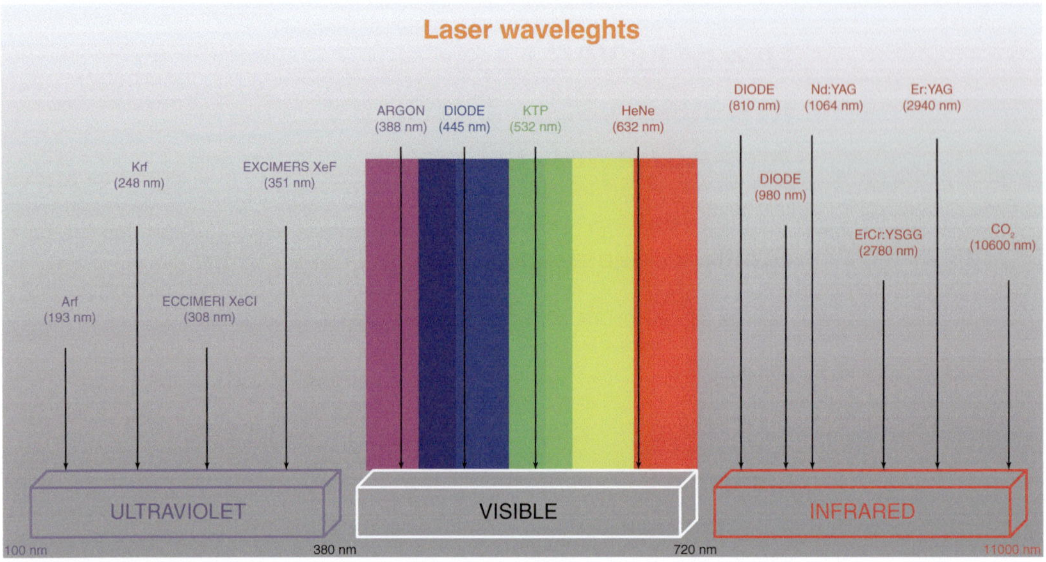

Fig. 7.1 Spectrum of light

tissue and the use of selective long-wave laser for tissues with a greater water density may be useful in minimizing the sacrifice of healthy tissue during the process of ablation in order to preserve the architectonic structure of the tooth.

3. *Restoration of lost tissue:* the adhesive techniques that have now become part of the normal routine in our work allow and, indeed, oblige us to exploit any portion of healthy tissue remaining in order to ensure the preservation and restoration of the tooth. The use of laser and ER:YAG in order to improve the process of adhesion and micro-infiltration at a marginal level both on the enamel and the dentine.
4. *Maintenance of dental health:* checking up on the maintenance of the suitable margins of the reconstructions, the physiological wear and tear that result from chewing, and the duration of the adhesive interface in subsequent years is a fundamental step in the mechanical maintenance of conservative restoration [1].

The definition of an adequate plan of conservative treatment entails certain fundamental steps, the first of which is the identification of the major problems involved in the conservation; subsequently, it is necessary to treat urgent problems as quickly as possible to obviate the progression of penetrating tooth decay, deep-rooted dentine traumas, etc.; the use of X-rays for an early diagnosis of interproximal tooth decay is still a fundamental step in any complete and precise intervention; a periodontal evaluation concludes the total diagnostic process following the restoration project (Fig. 7.1).

At this point, the optimal characteristics of a laser instrument should be:

- Cutting precision,
- Interactive selection with the tissue,
- Mini-invasiveness,
- Safety,
- Patient comfort,
- Compatibility with state-of-the art adhesive systems.

In order to make a cautious choice, we need to know the different wavelengths of the lasers so as to decide which is the most suitable for the abovementioned parameters.

In order to satisfy these requirements, we need to use a laser in which the predominant feature is the absorption of the rays on the tissue. In this respect, the wavelengths that best fit this requirement are ultraviolet wavelengths of between 190 and 300 nm, such as the excimer lasers used in ophthalmology because of their high rate of energy or infrared lasers such as CO_2, Ho:YAG, Er:YAG, and Er-Cr:YSGG of between 2000 and 11,000 nm.

The penetration depth of these lasers is very slight, between 1 and 100 μm; the diffusion element is basically irrelevant, and there is no retro-diffusion.

In light of these considerations in the course of our work, we have chosen the Er:YAG 2940 nm laser for work on the hard tissue of the tooth.

To obtain a correct photo-ablative alignment, the choice of the parameters is absolutely fundamental. The relation between power density, exposure time, and length of pulsation makes a significant difference in the efficacy of our operation. As shown in Fig. 7.2, it is only a correct balancing of these parameters that will lead to obtaining a process of real photo-ablation, called by some authors "cold-ablation" (Fig. 7.2).

The removal of the decayed tissue is facilitated by the use of the Er:YAG laser because the central parts of the decayed area contain more water than the surrounding tissue. Given the physical properties of the erbium laser for the absorption of water, we can verify clinically a certain selectivity for the decayed tissue (Fig. 7.3).

Considering the various anatomical components that make up the tooth, the action of the laser will differ according to the work to be done on enamel or dentine tissue.

Enamel: a mineralized acellular secretion with a very high component of inorganic material (96%), a very low organic component (1%), and a low water content (3%) (Fig. 7.4).

Dentine: a mineralized cellular tissue made up of three phases:

- A mineral phase composed of around 50% apatite.
- An organic phase of around 30% represented for 90% by type 1 collagen and 10% by non-collagen proteins as well as lipids.
- A watery phase of 20%, 75% of which is present within the dentine tubes and 25% mineralized matrix that varies according to the anatomical area [2].

The dentine tubules, hollow structures that run through the dentine tissue in a centripetal direction toward the pulp chamber, represented by a number between 20 and 45,000/mm², with a diameter comprising from 1 to 3 μm, contain the processes of

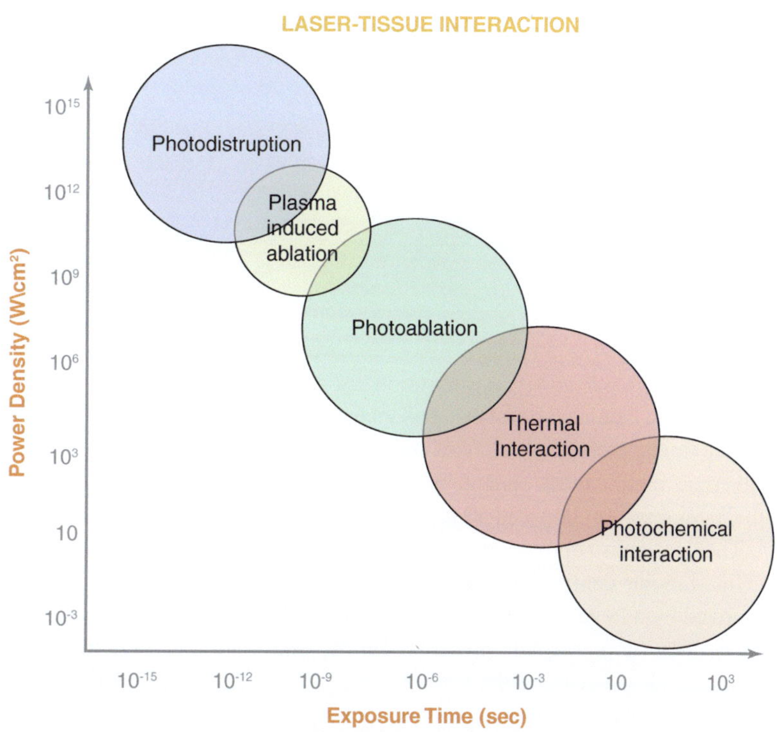

Fig. 7.2 Laser–tissue interaction on power density and time of exposure

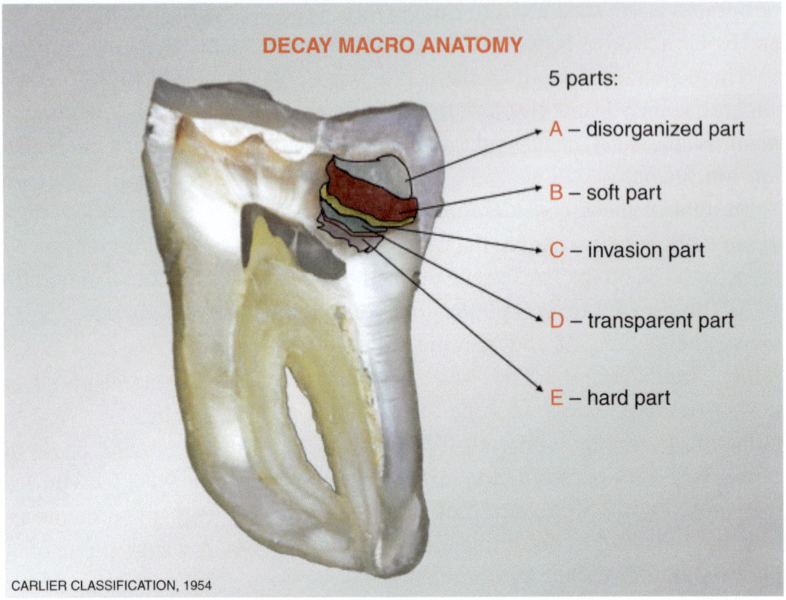

Fig. 7.3 Macro anatomy of decay lesion

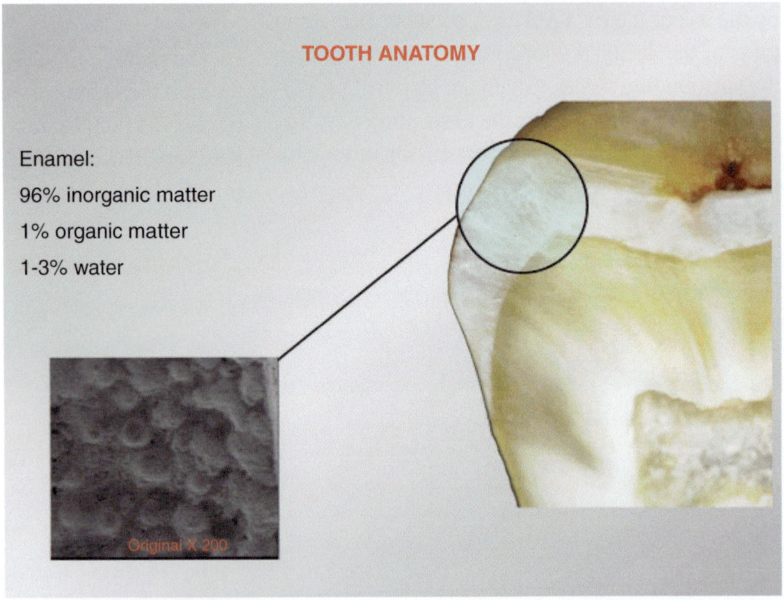

Fig. 7.4 Enamel structure anatomy

odontoblasts, lamina sslimitans, collagen, fibers, dentine fluids, proteins, etc. There are also present numerous ramifications and anastomosis with a smaller diameter of between 50 nm and 1 μm.

The dentine is subdivided into three parts:

Intertubular dentine within the tubules: characterized by a large quantity of water, type 1 collagen fiber, non-collagen proteins, lipids, and odontoblastic processes (Fig. 7.5).

Intratubular dentine: characterized by presence of type 1 collagen fiber, crystalline structure, non-collagen proteins, lipids, and water.

Peritubular dentine: hyper-mineralized dentine, around 40 times more mineralized than the preceding examples, characterized by a thickness that varies between 1 and 3 μm and a dense, homogenous structure characterized by hydroxyapatite crystals and no collagen (Fig. 7.6).

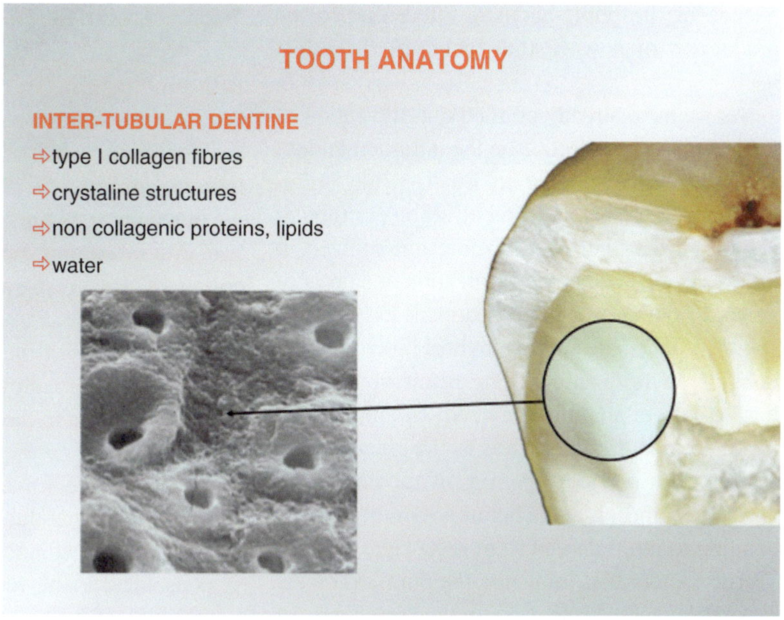

Fig. 7.5 Intertubular dentine and its composition

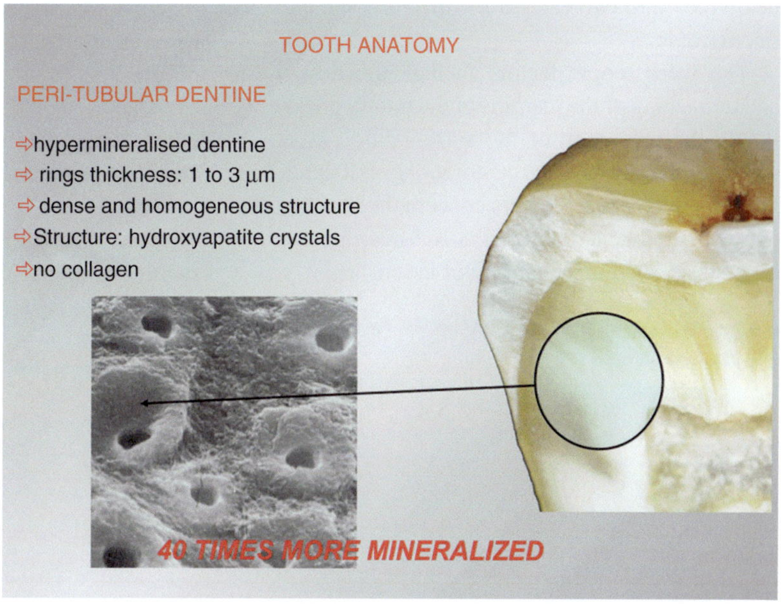

Fig. 7.6 Peritubular dentine, hyper-mineralized tissue

The iteration of the LASER on the tooth possesses an average absorption of around 85% thanks to the presence of water in the spray of the maniple and of hydroxyapatite [3].

On the dentine in particular, the efficacy of absorption is around ten times greater compared to the enamel, thanks to the larger quantity of water present in that tissue. This action can be considered as having a thermomechanical effect insofar as the ray hits the surface of the tooth creating a volumetric expansion and an increase of the internal pressure of the water with the creation of micro explosions that lead to the elimination of the substance in the form of "micro-drops" (ablation). We should also bear in mind that the quantity of the ablative water is also a consequence of the photo-acoustic effect due to the production of a wave that increases the effect itself.

As we have already pointed out, the action of the laser is more effective on the intratubular dentine because it is richer in water, while orthophosphoric acid has a greater effect on peritubular dentine in that the latter is more mineralized. It follows from this that the application of acid or of an acid primer after laser treatment exposes the collagen fibers and forms a hybrid layer with the bonding (hybridization). The result obtained is that the combination between chemical acid treatment and the laser leads to the creation of a surface with a wider opening of tubules, more open anastomoses, and a better possibility for the bonding to infiltrate and form resin tags.

The factors that influence the duration of the restoration, taking into account the correctness of the adhesive procedures and the use of lasers, can be divided into two categories: macroscopic and microscopic.

The macroscopic factors include the design and refinishing of the margins of the mouth preparation, the protection of the surrounding tissue, and the precision of the restoration/tooth interface; the microscopic factors concern the iteration between superficial hydrophilia and hydrophobia of the resin and the wettability of the surface.

7.2 Laser Er:YAG and Adhesion

Adhesion, defined as the tendency of some dissimilar substrata to join together thanks to the formation of forces of attraction, is still today a cornerstone of everyday dentistry, and we consider it as one of the most fundamental and crucial stages which can affect the outcome of the restoration (Ferrari, Breschi) (Fig. 7.7).

The functions of the adhesive system are:

Create a seal to allow the correct maintenance of the restoration in the course of time.

1. Distribute the forces to guarantee a correct functional rehabilitation of the tooth.
2. Prevent the characteristic separation indispensable for the retention of the restorative material, and impede polymerization contraction.

The aims of enamel-dentine adhesion according to Lutz et al. [4] are:

- Retention and stability of the restoration,
- Prevention and absorption of the stresses of contraction,
- Perfect marginal adaptation in the absence of fissures and micro-infiltrations,

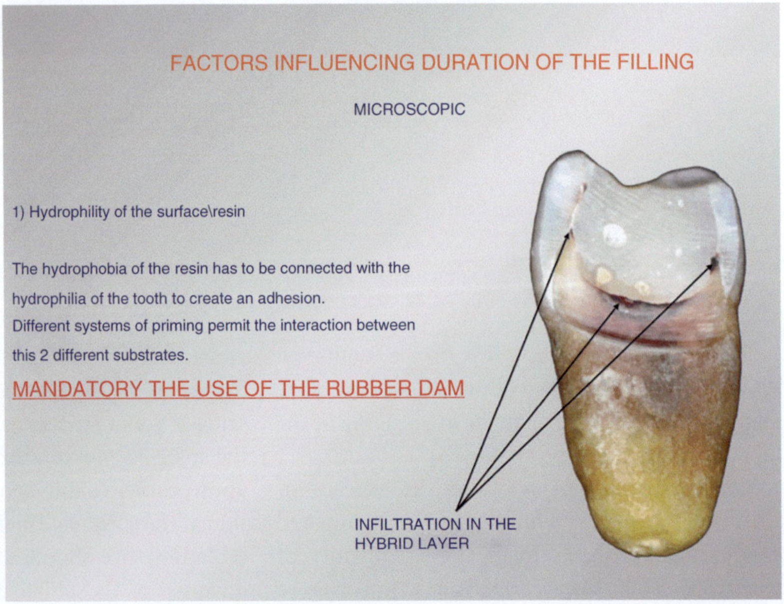

Fig. 7.7 Factors influencing adhesion

- Hermetic sealing of the dentine pulp complex,
- Reduction of post operation sensitivity,
- Strengthening of the restored tooth.

On the dental substratum, two types of adhesion occur: micromechanical and chemical.

Micromechanical adhesion which is created thanks to the forces of attrition between the surface and the bonding occurs both on enamel and dentine. On enamel, the roughness of the surface that we obtain by the use of laser and mordant acid increases the area of interaction between the parts. On dentine, the penetration of the resinous bonding within the tubules and the formation of resin tags produce an increase in the mechanical attrition between the resin and the tubular walls and an increase in adhesion (Fig. 7.8).

Chemical adhesion which only occurs on dentine is due to dentine priming and the process of hybridization. By means of the creation of a hybrid layer (collagen fiber + resinous bond joined together by van der Waals electrostatic forces), the strength of adhesion increases and microfiltration diminishes.

According to the classification of Silverstone of 1975, enamel can present four microscopic aspects of erosion depending on the type of stimulus applied. Specifically, type 1, which presents preferential erosion at the core of the prism (the most mineralized part) and to a lesser extent on the periphery which shows up after mordanting with a 35% solution of orthophosphoric acid, turned out to be the most suitable for subsequent adhesive interventions (Fig. 7.9).

The treatment of the enamel surface with laser creates the aspect seen in type 3, in other words of undifferentiated erosion, less suitable for adhesion systems. From this, there emerged the necessity of always using a mordanting acid after laser treatment on enamel in order to clean the surface treated of the residue of the micro explosions and bring it back to the aspect of type 1 (Fig. 7.10).

The differences observed between a surface of type 1 that was only treated with a mordant acid and a surface that was treated with laser and acid are the presence in the latter of micro and macro cracks within the enamel that create an interface of contact with the bonding that is not rectilinear but of an irregular sinusoidal type, increasing exponentially the surface contact between the enamel and the bonding and reducing the micro-infiltration of the preservative restoration in the course of time. In fact, studies have shown that the strength of the bond is basically identical but that there is a notable increase in marginal impermeability.

The effect of laser on dentine, as we have already mentioned, creates a larger opening at the entrance of the tubules and anastomoses.

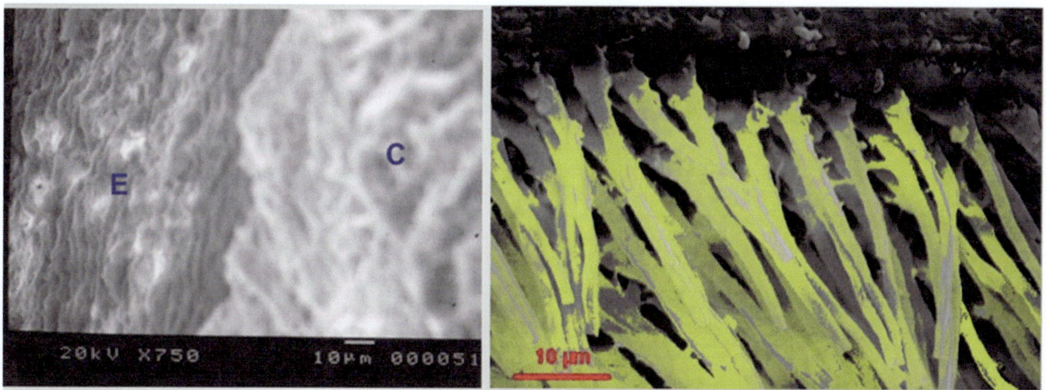

Borderline between surface cavity on enamel.
C = Composite resin,
E = enamel

Tags formation after bur and acid traditional preparation of the dentine. Micromechanic adhesion

Fig. 7.8 Resin tags penetrating into dentine tubules

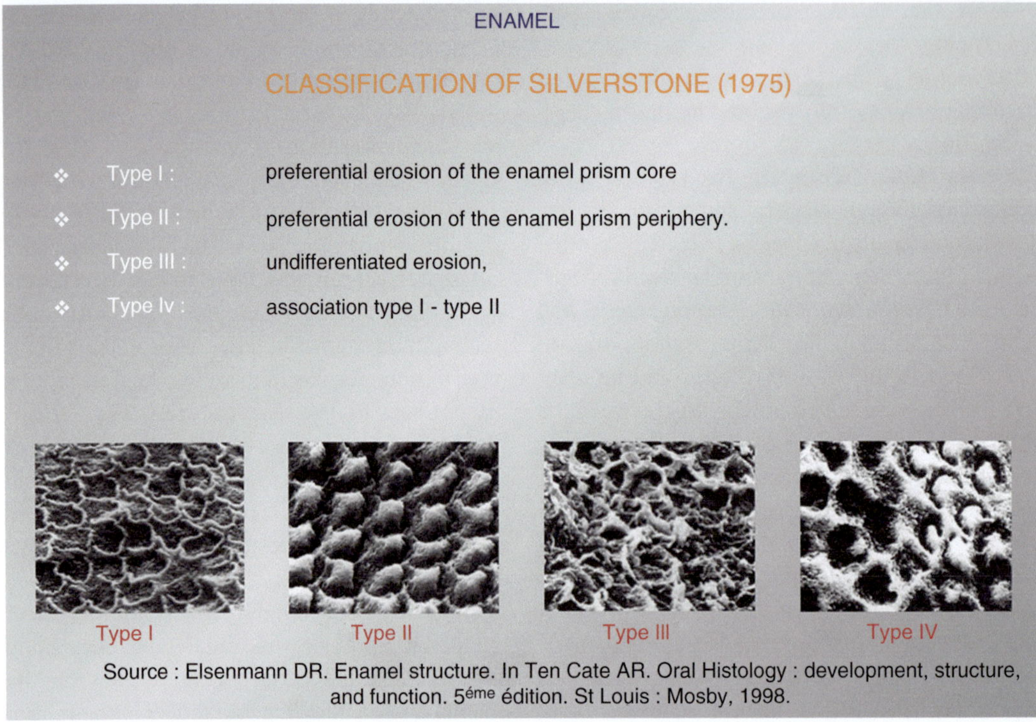

Fig. 7.9 Silverstone classification of enamel SEM aspect depending on erosion stimulus

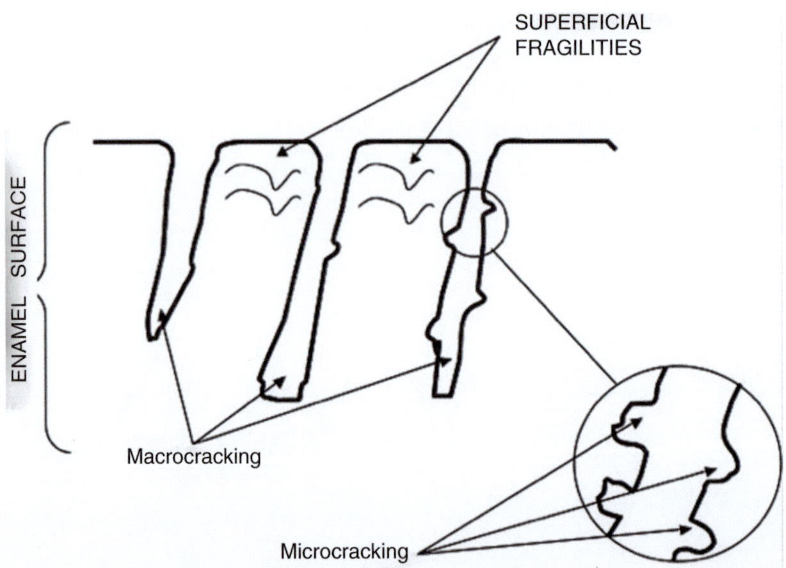

Fig. 7.10 Enamel cracks after laser irradiation

This characteristic allows a greater and better penetration of the resinous bonding within them and creates peculiar tags characterized by their longer length and thickness, numerous anastomoses, and a base of insertion that is longer and more represented, called "champagne cork" because of its shape compared to the traditional system where the tags are longer but thinner with fewer anastomoses and a short base in the typical shape of a "string of spaghetti" [5–7].

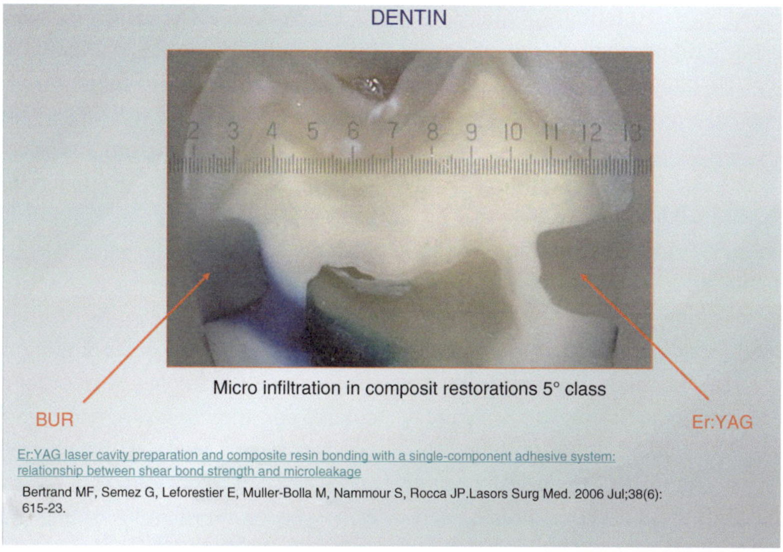

Fig. 7.11 Micro leakage after laser treatment alone and laser + acid treatment

The combined treatment of laser and etching acid both on enamel and dentine does not change substantially the absolute values of bond strength, but it has a considerable influence on the improvement of the prevention of micro-infiltration of the adhesive restoration carried out directly on cavities prepared and treated by laser (Fig. 7.11) within suitable parameters [8, 9].

7.3 Clinical Cases and Protocols for Laser Conservative Dentistry

In the light of all that has been said until now, it will have become clear how important it is to integrate the use of laser in everyday clinical practice.

For this reason, the authors, since as far back as 2009, consider it of fundamental importance to adopt a "laser-integrated" approach to dentistry in which laser instruments and techniques should be integrated within traditional protocols in order to obtain clinical advantages as regards:

- Comfort of patients,
- Reduction of healing time,
- Improved quality of the surfaces and tissues treated,
- Decontaminated operating area,
- Less possibility of intra- and postoperative complications.

Our experience has led us to draw up, on the basis of scientific studies and guidelines, some clinical protocols to use in daily practice.

We advise therefore keeping to hand the following checklist for laser-integrated conservative restoration:

1. Pinpoint the lesion (above/below gum, above/below crest).
2. Evaluate the seriousness and eventual pulp involvement (capping or endodontic treatment).
3. Local anesthetic (if necessary).
4. Protection of adjacent tissue.
5. Removal of undermined enamel.
6. Removal of infected dentine.
7. Adhesion procedures.
8. Incremental technique of reconstruction.

Case 1 Hypo-mineralization of enamel-dentine with a history of hyper fluorosis. The patient reported an esthetic deficit of 4.1, clearly revealed by and/or a lack of enamel integrity, a central hyperchromic area of the tooth at a lingual level in respect of the arch.

It was decided, after isolating the area to be operated on using a rubber dam, to proceed with the ablation of the damaged tissue using laser (Fig. 7.12).

With a view to improving the precision of the intervention, it was decided to use a mirror handpiece (Fotona) with a 0.5 mm spot.

This handpiece, since it bears no physical resemblance to the bur as regards proximity to the surface, is difficult for novices to use, so we decided to protect the adjacent teeth by positioning rough interproximal matrices (to fragment the reflected ray and reduce the risk to the people present). The assistant was asked to position the aspiration tube not very close to the air/water spray supply since the aiming beam on the mirror handpiece is visualized by the operator thanks to the drops of water which, in turn, could be deviated by the aspiration tube itself when we reduce significantly the water ratio. We should keep in mind that the Er:YAG laser is an IR laser and so not visible to the naked eye. Having evaluated the integrity of the enamel, it was decided to use a suitable setting of 250 mJ, 20 Hz, and air 6/water 3.

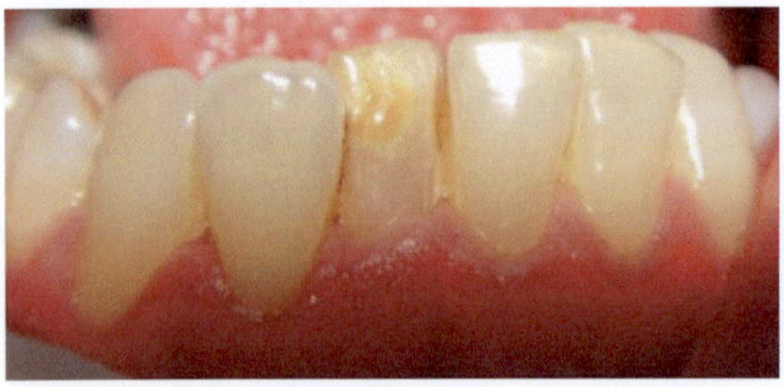

Fig. 7.12 Initial clinical view

It was decided to reduce the spray of water in order to have a greater ablative effect on the enamel which was very mineralized. By reducing the water, there is a risk of creating superficial carbonization, and so the duration of the pulsation should not exceed 150 ms. Once the dentine has been reached, the parameters will be changed to 150 mJ, 20 Hz, and the water will be increased to 4/4. The movement must take into consideration an overlapping of the spots of around 50%. For the polishing of the enamel margins, we advise diminishing the frequency in order to have better control and moving away from the focal point in order to disperse the ablative energy over a wider surface. There then follows a differentiated total etch type of mordanting of the enamel-dentine with at least 30 s washing and gentle drying.

The spreading of the primer and bonding must take into consideration the sinusoidal surface created by the laser, and so the brushing movement must be very close shaved so as to enable the product to penetrate all the anfractuosities of the enamel and dentine in a complete three-dimensional way. This is important to obtain an optimum dentine hybrid layer (tags and no sensitivity) and to cancel marginal blemishes on the enamel (white streaks).

Finishing touches and remodelling of the restoration with finishing burs and polishing with pop-on discs (Fig. 7.13).

Case 2 The patient presented multiple, incongruous fillings in the lower teeth with marginal infiltrations and secondary decaying lesions (Fig. 7.14).

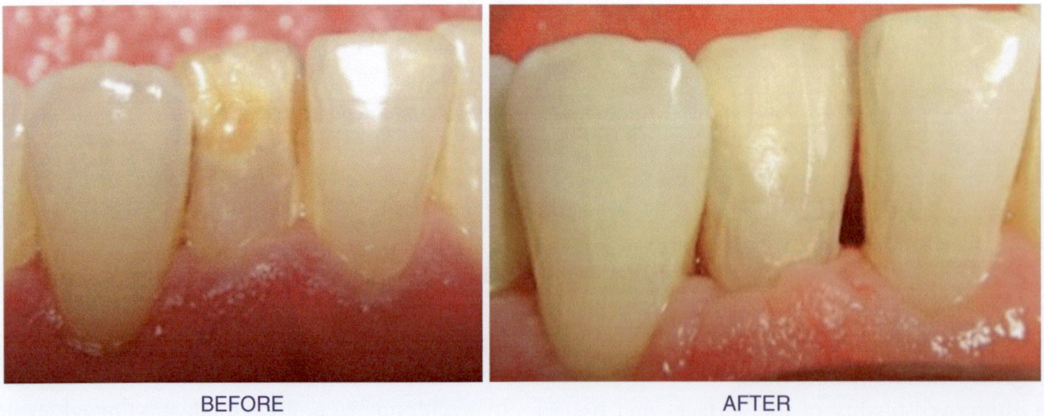

Fig. 7.13 Clinical before and after

After isolation, it was decided to use less energy, 150 mJ, 20 Hz, A/A 4/4, and pulsation 300 μs because the decaying tissue by reason of the fact that it is richer in water will absorb the ray more readily. In this case, we used a 0.8 mm spot and F = 30 J/cm^2 sapphire tip in order to have more control over the effect and avoid damage to the adjacent tissue.

The erbium laser is very useful in removing old compound restorations in that the photomechanic action directed on the hybrid layer, by vaporizing all the water, allows an easy removal of the filling without affecting the whole dental zone.

The use of the contact handpiece must take into consideration a minimum space between the area of the tip and the surface to be treated so as to allow the passage of water between the two and obtain both the photo-acoustic effect and not ruin the tip itself (Fig. 7.15).

NB: Never touch the surface of the tooth with the tip; otherwise, the damage will prevent the rectilinear emergence of the bundle and will produce what is called scattering effect [10].

The steps for acid etching, application of bonding, and polishing are the same (Fig. 7.16).

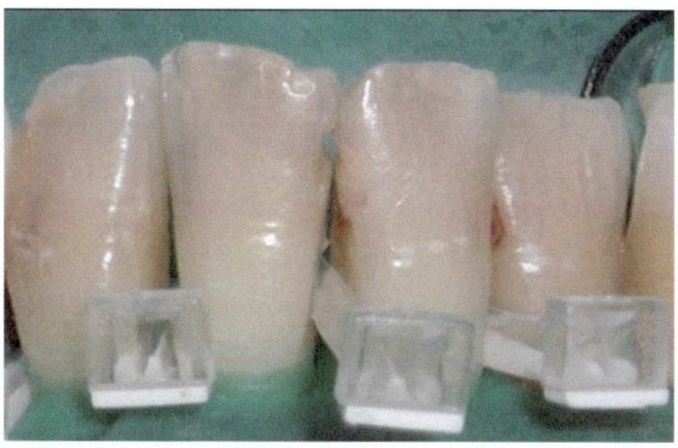

Fig. 7.14 Initial view

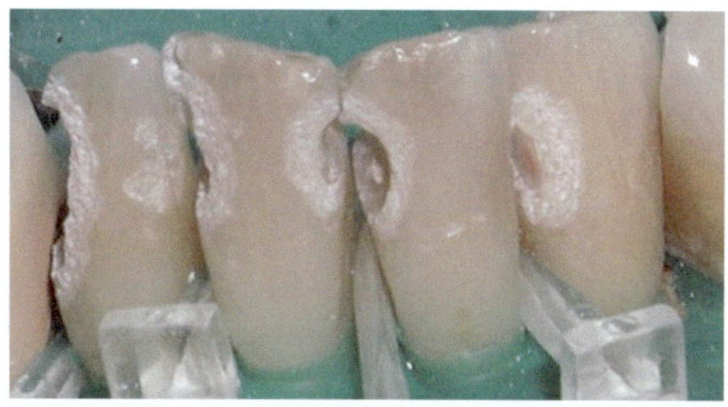

Fig. 7.15 Cavity preparation with Er:YAG laser

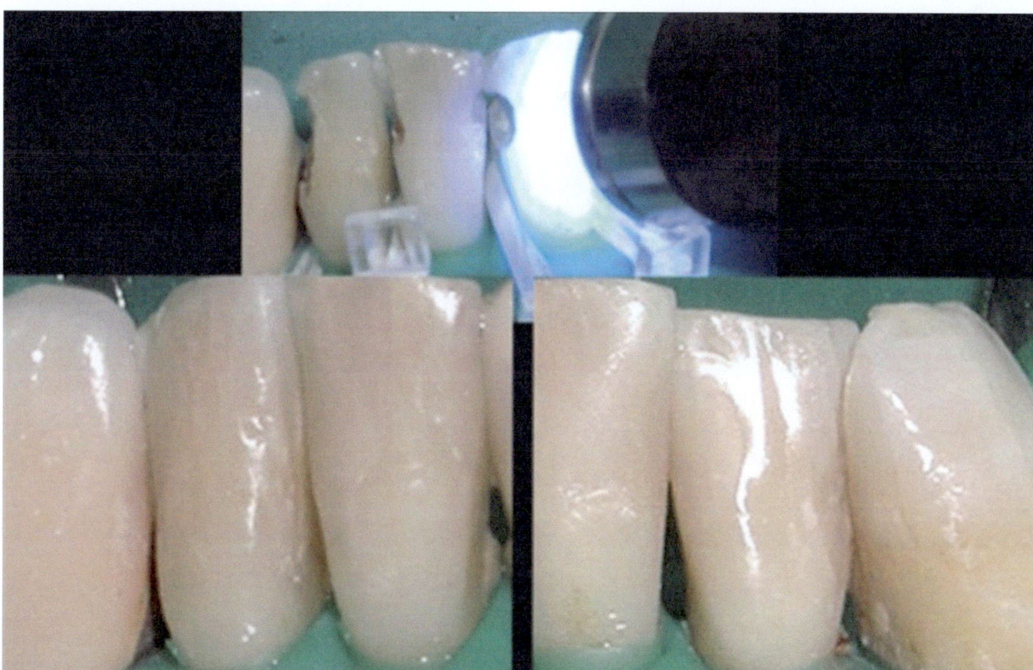

Fig. 7.16 Final result

Case 3 In this third clinical case, we take into consideration erbium not as regards the preparation of the teeth but simply as regards the treatment of the surface before applying adhesive cementing (Fig. 7.17).

The preparation is carried out according to the traditional rotating methods, and subsequently, the teeth are treated within the 150 mJ, 20 Hz at a distance, 150 μs pulse duration, and $F = 30$ J\cm^{2} parameters so that the surface contact with the adhesive will be increased.

Until today, it is not possible to treat ceramic facets and caps with laser, and so we must follow the traditional requirements of the producer (Fig. 7.18).

Traditional chemical treatment of ceramic surface to improve the micro leakage (Fig. 7.19).

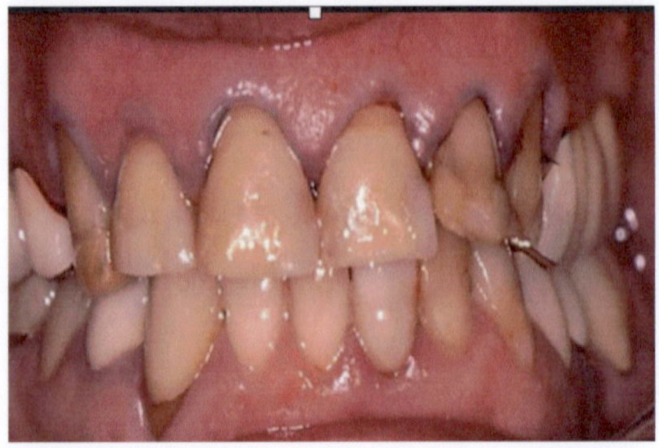

Fig. 7.17 Initial clinical view

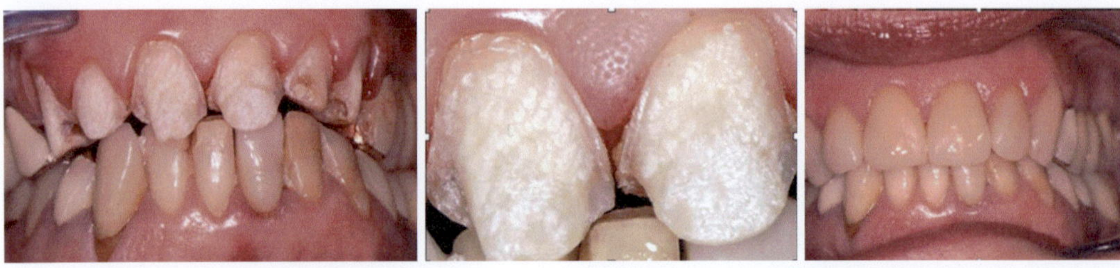

Fig. 7.18 Porcelain etching and cementation

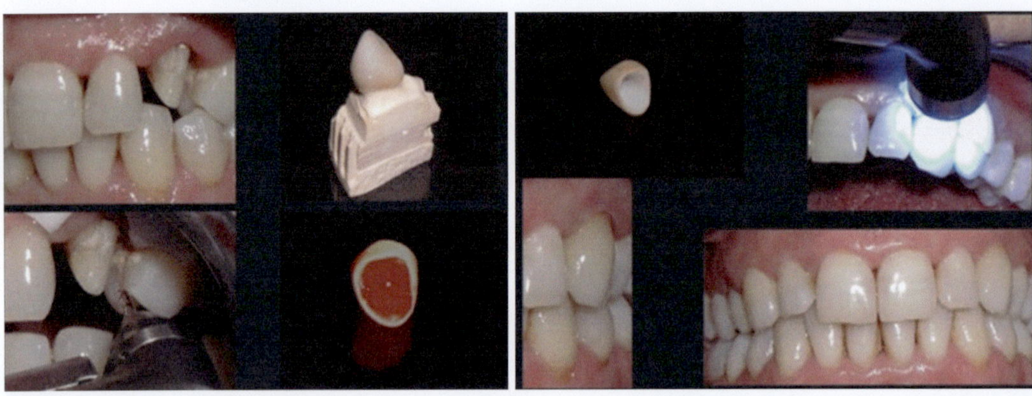

Fig. 7.19 Ceramic chemical etch on porcelain

References

1. Ferrari P. Odontoiatria restaurativa procedure di trattamento e prospettive future. Accademia Italiana di conservativa. Elsevier; 2009.
2. Meister J, Franzen R, Forner K, Grebe H, Stanzel S, Lampert F, Apel C. Influence of the water content in dental enamel and dentin on ablation with erbium YAG and erbium YSGG lasers. J Biomed Opt. 2006;11(3):34030.
3. Cvikl B, Lilaj B, Franz A, Degendorfer D, Moritz A. Evaluation of the morphological characteristics of laser-irradiated dentin. Photomed Laser Surg. 2015;33(10):504–8. https://doi.org/10.1089/pho.2015.3949.
4. Lutz F, et al. Restauri estetici nei settori posteriori - manuale operativo. Zurigo: Verlag PPK; 1996.
5. Hossain M, Yamada Y, Masuda-Murakami Y, Nakamura Y. Removal of organic debris with Er:YAG laser irradiation and microleakage of fissures sealants in vitro. Lasers Med Sci. 2012;27(5):895–902. https://doi.org/10.1007/s10103-011-0994-y.
6. Neves Ade A, Coutinho E, Cardoso MV, de Munck J, Van Meerbeek B. Micro-tensile bond strength and interfacial characterization of an adhesive bonded to dentin prepared by contemporary caries-excavation techniques. Dent Mater. 2011;27(6):552–62. https://doi.org/10.1016/j.dental.2011.02.008.
7. Attar N, Korkmaz Y, Ozel E, Bicer CO, Firatli E. Microleakage of class V cavities with different adhesive systems prepared by a diamond instrument and different parameters of Er:YAG laser irradiation. Photomed Laser Surg. 2008;26(6):585–91. https://doi.org/10.1089/pho.2007.2203.
8. Bahrololoomi Z, Razavi F, Soleymani AA. Comparison of micro-leakage from resin-modified glass ionomer restorations in cavities prepared by Er:YAG (Erbium-Doped Yttrium Aluminum Garnet) laser and conventional method in primary teeth. J Lasers Med Sci. 2014;5(4):183–7.
9. Navarro RS, Gouw-Soares S, Cassoni A, Haypek P, Zezell DM, de Paula Eduardo C. The influence of erbium:yttrium-aluminum-garnet laser ablation with variable pulse width on morphology and microleakage of composite restorations. Lasers Med Sci. 2010;25(6):881–9. https://doi.org/10.1007/s10103-009-0736-6.
10. Olivi G, Genovese MD, Maturo P, Docimo R. Pulp capping: advantages of using laser technology. Eur J Paediatr Dent. 2007;8(2):89–95.

Deep Lasers on Hard Tissue and Laser Prevention in Oral Health

8

Carlo Francesco Sambri and Gianfranco Semez

Contents

Abstract

The use of deep lasers on hard dental tissues to treat dental hypersensitivity and prevention by sealing with laser integrated procedures. Hypersensitivity is a common problem for many patients in our offices, and management is quite complex. Deep lasers such as Nd:YAG and diode laser can be used, with different techniques and different clinical approaches in our daily practice. The importance of using chromophore and desensitized chemical products, in addition to laser beam, seems to be strongly recommended. Results on clinical studies and medium-term evaluation show that these procedures are safe, efficient, and time-saving in expert hands.

Keywords

Nd:YAG · Diode laser · Dental hypersensitivity · Laser sealing · PDT

C. F. Sambri (✉) · G. Semez
Semez srl, Trieste, Italy

8.1 Laser and Hypersensitivity

Dental hypersensitivity (DH), defined as "a short sharp pain arising from physical or chemical stimuli which cannot be ascribed to dental pathologies" in 2003 by the Canadian Advisory Board, is a highly relevant and widespread problem among dental patients. Such pain, often described as short and sharp, can be ascribed to thermal stimuli, mechanical contacts, osmotic variations (e.g., drying of the surface of exposed dentine), or chemical stimulations (e.g., sugary or acid foods). According to the hydrodynamic theory already expounded at the beginning of the last century by Brannstrom, these stimuli would create a movement of the intratubular fluid that would stretch the nerve fibers within the processes of the odontoblasts contained in them.

Exposed dentine is often due to periodontal disease and is particularly related to gum recession in thin gingival biotypes, while it becomes a matter of resective periodontal surgery in patients undergoing such procedures for

S. Stübinger et al. (eds.), *Lasers in Oral and Maxillofacial Surgery*,
https://doi.org/10.1007/978-3-030-29604-9_8

the maintenance of the health of the periodontium. It is estimated that between 60% and 98% of patients are affected by periodontal disease with a loss of teeth, and undergoing resective therapies present varying degrees of dentine hypersensitivity.

Other situations that can be correlated to DH are the loss of dental tissue in the cervical region due to abrasions caused by mechanical traumas (e.g., incorrect brushing) or abfractions often found in patients affected by chewing parafunctions. Less common are pathologies linked to odontogenesis (e.g., *amelogenesis imperfecta*) or erosions due to chemical traumas (e.g., patients with eating disorders such as anorexia and/or bulimia).

For these reasons, nowadays, numerous systems are used with a view to obliterating the dentine tubules themselves so as to eliminate the movement of fluid and the consequent algic symptoms demonstrated by the affected teeth.

Following one of the various treatment protocols mentioned in previous studies, it is first of all important to identify and, where possible, to eliminate the root cause of DH. In the second place, chemical products such as KNO_3 and KCl are used in order to relieve the pain. If these preventive and curative measures should not produce satisfactory results, it is necessary to proceed with the obliteration of the dentine tubules.

There are numerous techniques proposed for this procedure including the following:

- **Gingival closing**: using the techniques of mucus-gingival surgery, the exposed dentine is corrected by repositioning the gingival margin.
- **Adhesive systems**: the enamel-dentine adhesive systems seem to be relatively effective in tubular obliteration.
- **Chemical sclerosis**: chemical products with the capacity to form weak links with the dental substratum are applied topically to the exposed surface. Some examples are CaOH2, fluoride, and HAp-based varnish and pastes.
- **Integrated laser techniques called LITS**: Laser integrated tubular sclerosis.

The light of the laser by transmitting energy under the form of photons (photonic energy) makes it possible, according to the characteristics of the laser itself, to have a direct effect on the exposed dentine or to activate an appropriately treated desensitizing chemical product.

8.1.1 Nd:YAG Laser: LITS Technique

The Nd:YAG laser is considered a high-energy laser in that the modality of the ray properly called a pulsate or super pulsate allows the built-up energy to be emitted in very high quantities (peak power of very high pulsations) in an extremely short time (short pulse duration). This binomial of energy and exposure time allows the wavelength to alter irreversibly the irradiated dentine surface without however transmitting the heat produced to the deep tissue and in particular to the pulp tissue which is extremely sensitive to rise in temperature.

This process, defined as the photothermal effect, consists in the absorption of the energy of a photon on the part of a target molecule which creates an increase in the molecular vibrations and is translated into the production of heat and a rise in temperature. The Nd:YAG laser, thanks to its type of pulsate emission, produces this effect, and thanks to the brief duration of the pulsation, the rise in temperature is not translated into the scattering of heat toward the pulp. This rise in temperature allows a permanent alteration of the architectonic structure of the irradiated dentine tissue, thus giving rise to dentine melting that obliterates the tubules very effectively. This process can be carried out clinically only in the presence of a suitable chromophore placed on the surface to be treated, in this specific instance on the graphite opportunely applied. The procedure we propose is the following (Fig. 8.1):

Clinical Protocol

1. Delicate washing of the surface with a rotating toothbrush.
2. Application of the graphite on the surface to be treated.

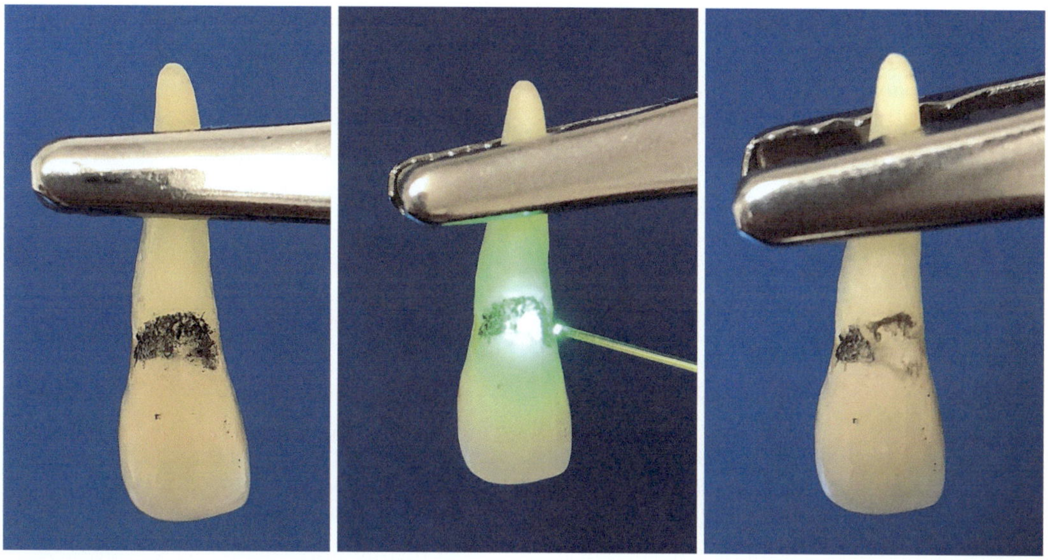

Fig. 8.1 Application of the graphite, fiber at an angle around 45°, graphite vaporization and superficial thermal structure modification

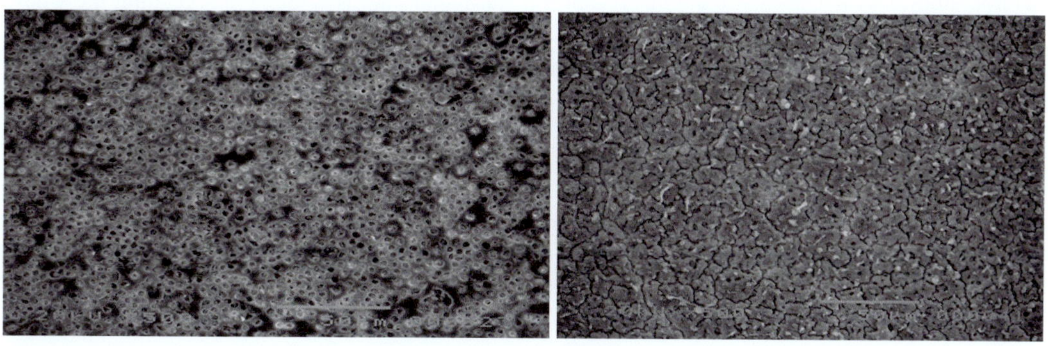

Fig. 8.2 SEM image before and after LITS treatment of dentine surface exposed

3. Application of the laser (Nd:YAG 0.5 W; 10 Hz; fiber 300 μ) with the fiber at an angle of around 45° in relation to the tooth.
4. Pause of 30 s (the time for thermal relaxation).
5. Application of the laser (Nd:YAG 0.5 W; 10 Hz; fiber 300 μ) with the fiber at an angle of around 45° in relation to the tooth.
6. Wash with air/water spray.
7. Test dentine sensitivity with air.
8. Polish gently with a toothbrush and fluorate paste.

We advise inclining the fiber to around 45° in order to reduce the phenomenon of refraction and diminish the concentration of energy deep down, above all at the level of the pulp chamber (Fig. 8.2). We recommend interrupting the treatment when the graphite has vaporized and resuming it only after having positioned a further layer of ophore. The sensitivity test with air allows us to evaluate the results obtained, and it is immediately felt by the patient. During the treatment, the patient may often feel a short sharp pain which is why we advise warning him/her about this before treatment begins. The duration of the treatment is extremely short, and so it fits well into daily clinical procedures [1].

8.1.2 Diode Laser

In order to carry out the same operation of desensitization using a diode laser, the procedure used must perforce include the application of an opportunely colored desensitizing product on the surface to be treated. The desensitizing product will absorb the energy of the laser light and prevent its diffusion downwards towards sensitive tissue and the heat produced within the substance itself by increasing the molecular kinetics will produce a form of activation of the product, not only tending to form a more homogenous layer of the treated surface but also leading to a greater penetration within the exposed dentine tubules with a desensitizing effect that is longer lasting over time. In a clinical study that we carried out on 44 treated teeth in the cervical portion we first provided the patient with a VAS/AVS test (Analogical Visual Scale) to evaluate the pre-operatory pain. The patients had to make a score from 0 (complete lack of pain) to 10 (highest level of pain) for the tooth in question. The stimulation was provided using a puff of air from the air/water pistol for about 2–3 s. Clinical protocol requires the delicate washing of the surface using ultrasound and gentle polishing using a rotating silicon toothbrush with soft, rounded bristles. Subsequently, after having isolated the area to be operated on with cotton rolls to soak up the excessive presence of saliva, we proceeded with the mixing of the product which is based on hydroxyapatite crystals and since they are white we added a blue food dye to them (Fig. 8.3).

The mixing time advised by the producer of the dye is 15 s but we prolonged it to 30 s to ensure the homogeneity of the final product. This was applied to the relevant surface of the teeth and particular care was taken in spreading the whole product smoothly even in the inter-proximal areas that were exposed [2]. For this operation we

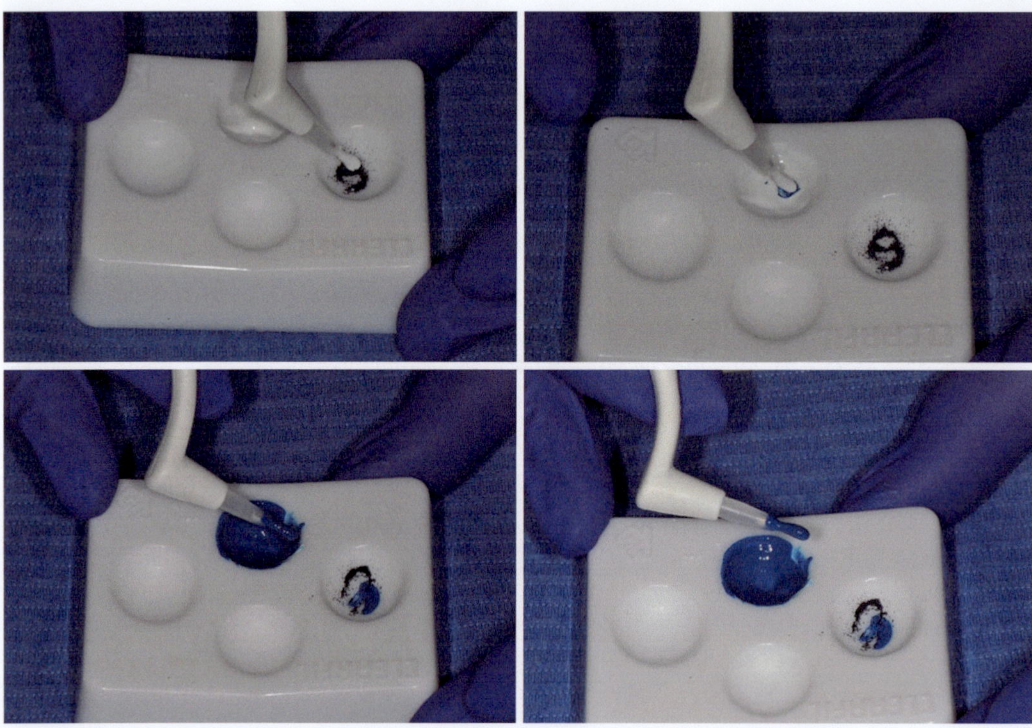

Fig. 8.3 Add the food dye to the desensitizing product

advise the use of a very fine brush. Once the colored desensitizing product has been positioned we began the process of irradiation with the laser (Fig. 8.4) using constant movements to brush the surface of the colored gel [3–5]. The protocol we used is the following:

Clinical Protocol

- Application of the colored paste on the surface to be treated.
- Application of the LASER (Diode 980 nm 0.5 W; CW; fiber 320 μ) about 20 s.
- Pause of 30 s (the time for thermal relaxation).
- Application of the LASER (Diode 980 nm 0.5 W; CW; fiber 320 μ) about 20 s.
- Washing with air/water spray.
- Dentine sensitivity test with air.

After laser irradiation the product is left in situ for about a minute and then rinsed off with water.

After completing the treatment, the sites were re-evaluated after 7 days, when necessary retreated, and then evaluated again 14 days and 3 months after the initial treatment.

The results that emerged from the operation were the following:

- No patient treated reported a worsening of their symptoms.
- No patient treated showed clinical signs of pain or pulp damage.
- All the patients experienced a clinical improvement in hypersensitivity during the treatment.
- No patient showed a return to his initial values after 3 months from the first application.
- 11 patients at 0 after 7 days and 1 application (25%).
- 17 patients at 0 after 14 days and 2 applications (38.6%).
- 17 patients at 0 after 90 days and 2 applications (38.6%).
- 28 patients with a score equal to or less than 2 after 90 days (63.6%).
- Average value at 3 months 1.63 against an initial value of 4.77.
- The average reduction in the scores is 3.14 points.

In the light of these results, we can confirm that the technique is safe and effective, simple to carry out, and devoid of discomfort for the patient during and after treatment [6].

The laser seems to allow a better formation of the isolating layer on the whole surface of the exposed dentine, but above all, it seems able to penetrate deeper into the hydroxyapatite crystals in the dentine tubules, thus forming longer intra-tubule tags. Longer tags are correlated with a more lasting desensitization over time with a prolonging of the therapeutic effect by almost 50% in patients treated with laser (Fig. 8.5).

This technique does not seem to undermine the adhesion maneuvers that may be required by the clinical situation itself, and consequently it can also be used on vital sensitive stumps before the adhesive cementation of metal-free-type prosthetic products.

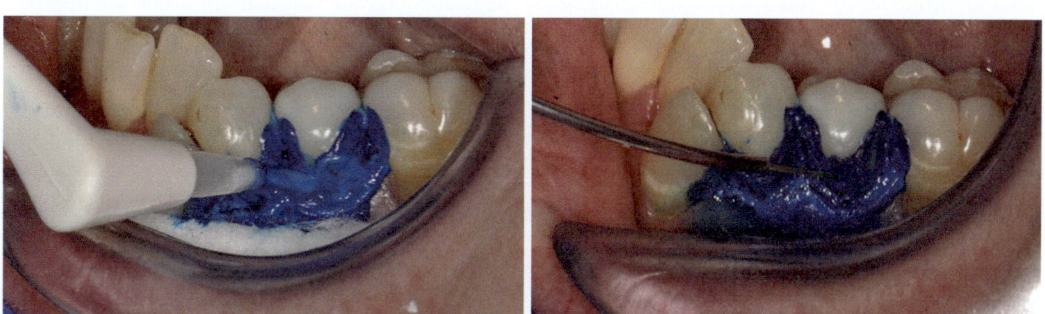

Fig. 8.4 Brushing homogeneous layer on the treated surface. Than laser diode irradiation following the protocol

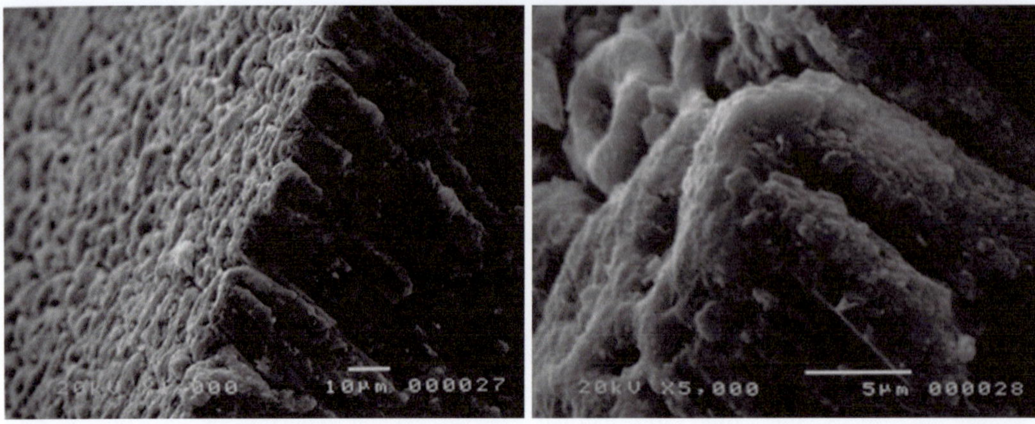

Fig. 8.5 Deeper tags formation inside dentinal tubules

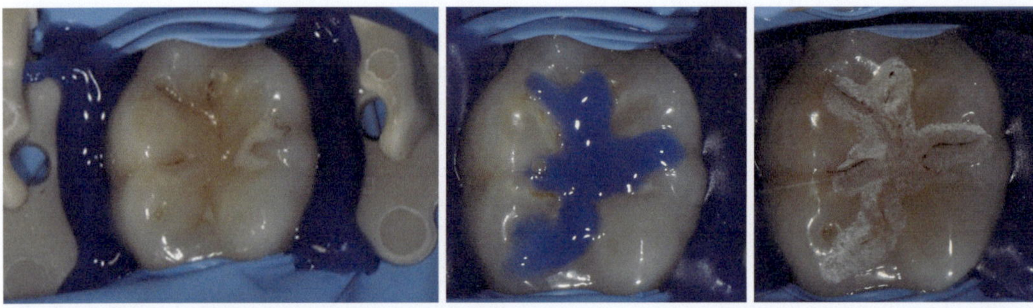

Fig. 8.6 Rubber dam positioning, laser treatment, acid etching

8.2 Er:YAG Sealing

The sealing of permanent teeth as soon as they erupt in young people is one of the prevention interventions that we habitually carry out in our surgeries. Permanent teeth when they have just erupted often present an unfavorable occlusal anatomy or, in other words, pits and furrows that are too pronounced and that compromise the health of the tooth. Furthermore, the vestibular pits of the lower molars and the dead holes on the upper central and lateral incisors are anatomical alterations with a greater possibility of becoming decayed.

For these reasons, it is considered important to treat these unfavorable anatomical defects especially in patients who are negligent in their oral hygiene.

The Er:YAG laser, with its characteristics of iteration with enamel tissue as described in the preceding chapter, is extremely useful in this technique. The microinvasive characteristics of the spot (0.5 mm diameter in the mirror handpiece) make it possible to work with great precision on the surfaces to be treated. What is more, by varying the fluence, it is possible to simply treat the enamel surface in order to improve the adhesive process or to be ablative and alter directly the anatomy of the tooth itself.

The procedure we used is the following.

After having inserted the rubber dam in order to isolate the operative area (Fig. 8.6), we proceeded with the laser, 150 mJ, 20 Hz, spot 0.5 mm, and pulse duration 50 μs therapy [7].

The treatment of the furrow was carried out using air/active water (ratio 3/6) until all detritus

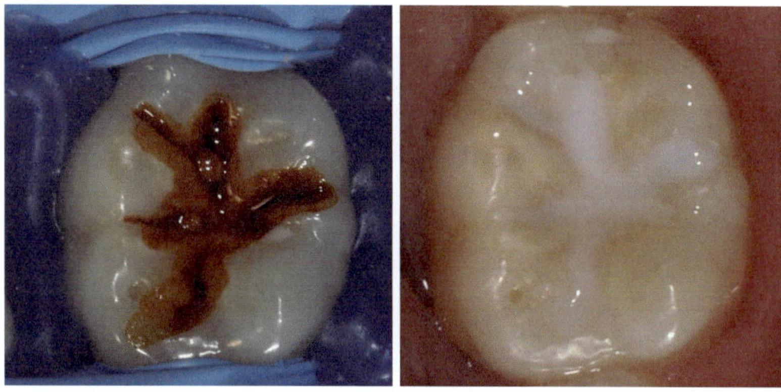

Fig. 8.7 PDT treatment and final sealing with resin

had been eliminated. Some authors have advised that subsequently a photodynamic therapy (PDT) should be carried out in order to decontaminate the site before positioning the resin sealant [8] (Fig. 8.7).

For the PDT, a wavelength of 645 nm, 500 mW, 60 s, is used after having positioned a specific product called a photosensitizer (e.g., indocyanine green). At the conclusion of this phase, the process continues with micro-acid etching using a 37% solution of orthophosphoric acid for 30 s. The chemical micro- acid etching is indispensable after the use of laser in order to remove the micro-cracks that are formed from the photo-acoustic effect of the erbium laser. Finally, the operation proceeds, as usual, with the positioning of the resin sealant and the subsequent polymerization of the same.

References

1. Farmakis ET, Kozyrakis K, Khabbaz MG, Schoop U, Beer F, Moritz A. In vitro evaluation of dentin tubule occlusion by Denshield and Neodymium-doped yttrium-aluminum-garnet laser irradiation. J Endod. 2012;38(5):662–6. https://doi.org/10.1016/j.joen.2012.01.019. Epub 2012 Mar 11.
2. Reddy GV, Akula S, Malgikar S, Babu PR, Reddy GJ, Josephin JJ. Comparative scanning electron microscope analysis of diode laser and desensitizing toothpastes for evaluation of efficacy of dentinal tubular occlusion. J Indian Soc Periodontol. 2017;21(2):102–6. https://doi.org/10.4103/jisp.jisp_153_17.
3. Gojkov-Vukelic M, Hadzic S, Zukanovic A, Pasic E, Pavlic V. Application of diode laser in the treatment of dentine hypersensitivity. Med Arch. 2016;70(6):466–9. https://doi.org/10.5455/medarh.2016.70.466-469.
4. Yaghini J, Mogharehabed A, Safavi N, Mohamadi M, Ashtiju F. Evaluation of the effect of low level laser therapy toothbrush in treatment of dentin hypersensitivity. J Lasers Med Sci. 2015;6(2):85–91.
5. Saluja M, Grover HS, Choudhary P. Comparative morphologic evaluation and occluding effectiveness of Nd: YAG, CO_2 and diode lasers on exposed human dentinal tubules: an in vitro SEM study. J Clin Diagn Res. 2016;10(7):ZC66–70. https://doi.org/10.7860/JCDR/2016/18262.8188. Epub 2016 Jul 1.
6. Cury MS, Silva CB, Nogueira RD, Campos MGD, Palma-Dibb RG, Geraldo-Martins VR. Surface roughness and bacterial adhesion on root dentin treated with diode laser and conventional desensitizing agents. Lasers Med Sci. 2018;33(2):257–62. https://doi.org/10.1007/s10103-017-2356-x. Epub 2017 Oct 14.
7. Bortolotto T, Mast P, Krejci I. Laser-prepared and bonding-filled fissure sealing: SEM and OCT analysis of marginal and internal adaptation. Dent Mater J. 2017;36(5):622–9. https://doi.org/10.4012/dmj.2016-025. Epub 2017 Aug 24.
8. Ozel E, Tuna EB, Firatli E. The effects of cavity-filling techniques on microleakage in class II resin restorations prepared with Er:YAG laser and diamond bur: a scanning electron microscopy study. Scanning. 2016;38(5):389–95. https://doi.org/10.1002/sca.21282. Epub 2015 Nov 5.

Laser in Bone Surgery

9

Lina M. Beltrán Bernal, Hamed Abbasi, and Azhar Zam

Contents

Abstract

During the past half-century, laser osteotomy has been studied for a broad range of lasers, which almost covers the entire range of available laser systems in the market, from early unsuccessful experiments with CW lasers to newly developed ultrashort pulse lasers. Although a large variety of laser parameters including wavelength, pulse energy, pulse duration, and repetition rate have been investigated to find an optimum laser system as an alternative osteotomy tool, there is not a universal agreement on a specific type of laser to replace conventional mechanical saws. The only universal agreement is on the speed of cutting (ablation rate) which went to long-pulse Er:YAG and CO_2 lasers. Microsecond pulse Er:YAG and CO_2 lasers perform osteotomy by inducing efficient photothermal effect to the bone with the help of high absorption peak of water in the bone. However, having a speedy cut is not the only effective parameter to pave the way for transferring lasers to the operating room. Other parameters including cutting with the lowest thermal damage, ability for deep cutting, and compatibility with integrating sensors are among the other determinant parameters. Moreover, being able to be delivered through the fiber optic and as a consequence fit inside the endoscope channel could extend their application from the open surgery to minimally invasive ones. This chapter besides proving the necessary information on the physics behind the laser–bone interaction provides a short review on the history of bone surgery with laser and state-of-the-art studies in this field.

L. M. Beltrán Bernal · H. Abbasi · A. Zam (✉)
Department of Biomedical Engineering, University of Basel, Allschwil, Switzerland
e-mail: lina.beltran@unibas.ch; hamed.abbasi@unibas.ch; azhar.zam@unibas.ch

S. Stübinger et al. (eds.), *Lasers in Oral and Maxillofacial Surgery*,
https://doi.org/10.1007/978-3-030-29604-9_9

Keywords

Laser osteotomy · Bone cutting · Hard bone Er:YAG · CO_2 · Nd:YAG · Irrigation Carbonization · Ablation efficiency · Pulse duration

9.1 Introduction

Bone surgery has been a challenge since ancient times due to the difficulties for performing free and precise shapes and trying to preserve, at the same time, the surrounding tissues. However, the conventional tools have not changed according to the new challenges and needs in the operating rooms [1]. The surgeons still are feeling more comfortable using the classical mechanical saws and drills despite the collateral effects those procedures have on the patients. The vibrations and heat generated by those mechanical tools provoke damage of soft tissue and delayed healing process for the cut area [2].

The main areas in which laser technology has achieved the best results in terms of less damage, more flexibility to perform the cuts, and better healing process for the patient are dermatology [3], ophthalmology [4], otolaryngology [5], and dentistry [6]. All those areas are mainly focused in soft tissue rather than in hard tissue. The only clinical application in which lasers like erbium, Nd:YAG, and CO_2 have been used to ablate hard tissue, like enamel and cementum, is in dentistry [7]. However, no deep cuts have been yet achieved. In the last decades, the use of laser for ablating oral tissues has shown a better performance because the laser provides small and flexible cuts and contact-free interaction with the cut area. Therefore, the collateral damage is reduced [7–10], and the healing process is much faster and easier for the patient.

9.2 History of Hard Tissue Laser Ablation

Bone surgery is found to be more challenging when fragile, and small bone parts (like in the maxilla and mandible) are under high pressure and vibration due to the contact with the mechanical tools (osteotomes). Also, the difficulties are found when cutting bones which are surrounded by delicate tissue like the spine or bones which require an invasive surgery to be reached, like in the partial or complete replacement of the knee. All those procedures require precision, less contact pressure and vibrations, and free shape cuts. Additionally, it is needed to reduce the bacterial contamination risk, which is very high when using the conventional osteotomes like drills and saws because sometimes there is deposition of metal material in the cut areas [7].

Right after the invention of the laser by Maiman in 1960 [11], many more types of lasers were launched [12]. Moreover, pulsed lasers were studied as potential tools in biomedical applications [13, 14], and only 5 years after its invention, the laser was used for precise tissue coagulation [15].

On the contrary, laser ablation of hard tissue was also investigated as early as other biomedical applications. The first studies were performed by hitting molar and incisor teeth using a ruby laser at the wavelength $\lambda = 694.3$ nm [16]. In 1964, the Nd:YAG and the CO_2 lasers were developed at the Bell Telephone Laboratories [17, 18]. Those lasers have been mostly used in dentistry applications for ablating soft and hard tissue, especially the CO_2 laser has been highly used since then. However, the ablation processes using the CO_2 laser showed that the tissues were getting carbonized due to the action of the laser [19, 20], and these carbonization effects led to delayed bone healing in comparison with the effect of the conventional mechanical tools. Even when changing the laser parameters, similar results were obtained [21, 22]. Studies of temperature rise and its effects while ablating the bone [23] showed that temperatures between 44 °C and 47 °C are critical and the consequences are the tissue presents thermal damage, which makes the healing process much more difficult, and, in some cases, the complete death of tissue in the surroundings of the ablated area.

The first studies in bone ablation using a pulsed Er:YAG laser were performed by Nuss [24] in 1988 and Hibst and Keller [25, 26] in 1989, where the interaction of middle-infrared wavelength laser with hard tissue was starting to be understood. Ten years after, deeper research in the interaction of the laser with the hard tissues showed that the most efficient wavelengths for ablating bone were 2.9, 3.0, and 5.9–6.45 μm [27]. When additional and proper amount of water spray was used together with the erbium laser to ablate the bones, the thermal damage was dramatically reduced [28]. In general, erbium laser wavelengths like 2.94 μm from the Er:YAG laser and 2.78 μm from the Er,Cr:YSGG laser were used and proven to be very efficient for dental hard tissue ablation [29, 30]. Nowadays, the lasers which are mainly used for hard tissue ablation are the Nd:YAG, the CO_2, and the erbium lasers.

9.3 The Physics Behind the Laser–Bone Interaction

The tissue properties involved in the interaction with the laser are absorption, scattering, anisotropy, and refractive index. The properties of the laser irradiation which might affect the tissues are wavelength, exposure time, pulse frequency, pulse duration, spot size, power, and energy density. There are two main types of laser–tissue interaction: Once the laser impinges the tissue, the light can be affected by the tissue properties, or the tissue can be affected by the laser parameters. In both cases, the laser parameters affect the result as well as the tissue properties. The first type of interaction is related to the field of diagnosis, imaging, and spectroscopy. All those methods are used basically to understand what is happening inside the tissues, what are their components, etc., by measuring the light properties after the interaction with the tissues. In the second type, the light affects the tissues because it is changing their properties; the laser can be used for surgical and therapeutic ablation, coagulating, and welding. Here we are interested in the second type. When the tissues are affected by the laser light, three main phenomena can occur: photochemical, photothermal, or photomechanical interactions [31]. Photodynamic therapy is a well-known procedure in which the photochemical interaction takes part. In this process, a photon interacts with a photosensitive dye and oxygen; from this reaction, a toxic material is produced, and therefore, the cancer cells are killed [31]. The photothermal interaction is the vaporization of tissue caused when the tissue absorbs the laser energy [32]. In the photomechanical interaction, the tissue is expelled, for instance, by explosions or the formation of plasma, in which the absorption properties of the tissues are not the main causes of tissue ablation [33]. In the following sections, we discuss the two main mechanisms used to ablate hard tissue: photothermal and photomechanical ablation.

Along the history of hard tissue laser ablation, the lasers which have been more used are the Nd:YAG, Ho:YAG, Er,Cr:YSGG, Er:YAG, CO_2, and ultrashort pulsed lasers. In the following, we discuss the ablation process driven by the interaction of those lasers and the hard tissues.

9.3.1 The Middle-Infrared Lasers

9.3.1.1 The Effect of Water Absorption

Water has the highest peaks of absorption at the middle-infrared wavelengths (2–10 μm) [33, 34]; this is the key point of working principle of the middle-infrared lasers to ablate the tissues better compared to other wavelengths, but that is not the only reason. In the case of hard tissues like enamel, cementum, dentin, and bone, the ablation process is driven by a thermomechanical event, which involves photothermal and photomechanical ablation [35, 36]. When the laser impinges the hard tissue surface, the energy is absorbed by the tissue and transferred into heat energy to the interstitial matrix inside the bone, the heat yields very high pressures in the water molecules of the tissue, and therefore, the ejection of the tissue occurs by explosive vaporization [7, 36, 37]. Therefore, the higher the absorption of water, the faster the ablation is [27], and this is the reason why under proper water cooling conditions, the Er:YAG laser working at $\lambda = 2.94$ μm (water has the highest absorption in the spectrum [33, 34]) is up to now the best laser known which is able to ablate bone very efficiently [36, 38–42]. Studies have shown that the Er:YAG working at the wavelength 2.94 μm is more efficient in ablating hard tissue at higher speeds compared to

Er,Cr:YSGG working at 2.78 μm [40, 43], and the main reason is that the absorption coefficient of Er:YAG is 1200 mm^{-1}, three times more than the one for Er,Cr:YSGG (400 mm^{-1}). The Ho:YAG laser has been also used to ablate bone; however, it has shown low ablation efficiency compared to Er:YAG lasers. The Ho:YAG laser works at the wavelength $\lambda = 2.1$ μm, in which water has *ca.* 120 times less absorption (10 mm^{-1}); this explains why this laser is not sufficiently efficient for bone ablation [44]. The CO_2 laser works at the wavelength 10.6 μm; the water absorption coefficient is 79 mm^{-1} [33, 45], approximately 15 times lower than the water absorption at Er:YAG wavelength. This laser has also been used for ablating hard and soft tissue, and the results show that its ablation efficiency is also very low in comparison with Er:YAG laser [46, 47].

9.3.1.2 The Effect of Pulse Duration

Not only the water absorption of the laser energy should be considered in order to ablate hard tissue more efficiently, but also it has been shown that, by shortening the pulse duration of CO_2 and Er:YAG lasers, for instance, from μs to ns regime, the damage zone is reduced [46–49]. To predict the depth of damaged tissue by thermal effects, there are two models based on the threshold amount of energy deposited at the surface of the target tissue [48]; this model applies to both soft and hard tissue. When the energy deposited in the tissue is above the ablation threshold (specific for every kind of tissue), the tissue is ablated. When the energy rise in the surroundings exceeds a critical value, e.g., 65° for tissues which contain high amounts of collagen like the cornea or the skin and 44–47° for the bone, the tissue is thermally damaged. The first model is based on Beer's law; it predicts the damage caused by the energy distribution at the end of the laser pulse; the width of damage D_d is given by:

$$D_{\mathrm{d}} = (1/\alpha)\ln\left[F_{\mathrm{th}}\alpha/(T_{\mathrm{c}} - T_0)\rho_{\mathrm{c}}\right],$$

where α is the absorption coefficient of the material at the specific wavelength of the laser used, F_{th} is the threshold fluence for ablation, T_c is the critical temperature for the denaturation of the tissue, T_0 is the initial tissue temperature before irradiation, and ρ_c is the volumetric-specific heat of the tissue [46].

In the second model, it is assumed that all the energy left at the end of the pulse is distributed uniformly in the tissue; the width of damage is:

$$D_{\mathrm{d}} = F_{\mathrm{th}}/(T_{\mathrm{c}} - T_0)\rho_{\mathrm{c}}.$$

The results reported in [48] using a Q-switched Er:YAG for ablating pig skin, aorta, and bone give damaged widths bigger than the predicted by the first model and smaller than the predicted by the second model. In that study, they show that the damage created by ns laser pulses is less than for the μs laser pulses. Similar results are shown when using a CO_2 laser [46].

9.3.1.3 The Effect of Water Cooling

The thermal damage caused by the ablation with middle-infrared lasers is due to the excess of temperature rise in the surroundings of the ablated tissue. To rehydrate the tissues and prevent damage like carbonization, water cooling is needed. As we have seen before, the higher the water absorbs the energy of the laser, the more efficient the ablation is. While using water during the ablation process, this water is also absorbing the energy of the laser; therefore, the ablation process becomes slower or completely stopped depending on the amount of water and the spray method used [50–53]. The Er:YAG and Er,Cr:YSGG lasers are commercially available as dental lasers, and they have their own continuous spray system. These lasers work very good for dentistry applications in which dentin, enamel, and cementum have to be superficially ablated [51]. For ablating deeper, the current irrigation system of the erbium lasers does not work as good as for superficial cuts because the water goes inside the ablated areas and it gets trapped preventing ablation to happen even when using pulsed water jet [53]. A different water cooling system should be used to be able to control precisely the amount of water on the tissue such that the ablation is optimal and no thermal damage

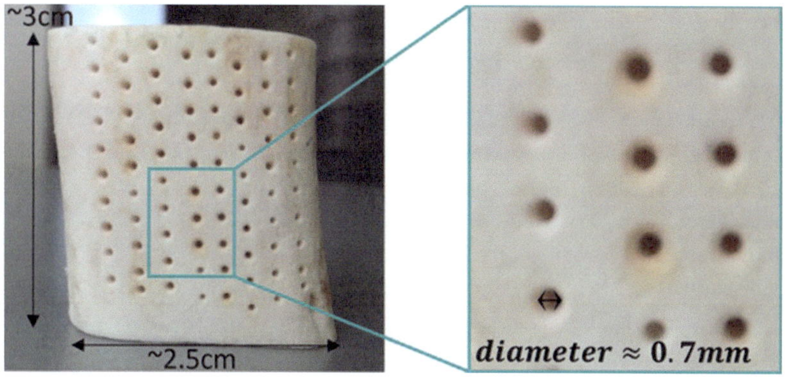

Fig. 9.1 Result of Er:YAG bone ablation holes with different water jet cooling conditions. A yellowish partial carbonization around the hole is observable (the darkness inside the hole in the picture is because of lack of light inside the hole). This figure was taken from [53] with permission

occurs. In Fig. 9.1, there are several holes made using an Er:YAG laser, and they have different water jet cooling conditions. The water cooling system used is an ESI Elveflow pulsed water jet which has a pneumatic pressure controller, a water reservoir of 80 mL capacity, and a Tygon tubing coil of 500 μm inner diameter. The pressure was set at its maximum capacity of 2 bar, which provided a flow rate of 14 mL/min and a velocity of 1 m/s. The system was used at different time of water on and water off sequences [53]. The fine water jet of similar size as the crater created by the laser (*ca.* 500 μm) provided a very good distribution of water inside and in the surroundings of the ablated area. However, the maximum depth achieved was 1 cm. Still several improvements should be implemented; for instance, having a suction system to avoid the excess of water inside the tissue, a finer water jet beam to direct more precisely the water inside the crater could be integrated as well.

In [53], it was confirmed, as in previous studies [50], that the ablation of hard tissue using middle-infrared lasers like erbium is very sensitive to the water spray system and amount of water used.

9.3.1.4 The Effect of Beam Quality

As expected, other laser parameters also affect the result of ablation. When the beam is not an ideal Gaussian beam (quality factor for ideal beam $M^2 = 1$), the Rayleigh length (Z_R) which provides the depth of focus ($D_{Focus} = 2Z_R$) is smaller as it should be:

$Z_R = \frac{\pi\omega_0^2}{M^2\lambda}$ where ω_0^2 is the beam radius of the focused beam at the surface of the tissue. Many commercially available Er:YAG lasers have a quality factor which is much higher ($15 < M^2 < 30$) than for an ideal Gaussian beam. Therefore, the depth of focus is dramatically reduced, reducing as well the depth of ablation.

9.3.2 Neodymium-Doped Lasers

As it has been mentioned before, in order to successfully replace conventional mechanical osteotomy tools with lasers, two main difficulties should be overcome: speedy cut and inducing less thermal damage to the bone as compared to mechanical saws and burrs. The first one was achieved with the help of high absorption of Er:YAG and CO_2 lasers in water and hydroxyapatite, which are the main component of the bone. The later one is also accessible, but it needs a proper cooling system. Otherwise it would lead to delayed healing process. Since the water is well absorbed in 3 and 10 μm, the amount of water that can be applied to the bone is very limited in both Er:YAG [54] and CO_2 lasers [55]. It has been shown that the maximum thickness of the water which a typical Er:YAG laserosteotome can pass through it is in order of *ca.* 1 mm (fluctuating depends on the laser parameters specially the peak power) [52]; otherwise the Er:YAG laser beam will be absorbed by the cooling water and cannot reach the tissue. Similar numbers are reported for both Er,Cr:YSGG and CO_2 lasers [56]. Therefore, when bleeding occurs and the target area needs to be flushed, the ablation process will be dramatically prolonged. Also if the bone cut needs to be performed in the presence of bulk water, then a laser with less absorption in water is necessary. Neodymium-doped lasers, including Nd:YAG (neodymium-doped yttrium aluminum garnet) and Nd:YVO4 (neodymium-doped yttrium orthovanadate), which emit 1064 nm as a primary harmonic and 532 nm as a second harmonic, with very low absorption in water are appropriate candidates to ablate the bone in the presence of water.

A damage-free bovine cortical bone ablation submerged under 15 mm of water with a frequency-doubled Nd:YVO4 laser has been demonstrated [42, 57]. The reported ablation rate is around 0.2 mm^3/s. Also, they reported the observation of 30% reduction in ablation rate when some bovine serum albumin was mixed with the water. There are also some studies about bone ablation with 1064 and 532 nm laser beams without cooling water [58, 59]. Without applying cooling water, full carbonization is reported during MHz bone ablation with mode-locked Nd:YVO4 laser oscillator [58] and carbonization-free kHz bone ablation using principal harmonic of picosecond Nd:YVO4 laser [59]. Repetition rate plays a key role in ultrashort laser ablation, which is discussed in the next section of this chapter. The authors' own unpublished results using a nanosecond Nd:YAG at 532 nm also support these findings. Figure 9.2 shows the hole made by a 5 ns laser beam with an energy of 200 mJ at 20 Hz repetition rate without any irrigation.

In addition, it is reported that Nd:YVO4 laser can ablate and remove the carbonized bone as well [58]. Thus, the carbonization detection with the beam Nd:YAG laser through laser-induced breakdown spectroscopy (LIBS) was possible [60]. Another advantage of neodymium-doped lasers is that they are compact, turnkey, affordable, and allow for high powers. Also, its optical components are easily available in the market, and water-jet-guided delivery is possible within neodymium laser wavelengths [61, 62]. One disadvantage of neodymium laser as compared to the middle-infrared laser is that their safety goggles have a less visible light transmission which could make it a bit uncomfortable for the surgeon. To sum up, while neodymium-doped laser showed ablation without thermal damage, they still suffer from low ablation rate which is one order of magnitude lower than reported ablation rate of Er:YAG or CO_2 laserosteotomes. Further experiments with neodymium-doped lasers with higher average power may lead to comparable ablation rate with erbium-doped lasers.

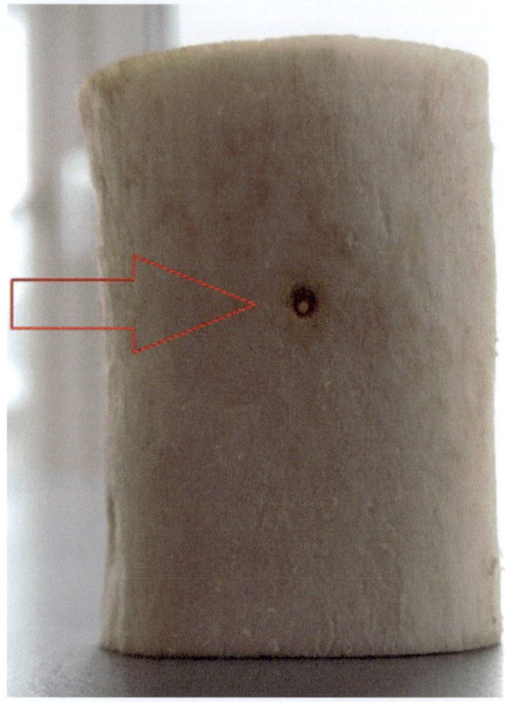

Fig. 9.2 Result of nanosecond Nd:YAG bone ablation without any cooling. A yellowish partial carbonization around the hole is observable (the darkness inside the hole in the picture is because of lack of the light inside the hole)

9.3.3 Ultrashort Pulsed Lasers

As it has been mentioned at the beginning of this chapter, the high power density of laser lights leads to photomechanical interactions of light with the tissue through plasma formation (so-called plasma-mediated ablation). Achieving high power density of laser light requires short (nanoseconds) and ultrashort (picoseconds and femtoseconds) pulse duration. Due to the nonlin-

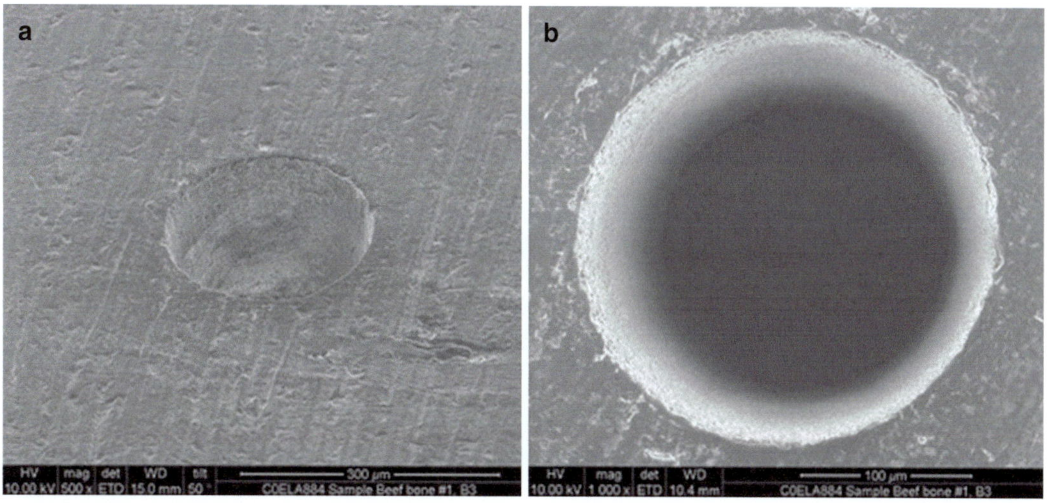

Fig. 9.3 The SEM image of a microhole generated with a femtosecond laser: (**a**) Overview and (**b**) top view, taken from [74] with permission

ear optical phenomena in ultrashort pulse regime, the absorption properties of the tissues are not the main causes of tissue ablation [33]. In this timescale, a picosecond or femtosecond laser beam ablates a dielectric material through multiphoton absorption of light and avalanche ionization or hydrodynamic expansion of plasma induced by the very high electric field in the focal spot of the laser line [58].

One of the difficulties of working with short and ultrashort lasers is that it becomes more challenging to couple them into the fiber for minimally invasive surgeries due to plasma formation in the environment air and it needs a vacuum chamber or an optical homogenizer to prevent this breakdown [63]. The generated plasma in the air could become much bigger than the actual spot size of the laser beams over time, due to the expansion of the ionized area. It has been shown that the generated plasma in the air using a typical nanosecond Nd:YAG laser could be a bit smaller than generated plasma in the surface of the bone but still in millimeter scale [64]. The generated plasma expands in both lateral and axial directions [65]. Also, it has been demonstrated that the generated plasma could last up some hundreds of microseconds (fluctuating depending on laser parameters) [64]. Therefore, such a laser with the repetition rate of more than 10 kHz could result in plasma shielding effects and as a result reducing the ablation rate due to the absorption of the laser line by the plasma itself. However, the generated plasma in liquids [66–68] or with shorter laser pulse duration [33, 69, 70] could result in shorter ionization lasting time and smaller plasma formation (very localized) in size which allow using higher repetition rates without suffering from shielding effect and doing microsurgeries (fine cuts), respectively [33, 71, 72]. Also, accelerated bone healing after the femtosecond laser ablation of cranial bone has been reported [73]. Figure 9.3a, b shows the SEM image of a microhole generated with a femtoseconds laser. Figure 9.4 shows the SEM image of a trench made with the same laser in cross-sectional view (Fig. 9.4a) and side wall view (Fig. 9.4b). As shown in Figs. 9.3 and 9.4, there is no visible cracks or thermal damage around the edges of the ablated part. Both figures are taken from [74] with permission.

One of the main advantage of ultrashort laser pulses to ablate the bone is that they transfer their energy to the tissue in a very short timescale, and as a result, thermal energy dissipation is faster than thermal energy accumulation which could prevent carbonization. The effect of laser repetition rate on femtosecond laser ablation of dry bone has been investigated [75]. They have found that heat accumulation exceeds heat dissipation which results in carbonization of the sample. Therefore, in a nutshell, ultrashort laser

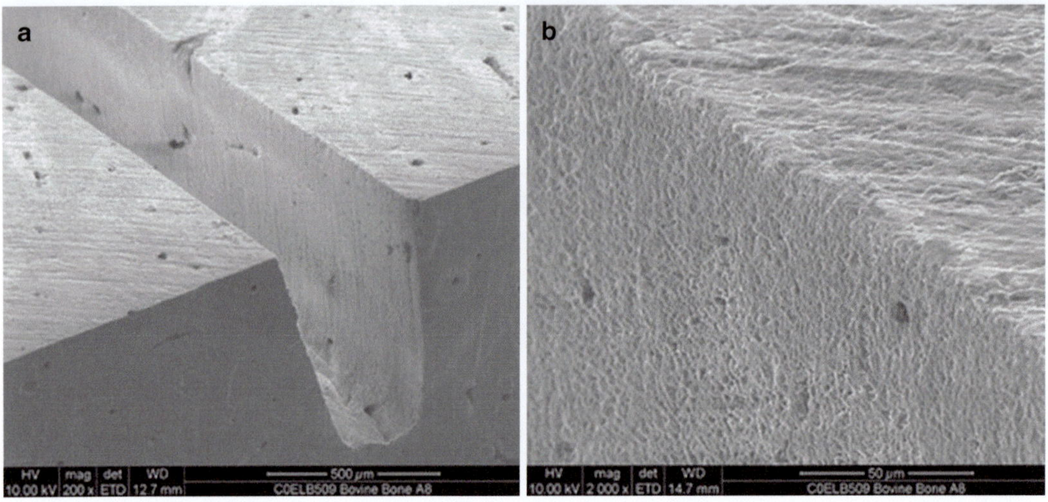

Fig. 9.4 The SEM image of a trench made with a femtosecond laser in cross-sectional view (**a**) and side wall view (**b**), taken from [74] with permission

ablation is temperature limited [76]. Their finding is in line with other reports, where kHz osteotomy led to carbonization-free result [59] and MHz osteotomy led to full carbonization [58]. The other advantage of plasma-mediated ablation over photothermal one is that by monitoring the plasma-emitted light (breakdown light) and also plasma-produced sound (shock wave), detecting type of the ablating tissue is possible [74, 77–82].

It has been shown that in the photothermal osteotomy, the bone ablation rate is mainly determined by the average power of the laser and not the peak power [83]. Therefore, changing the pulse duration (changing the peak power), while the repetition rate and pulse energy (entirely as average power) are the same, has not any significant effect on the ablation rate. However, if the pulse duration is changed too much, which could change ablation mechanism from photothermal to photomechanical ablation (plasma-mediated), then the ablation efficiency is dramatically reduced due to energy losses in the plasma formation process. Thus, very low ablation rate in short and ultrashort laser osteotomy is yet the main disadvantage in the state-of-the-art nano-, pico-, and femtosecond laser system for cutting bones. Moreover, the effect of using the ionizing beam on the biological samples is not clear enough yet [58, 59, 84, 85].

To conclude, even short and ultrashort pulse laser bone ablation provide some advantages including information on the type and properties of the ablated tissue, finer cut, and also carbonization-free ablation even without applying cooling water (by using a suitable repetition rate); they cannot find a way to be used instead of long-pulse Er:YAG laser when their ablation rate is highly below them. However, in special kind of surgeries, like tissue-specific surgeries and microsurgeries, where having finer cut on a particular type of tissue is more important than speed of the cut, they can be used efficiently. Employing higher average power ultrashort lasers may lead to higher ablation rate in the future. Combination of laser bone cutting and providing a baseline for LIBS- or shockwave-based sensors could result in a novel, fast, and safe osteotomy tool.

References

1. Lawrence C. The evolution of surgical instruments: An illustrated history from ancient times to the twentieth century. Bull Hist Med. 2007;81(3):661–2.
2. Eriksson AR, Albrektsson T, Albrektsson B. Heat caused by drilling cortical bone: temperature measured in vivo in patients and animals. Acta Orthop Scand. 1984;55(6):629–31.

3. Steiner R, Raulin C, Karsai S. Laser and ipl technology in dermatology and aesthetic medicine. Berlin Heidelberg: Springer-Verlag; 2011.
4. Soong HK, Malta JB. Femtosecond lasers in ophthalmology. Am J Ophthalmol. 2009;147(2):189–97.
5. Shapshay SM, Hybels RL, Beamis JF Jr, Bohigian RK. Endoscopic treatment of subglottic and tracheal stenosis by radial laser incision and dilation. Ann Otol Rhinol Laryngol. 1987;96(6):661–4.
6. Berlien H-P, Breuer H, Müller GJ, Krasner N, Okunata T, Sliney D. Applied laser medicine. New York: Springer Science & Business Media; 2012.
7. Stübinger S. Advances in bone surgery: the Er:Yag laser in oral surgery and implant dentistry. Clin Cosmet Investigat Dentist. 2010;2:47.
8. Parker S. Surgical lasers and hard dental tissue. Br Dent J. 2007;202(8):445.
9. Jowett N, Wöllmer W, Reimer R, Zustin J, Schumacher U, Wiseman PW, Mlynarek AM, Böttcher A, Dalchow CV, Lörincz BB, et al. Bone ablation without thermal or acoustic mechanical injury via a novel picosecond infrared laser (pirl). Otolaryngol Head Neck Surg. 2014;150(3):385–93.
10. Rajitha Gunaratne G, Khan R, Fick D, Robertson B, Dahotre N, Ironside C. A review of the physiological and histological effects of laser osteotomy. J Med Eng Technol. 2017;41(1):1–12.
11. Maiman T. Stimulated optical radiation in ruby. Nature. 1960;187(4736):493–4.
12. Rawicz AH. Theodore harold maiman and the invention of laser. Photon Device Syst IV. 2008;7138:713802, International Society for Optics and Photonics
13. Solon LR, Aronson R, Gould G. Physiological implications of laser beams. Science. 1961;134(3489):1506–8.
14. Goldman L. Effect of the laser beam on the skin, preliminary report. J Invest Derm. 1963;40:121–2.
15. Zweng H, Flocks M, Kapany N, Silbertrust N, Peppers N. Experimental laser photo-coagulation. Am J Ophthalmol. 1964;58(3):353–62.
16. Goldman L, Gray JA, Goldman J, Goldman B, Meyer R. Effect of laser beam impacts on teeth. J Am Dent Assoc. 1965;70(3):601–6.
17. Geusic J, Marcos H, Van Uitert L. Laser oscillations in nd-doped yttrium aluminum, yttrium gallium and gadolinium garnets. Appl Phys Lett. 1964;4(10):182–4.
18. Patel C. N continuous wave laser action on vibrational-rotational transitions of co2. Phys Rev A. 1964;136:1187.
19. Horch H, McCord R, Keiditsch E. Histological and long term results following laser osteotomy. In: Laser Surgery II. Jerusalem. Israel: Academic Press; 1978. p. 318.
20. Horch H. Current status of laser osteotomy. Der Orthopade. 1984;13(2):125–32.
21. Clayman L, Fuller T, Beckman H. Healing of continuous-wave and rapid superpulsed, carbon dioxide, laser-induced bone defects. J Oral Surg. 1978;36(12):932–7.
22. Gopin BW, Cobb CM, Rapley JW, Killoy WJ. Histologic evaluation of soft tissue attachment to co 2 laser-treated root surfaces: an in viva study. Int J Periodont Restorat Dentist. 1997;17(4)
23. Eriksson A, Albrektsson T. Temperature threshold levels for heat-induced bone tissue injury: a vital-microscopic study in the rabbit. J Prosthet Dent. 1983;50(1):101–7.
24. Nuss RC, Fabian RL, Sarkar R, Puliafito CA. Infrared laser bone ablation. Lasers Surg Med. 1988;8(4):381–91.
25. Hibst R, Keller U. Experimental studies of the application of the er: Yag laser on dental hard substances: I. measurement of the ablation rate. Lasers Surg Med. 1989;9(4):338–44.
26. Keller U, Hibst R. Experimental studies of the application of the er: Yag laser on dental hard substances: Ii. light microscopic and sem investigations. Lasers Surg Med. 1989;9(4):345–51.
27. Peavy GM, Reinisch L, Payne JT, Venugopalan V. Comparison of cortical bone ablations by using infrared laser wavelengths 2.9 to 9.2 μm. Lasers Surg Med. 1999;25(5):421–34.
28. Hibst R, Keller U. Effects of water spray and repetition rate on the temperature elevation during Er: Yag laser ablation of dentine. Med Applicat Lasers III. 1996;2623:139–45, International Society for Optics and Photonics
29. Convissar RA. The biologic rationale for the use of lasers in dentistry. Dental Clinics. 2004;48(4):771–94.
30. Iaria G. Clinical, morphological, and ultrastructural aspects with the use of Er:Yag and Er, Cr:Ysgg lasers in restorative dentistry. General Dentist. 2008;56(7):636.
31. Jacques SL. Laser-tissue interactions: photochemical, photothermal, and photomechanical. Surg Clin N Am. 1992;72(3):531–58.
32. Lowery AR, Gobin AM, Day ES, Halas NJ, West JL. Immunonanoshells for targeted photothermal ablation of tumor cells. Int J Nanomedicine. 2006;1(2):149.
33. Vogel A, Venugopalan V. Mechanisms of pulsed laser ablation of biological tissues. Chem Rev. 2003;103(2):577–644.
34. Matos AB, de Azevedo CS, da Ana PA, Botta SB, Zezell DM. Laser technology for caries removal. In: Contemporary approach to dental caries. London: InTech; 2012.
35. Hibst R, Keller U. Mechanism of Er: Yag laser-induced ablation of dental hard substances. Lasers Orthop Dent Vet Med II. 1993;1880:156–63, International Society for Optics and Photonics
36. Selting WJ. Fundamental erbium laser concepts: Part I. J Laser Dent. 2009;17(2):87–93.
37. Tuchin VV. Tissue optics and photonics: light-tissue interaction II. J Biomed Photon Eng. 2016;2:3.
38. Stock K, Hibst R, Keller U. Comparison of er: Yag and er: Ysgg laser ablation of dental hard tissues. Med Appl Lasers Dermatol Ophthalmol Dentist Endosc.

1997;3192:88–96, International Society for Optics and Photonics
39. Spencer P, Payne JM, Cobb CM, Reinisch L, Peavy GM, Drummer DD, Suchman DL, Swafford JR. Effective laser ablation of bone based on the absorption characteristics of water and proteins. J Periodontol. 1999;70(1):68–74.
40. Perhavec T, Diaci J. Comparison of er: Yag and er, cr: Ysgg dental lasers. J Oral Laser Applicat. 2008;8:2.
41. Selting WJ. Fundamental erbium laser concepts: part ii. J Laser Dent. 2010;18(3):116–22.
42. Tulea C-A, Caron J, Gehlich N, Lenenbach A, Noll R, Loosen P. Laser cutting of bone tissue under bulk water with a pulsed ps-laser at 532 nm. J Biomed Opt. 2015;20(10):105007.
43. Diaci J, Gaspirc B. Comparison of er: Yag and er, cr: Ysgg lasers used in dentistry. J Laser health Acad. 2012;1(1):1–13.
44. Trauner K, Nishioka N, Patel D. Pulsed holmium: yttrium-aluminum-garnet (ho: Yag) laser ablation of fibrocartilage and articular cartilage. Am J Sports Med. 1990;18(3):316–20.
45. Robertson CW, Williams D. Lambert absorption coefficients of water in the infrared. JOSA. 1971;61(10):1316–20.
46. Walsh JT Jr, Flotte TJ, Anderson RR, Deutsch TF. Pulsed co2 laser tissue ablation: effect of tissue type and pulse duration on thermal damage. Lasers Surg Med. 1988;8(2):108–18.
47. Walsh JT, Deutsch TF. Pulsed co2 laser tissue ablation: measurement of the ablation rate. Lasers Surg Med. 1988;8(3):264–75.
48. Walsh JT, Flotte TJ, Deutsch TF. Er: Yag laser ablation of tissue: effect of pulse duration and tissue type on thermal damage. Lasers Surg Med. 1989;9(4):314–26.
49. Walsh JT. Pulsed laser ablation of tissue: analysis of the removal process and tissue healing. PhD thesis, Massachusetts Institute of Technology, 1988.
50. Visuri SR, Walsh JT, Wigdor HA. Erbium laser ablation of dental hard tissue: effect of water cooling. Lasers Surg Med. 1996;18(3):294–300.
51. Kuščer L, Diaci J. Measurements of erbium laser-ablation efficiency in hard dental tissues under different water cooling conditions. J Biomed Opt. 2013;18(10):108002.
52. Abbasi H, Beltrán L, Rauter G, Guzman R, Cattin PC, Zam A. Effect of cooling water on ablation in er: Yag laserosteotome of hard bone. Third Int Conf Applicat Opt Photon. 2017;10453:104531I, International Society for Optics and Photonics
53. Bernal LMB, Shayeganrad G, Kosa G, Zelechowski M, Rauter G, Friederich N, Cattin PC, Zam A. Performance of er: Yag laser ablation of hard bone under different irrigation water cooling conditions. Opt Interact Tissue Cells XXIX. 2018;10492:104920B, International Society for Optics and Photonics
54. Stock K, Diebolder R, Hausladen F, Wurm H, Lorenz S, Hibst R. Primary investigations on the potential of a novel diode pumped er: Yag laser system for bone surgery. Photon Therapeut Diagn IX. 2013;8565:85656D, International Society for Optics and Photonics
55. Zhang X, Zhan Z, Liu H, Zhao H, Xie S, Ye Q. Influence of water layer thickness on hard tissue ablation with pulsed co 2 laser. J Biomed Opt. 2012;17(3):038003.
56. Kang H, Oh J, Welch A. Investigations on laser hard tissue ablation under various environments. Phys Med Biol. 2008;53(12):3381.
57. Tulea C, Caron J, Wahab H, Gehlich N, Hoefer M, Esser D, Jungbluth B, Lenenbach A, Noll R. Highly efficient nonthermal ablation of bone under bulk water with a frequency- doubled nd: Yvo 4 picosecond laser. Photon Therapeut Diagn IX. 2013;8565:85656E, International Society for Optics and Photonics
58. Lee Y-M, Tu R, Chiang A, Huang Y-C. Average-power mediated ultrafast laser osteotomy using a mode-locked nd: Yvo 4 laser oscillator. J Biomed Opt. 2007;12(6):060505.
59. Plötz C, Schelle F, Bourauel C, Frentzen M, Meister J. Ablation of porcine bone tissue with an ultrashort pulsed laser (uspl) system. Lasers Med Sci. 2015;30(3):977–83.
60. Abbasi H, Rauter G, Guzman R, Cattin PC, Zam A. Laser-induced breakdown spectroscopy as a potential tool for autocarbonization detection in laser osteotomy. J Biomed Opt. 2018;23(7):071206.
61. Porter JA, Louhisalmi YA, Karjalainen JA, Füger S. Cutting thin sheet metal with a water jet guided laser using various cutting distances, feed speeds and angles of incidence. Int J Adv Manuf Technol. 2007;33(9–10):961–7.
62. Li C-F, Johnson D, Kovacevic R. Modeling of water-jet guided laser grooving of silicon. Int J Mach Tools Manuf. 2003;43(9):925–36.
63. Schmidt-Uhlig T, Karlitschek P, Marowsky G, Sano Y. New simplified coupling scheme for the delivery of 20 mw nd: Yag laser pulses by large core optical fibers. Appl Phys B Lasers Opt. 2001;72(2):183–6.
64. Abbasi H, Rauter G, Guzman R, Cattin PC, Zam A. Plasma plume expansion dynamics in nanosecond nd: Yag laserosteotome. High-Speed Biomed Imag Spectrosc III: Toward Big Data Instrument Manag. 2018;10505:1050513, International Society for Optics and Photonics
65. Nazeri M, Majd AE, Massudi R, Tavassoli SH, Mesbahinia A, Abbasi H. Laser-induced breakdown spectroscopy via the spatially resolved technique using non-gated detector. J Russ Laser Res. 2016;37(2):164–71.
66. Hammer DX, Jansen ED, Frenz M, Noojin GD, Thomas RJ, Noack J, Vogel A, Rockwell BA, Welch AJ. Shielding properties of laser-induced breakdown in water for pulse durations from 5 ns to 125 fs. Appl Opt. 1997;36(22):5630–40.
67. De Giacomo A, DellAglio M, De Pascale O. Single pulse-laser induced breakdown spectroscopy in aqueous solution. Appl Phys A Mater Sci Process. 2004;79(4–6):1035–8.

68. De Giacomo A, Dell'Aglio M, Colao F, Fantoni R. Double pulse laser produced plasma on metallic target in seawater: basic aspects and analytical approach. Spectrochim Acta B At Spectrosc. 2004;59(9):1431–8.
69. Verhoff B, Harilal S, Freeman J, Diwakar P, Hassanein A. Dynamics of femto-and nanosecond laser ablation plumes investigated using optical emission spectroscopy. J Appl Phys. 2012;112(9):093303.
70. Zeng X, Mao X, Greif R, Russo R. Experimental investigation of ablation efficiency and plasma expansion during femtosecond and nanosecond laser ablation of silicon. Appl Phys A Mater Sci Process. 2005;80(2):237–41.
71. Tsai PS, Blinder P, Migliori BJ, Neev J, Jin Y, Squier JA, Kleinfeld D. Plasma-mediated ablation: an optical tool for submicrometer surgery on neuronal and vascular systems. Curr Opin Biotechnol. 2009;20(1):90–9.
72. Cangueiro L, Vilar R. Influence of the pulse frequency and water cooling on the femtosecond laser ablation of bovine cortical bone. Appl Surf Sci. 2013;283:1012–7.
73. Lo DD, Mackanos MA, Chung MT, Hyun JS, Montoro DT, Grova M, Liu C, Wang J, Palanker D, Connolly AJ, et al. Femtosecond plasma mediated laser ablation has advantages over mechanical osteotomy of cranial bone. Lasers Surg Med. 2012;44(10):805–14.
74. Huang H, Yang L-M, Bai S, Liu J. Smart surgical tool. J Biomed Opt. 2015;20(2):028001.
75. Gill RK, Smith ZJ, Lee C, Wachsmann-Hogiu S. The effects of laser repetition rate on femtosecond laser ablation of dry bone: a thermal and libs study. J Biophotonics. 2016;9(1–2):171–80.
76. de Menezes RF, Harvey CM, de Martínez Gerbi MEM, Smith ZJ, Smith D, Ivaldi JC, Phillips A, Chan JW, Wachsmann-Hogiu S. Fs-laser ablation of teeth is temperature limited and provides information about the ablated components. J Biophotonics. 2017;10(10):1292–304.
77. Abbasi H, Rauter G, Guzman R, Cattin PC, Zam A. Differentiation of femur bone from surrounding soft tissue using laser induced breakdown spectroscopy as a feedback system for smart laser osteotomy. Biophoton: Photon Solution Better Health Care VI. 2018;10685:1068519, International Society for Optics and Photonics
78. Mehari F, Rohde M, Knipfer C, Kanawade R, Klämpfl F, Adler W, Stelzle F, Schmidt M. Laser induced breakdown spectroscopy for bone and cartilage differentiation- ex vivo study as a prospect for a laser surgery feedback mechanism. Biomed Opt Express. 2014;5(11):4013–23.
79. Rohde M, Mehari F, Klämpfl F, Adler W, Neukam F-W, Schmidt M, Stelzle F. The differentiation of oral soft- and hard tissues using laser induced breakdown spectroscopy–a prospect for tissue specific laser surgery. J Biophotonics. 2017;10(10):1250–61.
80. Kim B-M, Feit M, Rubenchik A, Mammini B, Da Silva L. Optical feedback signal for ultrashort laser pulse ablation of tissue1. Appl Surf Sci. 1998;127: 857–62.
81. Jeong DC, Tsai PS, Kleinfeld D. Prospect for feedback guided surgery with ultra-short pulsed laser light. Curr Opin Neurobiol. 2012;22(1):24–33.
82. Kenhagho HKN, Rauter G, Guzman R, Cattin PC, Zam A. Comparison of acoustic shock waves generated by micro and nanosecond lasers for a smart laser surgery system. Adv Biomed Clin Diagn Surg Guid Syst XVI. 2018;10484:104840P, International Society for Optics and Photonics
83. Beltrán L, Abbasi H, Rauter G, Friederich N, Cattin P, Zam A. Effect of laser pulse duration on ablation efficiency of hard bone in microseconds regime. Third Int Conf Applicat Opt Photon. 2017;10453:104531S, International Society for Optics and Photonics
84. Strassl M, Wieger V, Brodoceanu D, Beer F, Moritz A, Wintner E. Ultra-short pulse laser ablation of biological hard tissue and biocompatibles, na, 2008.
85. Cangueiro LT, da Silva Vilar RMC, do Rego AMB, Muralha VS. Femtosecond laser ablation of bovine cortical bone. J Biomed Opt. 2012;17(12):125005.

Utilization of Dental Laser as an Adjunct for Periodontal Surgery

10

Fernando Suárez López del Amo, Pimchanok Sutthiboonyapan, and Hom-Lay Wang

Contents

F. Suárez López del Amo
Private practice, Tacoma, WA, United States
e-mail: fsuarez@soundsurgicalarts.com

P. Sutthiboonyapan
Department of Periodontology, Faculty of Dentistry, Chulalongkorn University, Bangkok, Thailand
e-mail: pimchanok.s@chula.ac.th

H.-L. Wang (✉)
Graduate Periodontics, Department of Periodontics and Oral Medicine, University of Michigan School of Dentistry, Ann Arbor, MI, USA
e-mail: homlay@umich.edu

Abstract

While presenting with numerous indications, the long-term effectiveness of lasers has been repeatedly questioned. As such, laser usage for periodontal applications remains a topic of controversy. These devices can successfully replace and/or serve as an adjunct to conventional instruments in a variety of procedures providing also with certain advantages such as hemostatic and antibacterial effects. This chapter aimed at summarizing the characteristics and current available applications of lasers for periodontal surgical procedures.

S. Stübinger et al. (eds.), *Lasers in Oral and Maxillofacial Surgery*,
https://doi.org/10.1007/978-3-030-29604-9_10

Keywords

Lasers · Periodontics · Laser therapy · Periodontal surgery

10.1 Introduction

As defined by the *Glossary of Periodontal Terms*, periodontal surgery encompasses any surgical procedures aimed at the treatment of periodontal disease or the modification of the morphology of the periodontium [1]. Included in this category are procedures for correction of both mucogingival deformities and bone atrophies. This broad spectrum of operations grouped under the term "periodontal surgery" can also be accomplished by a great variety of different approaches. From traditional instruments and classic surgical techniques to more advanced tools and regenerative methods, periodontal surgery has significantly evolved with time. Similarly, materials and devices are constantly introduced in the periodontal arena aiming at facilitating and more predictably treating the complex scenarios that clinicians face routinely. Although not new to the periodontal field, laser therapy has recently gained major attention due to the promising results and broad range of clinical applications.

10.2 History of Lasers in the Periodontal Field

The use of lasers in the periodontal field has significantly evolved during the last decades. The development of new devices along with more applications and clearances from the Food and Drug Administration (FDA) have made the employment of lasers an integral part of today's practice in periodontal surgery. Initially, the first laser prototype (ruby crystal laser) was developed by Maiman in 1960 [2]. However, it wasn't until years later that lasers were first applied to dental tissues [3, 4]. Later on, in 1989, Myers suggested the use of lasers for oral soft tissue surgery, leading the way and establishing the foundation for the use of lasers in periodontics [5]. Today, lasers are used in multitude of different periodontal and peri-implant procedures including surgical and nonsurgical approaches [6, 7]. In spite of the increasing number of investigations in the periodontal arena, the utilization of lasers for periodontal surgery remains a topic of controversy.

10.3 Types of Lasers Used in Periodontics: Characteristics and Indications

The field of periodontology embraces multitude of different procedures with distinct objectives and methodologies. From classical nonsurgical therapies for bacterial elimination to more advanced procedures involving periodontal regeneration, flap mobilization, and implant dentistry, the periodontal arena gathers together a broad spectrum of procedures. Consequently, it is no surprise that these operations can be performed with great variety of instruments and devices. As such, lasers can be applied in multitude of different clinical scenarios. Depending on the lasers' characteristics, mostly determined by the wavelength, these devices can be applied to both periodontal nonsurgical and surgical procedures. Today, some of the most commonly used lasers in the periodontal field include argon; carbon dioxide (CO_2); diodes; erbium, chromium:yttrium-selenium-gallium-garnet (Er,Cr:YSGG); erbium:yttrium-aluminum-garnet (Er:YAG); neodymium:yttrium-aluminum-garnet (Nd:YAG); neodymium:yttrium-aluminum-perovskite (Nd:YAP); and holmium:yttrium-aluminum-garnet (Ho:YAG). Table 10.1 describes some of the most common applications of the lasers employed in the periodontal field; however, it is not intended to be a complete description of all possible indications. The following section summarizes the most relevant lasers used to date in periodontal surgery:

- *Carbon dioxide (CO_2):* 10,600 nm wavelength.
  - The CO_2 has gated or continuous waveform. It exhibits a high absorption coefficient in water. With its low scatter and penetration, it absorbs at the tissue surface and produces thin layer of coagulation. CO_2 laser is effective at ablating soft tissue but creates severe carbonization due to high heat production.

Table 10.1 Common clinical applications of lasers in periodontal field

Application / Type of laser	Soft tissue incision, ablation and coagulation	Aphthous ulcers	LANAP	Subgingival curettage	Bacterial elimination	Scaling of root surfaces (calculus removal)	Osteoplasty and ostectomy	Peri-implantitis
Argon	X							
CO_2	X	X	X	X				X
Diode	X	X		X	X			X
Er,Cr:YSGG	X	X		X		X	X	X
Er:YAG	X	X		X		X	X	X
Nd:YAG	X	X	X	X	X			X
Nd:YAP	X			X	X			
Ho:YAG	X			X	X			

CO_2 carbon dioxide, *Er:YAG* erbium:yttrium-aluminum-garnet, *Er,Cr:YSGG* erbium, chromium:yttrium-selenium-gallium-garnet, *Nd:YAG* neodymium:yttrium-aluminum-garnet, *Ho:YAG* holmium:yttrium-aluminum-garnet, *Nd:YAP* neodymium:yttrium-aluminum-perovskite

With the large amount of thermal change, this laser should be avoided in hard tissue procedures in order to prevent tissue damage.

  - FDA approved the use of CO_2 laser in intraoral soft tissue surgery, aphthous ulcer treatment, sulcular debridement, coagulation at extraction sites, and laser-assisted new attachment procedure (LANAP).

- *Diode*: 635–950 nm wavelength.
  - Diode lasers generated gated or continuous waveform. They mainly absorb in pigmented tissues due to less water absorption coefficients than CO_2 lasers. Their penetration is deep and produces the most coagulation effect with moderate carbonization. It has been shown to carbonize cementum only when blood is presented.
  - Diode lasers demonstrate good tissue cut ability. FDA approved the use of diode lasers in intraoral soft tissue surgery, aphthous ulcer treatment, sulcular debridement, coagulation of extraction sites, decontamination, subgingival calculus detection, and removal of inflamed pocket epithelium.
- *Neodymium:yttrium-aluminum-garnet (Nd:YAG):* 1064 nm wavelength.
  - Nd:YAG laser exhibits pulsed waveform. It also has less water absorption coefficients than CO_2 laser but is able to deeply penetrate into tissue. It produces a thick coagulation with moderate carbonization favoring hemostasis. Major thermal changes can occur when this laser is used on hard tissue and, thus, it should be avoided for these procedures.
  - FDA approved this laser for intraoral soft tissue surgery, aphthous ulcer treatment, and laser-assisted new attachment procedure (LANAP).
- *Erbium:yttrium-aluminum-garnet (ER:YAG):* 2940 nm.
  - Er:YAG laser is free-running pulsed. It has high absorption ability in both water and hydroxyapatite. This helps thermal effect on surrounding tissue. Er:YAG laser can ablate soft tissue with minimal coagulation and without carbonization. In addition, with water coolant, this laser is able to ablate hard tissue effectively.
  - This is the only FDA-approved laser for hard tissue procedure including osteotomy, osseous crown lengthening, and osteoplasty. Other indications include intraoral soft tissue surgery, aphthous ulcer treatment, sulcular debridement, and subgingival calculus removal.

10.4 Applications of Lasers in Periodontal Therapy

The employment of lasers in periodontal surgery is sustained by multiple potential indications and advantages (Table 10.2) when compared to traditional instrumentation. Depending on the charac-

Table 10.2 Advantages of using lasers in periodontal therapy

• Tissue ablation or vaporization
• Hemostasis
• Microbial inhibition and destruction
• Biological effect from biostimulation (photobiomodulation)
• Enhance wound healing
• Better access to narrow furcations and/or deep infrabony defects
• Alleviate patients' physical and mental stress and pain

Table 10.3 Limitations associated with the use of lasers for different periodontal therapies

• Treatment outcomes comparable to conventional therapies
• Lack of tactile sensitivity
• Limited visualization (nonsurgical therapy)
• More time-consuming
• Thermal damage
• Excessive ablation/thermal coagulation
• Carbonization/necrosis of the root, connective tissue, bone, pulp

teristics of the lasers, these devices can be used for multiple procedures including soft tissue incisions, ablation, and coagulation; treatment of aphthous ulcers; laser-assisted new attachment procedure (LANAP); subgingival curettage and sulcular debridement; disinfection of periodontal pockets; calculus removal; bone removal and recontouring; as well as a method for coagulation [6, 8, 9].

Lasers can provide additional benefits to conventional treatment modalities in several aspects. First, Laser therapy was shown to increase patient acceptance according to patient-reported outcomes (PRO). Similarly, their ability for tissue ablation and/or vaporization makes lasers to be a potential alternative to scalpel use. A laser can also provide with coagulation effect leading to hemostasis and better visualization during the procedure. Its photothermal effect results in microbial inhibition and destruction, thus creating a disinfected field during surgery, decreasing risk of infection, and promoting new tissue attachment. Most importantly, its photobiomodulation properties can provide biological effect to enhance wound healing [8, 9].

Although presenting with numerous advantages, the use of lasers could also lead to potential drawbacks and/or limitations, especially with high-energy-level lasers (Table 10.3). Irreversible thermal damage, excessive ablation and/or thermal coagulation, carbonization or necrosis of the root, the gingival tissue, the bone, and the pulp tissues represent some of the potential side effects of laser usage [10]. Therefore, the selection of proper laser type for the intented procedure is of paramount importance.

10.4.1 Treatment of Periodontal Diseases

10.4.1.1 Introduction to Gingivitis and Periodontitis

Gingivitis and periodontitis are both inflammatory conditions of the attachment apparatus surrounding the teeth. Gingivitis always precedes periodontitis and is characterized by soft tissue inflammation often including redness and swelling of the gingival tissues as well as tendency to bleed. On the contrary, periodontitis is defined by an initial inflammatory status of the periodontium which progresses to destruction of the alveolar bone. Although different forms of periodontitis could be described, all types share similar characteristics mainly determined by the presence of inflammation, bacterial plaque, and bone resorption. If left untreated, the progression of this chronic inflammatory condition will ultimately compromise the stability of the dentition leading to tooth loss.

10.4.1.2 Nonsurgical Therapy

Nonsurgical periodontal treatment targets the removal of the main etiologic agent responsible for periodontal disease, bacterial plaque. This nonsurgical therapy is performed through the supra- and sub- gingival instrumentation of the dental surfaces aiming at the complete elimination of both plaque and calculus attached to the tooth (Fig. 10.1). Different tools and devices have been used for this purpose including but not limited to curettes, files, hoes, sickles, chisels, burr, and lasers. While the removal of the etiologic

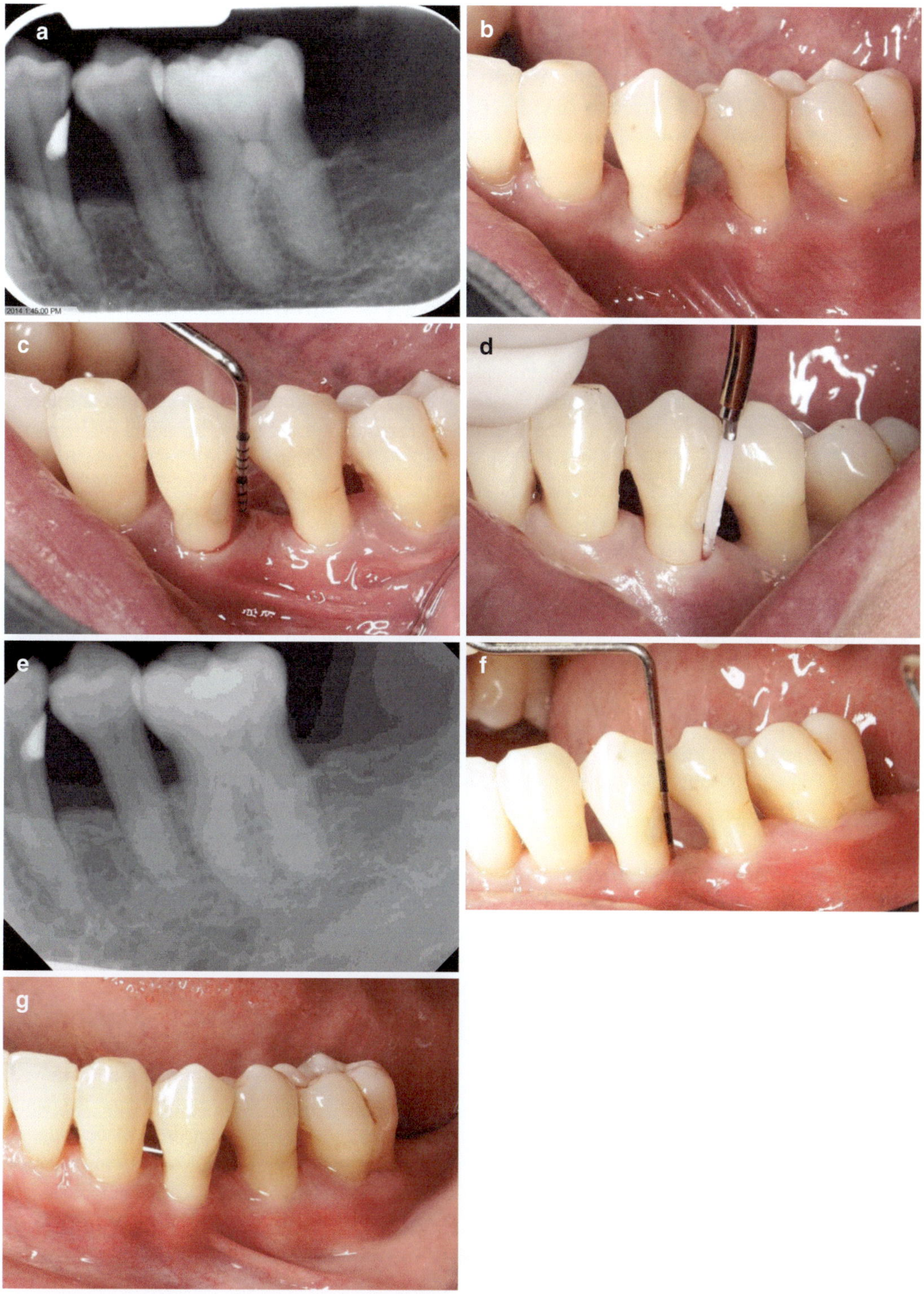

Fig. 10.1 Er:YAG laser in combination with scaling and root planing for treatment of chronic periodontitis on left posterior mandibular sextant. (**a**) Baseline radiograph. (**b**) Baseline clinical appearance. (**c**) Initial presentation demonstrating 6 mm PD and BOP. (**d**) Adjunctive use of laser therapy. (**e**) Radiograph at 9 months. (**f**) Final presentation at 9 months demonstrating reduced PD and no BOP. (**g**) 18 months follow-up

agents is of paramount importance for disease resolution, the method of bacterial decontamination seems not to play a significant role. As such, laser therapy has failed to demonstrate any significant benefit compared to conventional mechanical instrumentation.

During initial periodontal treatment, the laser can facilitate bacterial elimination and removal of inflamed tissues [11]. Nd:YAG laser was proposed to be used for removal of pocket epithelium during laser-assisted new attachment procedure (LANAP) [12]. Steps included in this procedure are measurement of pockets, removal of the inner pocket epithelial lining with laser, scaling and root planing, laser application again to allow for a stable fibrin clot formation, tissue readaptation, and finally occlusal adjustment. It has been demonstrated that the LANAP-treated teeth had greater mean probing pocket depth (PPD) reduction (4.7 mm vs. 3.7 mm) and greater clinical probing attachment level gain (4.2 mm vs. 2.4 mm) compared to the control teeth. All six LANAP-treated teeth showed new cementum and connective tissue attachment at 3 months postoperatively. These results were also in agreement with a recent study [13]. Although LANAP seems to provide favorable results, due to the small sample size investigated, no clinical significant difference was found.

Systematic reviews and meta-analysis demonstrated similar clinical attachment gain with the use of Er:YAG laser in combination with scaling and root planing, compated with scaling and root planing alone for treatment of chronic periodontitis. Similarly, When comparing the use of laser alone with scaling and root planing, inconclusive results were found at 6- and 12-month follow-ups [14]. Even though Er:YAG laser shows great potential for root debridement, there is insufficient evidence supporting the superior outcomes of lasers in nonsurgical periodontal treatment when compared to scaling and root planing alone [6, 15], p. 200 [16].

Another technique that can be used for antimicrobial purposes is photodynamic therapy. It is mainly composed of visible harmless light or lower-level laser and photosensitizer that aim to target specific bacteria without damaging the host tissue. Once the photosensitizer is activated, it produces high reactive state of oxygen that damages bacterial cell wall and cell membrane [8, 9, 11, 17]. This approach helps avoiding bacterial resistance compared to the use of chemotherapeutic agents. It is also shown to reduce periodontal pathogen by more than 95% in vitro, yet clinical outcomes are comparable to conventional treatment [17].

10.4.1.3 Surgical Therapy

Lasers can also be used as an adjunct to periodontal surgical therapy. Their small and various tip designs allow lasers to gain better access to narrow and/or deep infrabony defects as well as furcations with minimal tissue damage (Fig. 10.2). Additionally, the photobiomodulation effect may help promote wound healing and tissue regeneration [8, 9].

In deep pockets (>7 mm), the use of CO_2 laser with a coronally advanced flap showed more probing depth reduction and clinical attachment gain in comparison with a Modified Widman flap procedure. This result was stable over 15-year follow-up [18]. Currently, Er:YAG laser has been shown to be most effective for periodontal flap surgery as an alternative or adjunct to conventional therapy [8, 9]. However, there is still limited evidence showing significant advantages of this laser over conventional surgical approaches.

10.4.1.4 Regenerative Therapy

The field of periodontology could not be described today without mentioning the use of regenerative procedures. By means of grafting materials and barrier membranes, the reconstruction of the lost structures of the periodontium can be achieved. These regenerative procedures share the same principles that apply to nonsurgical periodontal therapy in which removal of the etiologic agent/agents is imperative for successful outcomes.

The use of lasers in regenerative procedures is mainly performed for root biomodification purposes. As mentioned previously, the antibacterial property of laser is beneficial in disinfecting the area. Moreover, the ability to remove the smear layer may also help promoting new tissue attachment on the root surface.

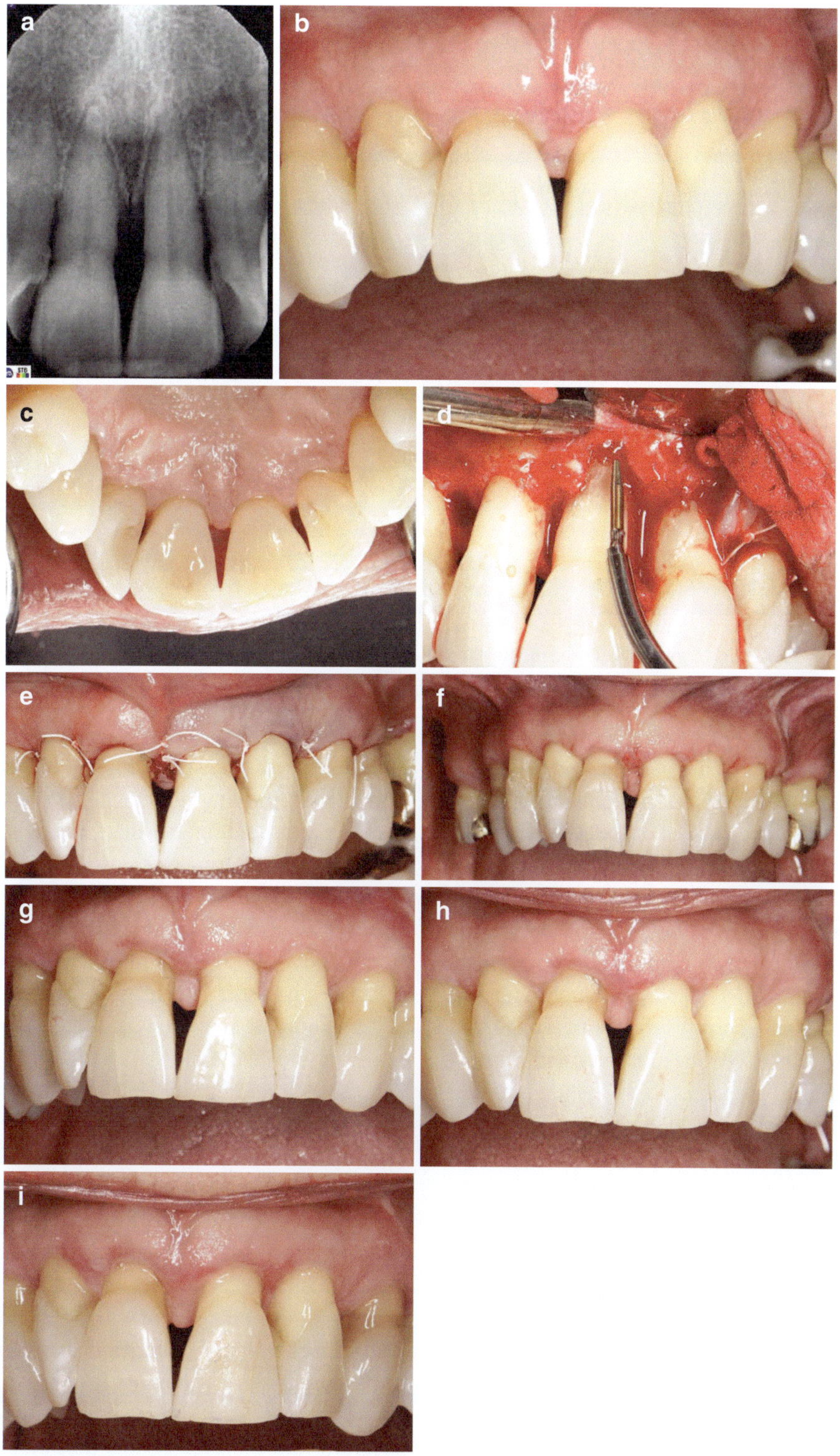

Fig. 10.2 (**a**) Baseline radiograph. (**b**) Baseline clinical appearance. (**c**) Baseline clinical appearance. (**d**) Bony architecture. (**e**) Flap closure. (**f**) Two weeks follow-up. (**g**) Six weeks follow-up. (**h**) Four months follow-up. (**i**) Twelve months follow-up

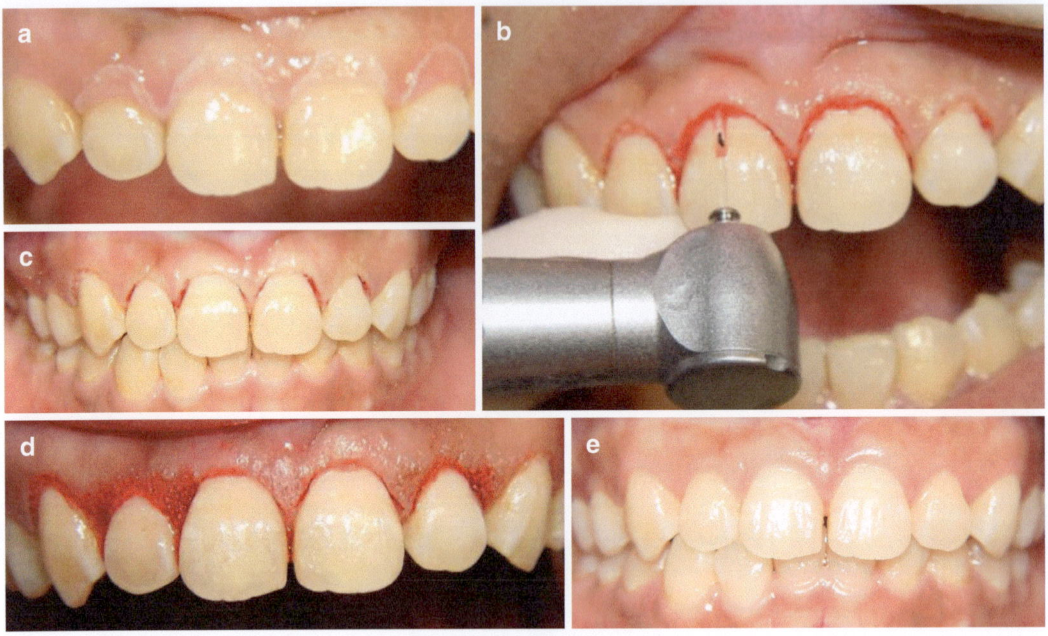

Fig. 10.3 (**a**) Preoperative view. (**b**) Laser therapy for tissue removal. (**c**) Postoperative view. (**d**) Early healing. (**e**) Final outcome

Yukna et al. were among the first to describe the benefit of LANAP for periodontal regeneration histologically. Two out of six LANAP-treated teeth exhibited new connective tissue attachment and new cementum within the intrabony defects next to new alveolar bone [12]. Later, Nd:YAG laser was evaluated in conjunction with enamel matrix proteins (EMP) and compared with EMP and EDTA alone (control) for the treatment of 42 intrabony defects. The results revealed improvement in clinical outcomes for both therapies without addition benefit of Nd:YAG over EDTA [19]. To date, there is still insufficient evidence to support the effectiveness of lasers as an adjunct to either resective or regenerative surgical periodontal therapy [20, 21].

10.4.2 Soft Tissue Applications

The correction of mucogingival deformities represents an integral part of periodontal therapy. Through the employment of different surgical techniques, soft tissue irregularities such as recession defects or excessive gingival display can be corrected improving function and esthetics while ultimately providing the dentition with a more favorable long-term prognosis. In this sense, lasers can be applied in different soft tissue applications such as crown lengthening (Fig. 10.3), frenectomy, biopsies (Fig. 10.4), removal of tumors, and soft tissue grafting procedures. When compared to conventional instrumentation, some of the major advantages of lasers for soft tissue surgeries are relatively easier ablation, hemostatic, and bactericidal effects, among others. In addition, lasers can often reduce bleeding, pain, and the need for suturing.

CO_2, Nd:YAG, and Er:YAG lasers have been approved by FDA for intraoral soft tissue procedures. Nd:YAG lasers have demonstrated good outcomes with depigmentation procedures as they have high ability to target melanin and dark pigments [8, 9]. However, it should be used carefully due to the high tissue ablation and thermal effects that may increase the risk of gingival recession and ulcerations in the thin gingiva area [22].

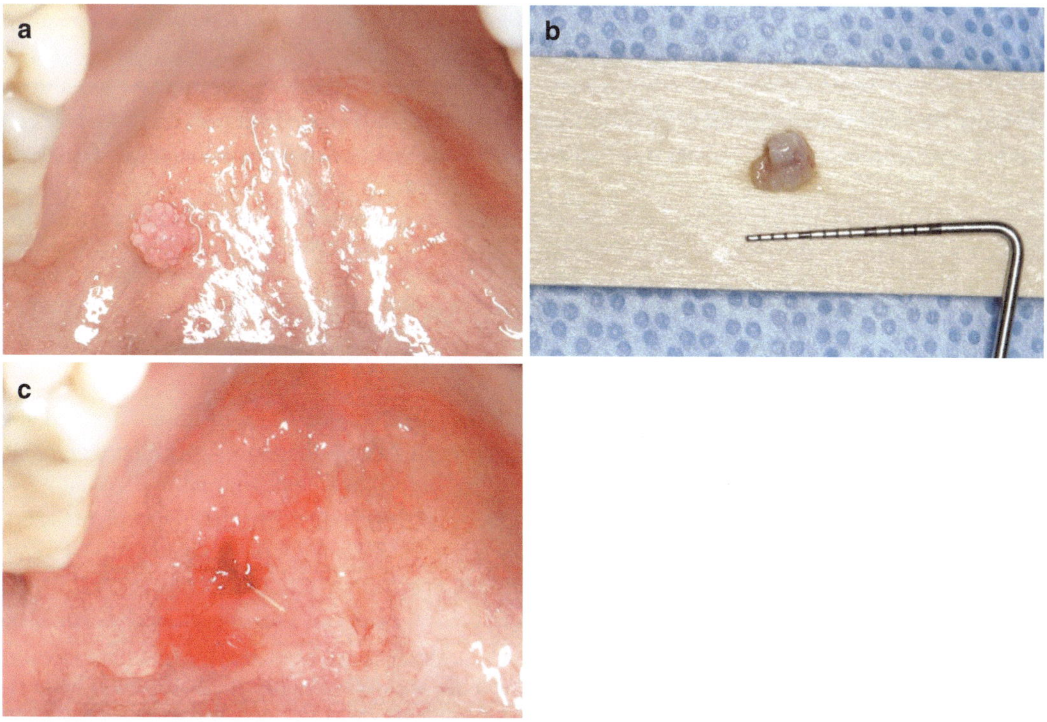

Fig. 10.4 (**a**) Initial clinical appearance. (**b**) Lesion after removal from palate. (**c**) Final postoperative view of the palate

Clinical studies have been conducted in order to evaluate the effects of lasers in root coverage procedures. The comparisons between subepithelial connective tissue graft and coronally advanced flap with or without Er:YAG or Nd:YAG were carried out. Results from these studies showed that Er:YAG laser did not enhance the outcomes of root coverage procedures [23]. Interestingly, Nd:YAG laser significantly decreased the percentage of root coverage from 77% to 33%. Percentage of complete root coverage also decreased from 65% to 18% [24]. On the other hand, a recent study demonstrated an increase in percentage of root coverage when using diode laser (660 nm) in combination to subepithelial connective tissue graft with coronally advanced flap after 6 months [25]. Thus, the use of lasers in soft tissue procedures for the treatment of gingival recessions may provide additional benefits related to root coverage. Nonetheless, less favorable outcomes appeared with the use of Nd:YAG laser [26].

10.4.3 Hard Tissue Indications

The removal of calculus and the reshaping of the alveolar bone represent the two of the main applications for laser therapy in the periodontal field. In addition, lasers have also been used for the treatment of dentinal hypersensitivity.

10.4.3.1 Calculus Removal

A suitable wavelength laser should be selected in order to remove calculus without damaging tooth surfaces. Typically, erbium lasers (Er:YAG and Er,Cr:YSGG) are capable of this purpose due to their high water and hydroxyapatite absorption [6]. They react to water within micropores and intrinsic component in calculus. This has been shown to be able to remove the smear layer and endotoxins resulting in root surface modification which promotes fibroblast attachment [8, 9]. Currently, Er:YAG laser can be used as an adunct to mechanical instrumentation for pocket reduction. However, there is no major additional benefits when compared to the conventional therapy. In addition, there are several limitations such as accessibility and lack of tactile sensation with the use of lasers.

10.4.3.2 Osseous Surgery

Er:YAG is the only type of laser that can be used in osseous tissue, according to the FDA. It has been shown to safely and effectively remove granulation tissue in osseous defects during periodontal surgery, unlike CO_2 and Nd:YAG lasers which produced carbonized surface that is toxic to cell proliferation and attachment. The use of Er:YAG laser demonstrated a significant improvement in clinical parameters after 6 months following treatment of intrabony defects [27]. It is also believed that the photobiomodulation effect of lasers such as bactericidal and detoxification can enhance wound healing and promote tissue regeneration. However, clinical evidence with this regard is still lacking.

Several drawbacks are found with laser-assisted osseous surgery. Weak bone remodeling between lased bone and new bone was noted in a histological study demonstrating that it may compromise the longevity of bone integration [28]. Delayed healing can also occur with thermal damage. Thus, profuse irrigation is important along with the use of lasers [29].

10.4.3.3 Dentinal Hypersensitivity

Dentinal hypersensitivity is a common phenomenon caused by exposure of the dentin. Lasers can be considered as an alternative treatment for this condition. One of the possible mechanisms for the favorable outcomes observed after laser application is the hyperactivation of cellular metabolism in odontoblasts leading to tertiary dentine production which ultimately blocks dentinal tubules. Another reason may be that the laser creates neural analgesia blocking pain transmission by depolarized C afferent fibers and reducing cell membrane action potential. Lastly, it can also be used as a placebo [7]. A recent study demonstrated the effectiveness of low-level laser therapy in reducing postoperative pain and hypersensitivity 7 days after periodontal surgery [30]. A novel low-level laser toothbrush was also investigated and showed to reduced dentinal hypersensitivity compared to Sensodyne toothbrush [31]. Yet, the effectiveness of lasers in reducing dentin hypersensitivity remains controversial [7].

10.5 Current Status

Today, laser therapy can be safely applied for nonsurgical periodontal treatment, hard and soft tissue procedures, and dentinal hypersensitivity. However, the long-term effectiveness of lasers when used in combintation to conventional treatment approaches remains controversial. There is limited evidence showing clinical benefits of Nd:YAG and Er:YAG lasers as an adjunct to scaling and root planing [6, 14] as well as periodontal surgery [20]. It may be recommended in the areas that do not respond to conventional therapy or medically compromised patients who are not candidates for periodontal surgery. Additionally, it can be proposed as an alternative

Table 10.4 Summary of laser evidence for periodontal therapies

Procedures	Evidence
Nonsurgical periodontal treatment	Limited evidence to support the superiority of lasers alone or in combination to scaling and root planing
Surgical periodontal treatment	Limited evidence supporting the clinical benefit of lasers as an adjunct to resective or regenerative procedures
Soft tissue surgery	
• Depigmentation	lasers can provide satisfactory outcomes
• Root coverage	Lack of evidence showing additional benefit to conventional root coverage outcomes Nd:YAG may impair root coverage outcomes
Desensitizer	The effectiveness of laser is still controversial

treatment option for higher patient acceptance. Table 10.4 summarizes the current understanding for the application of lasers in periodontal therapy. New randomized controlled studies with larger population and longer follow-up would be necessary to confirm the potential superior benefits of lasers.

10.6 Conclusions

Laser therapy has multitude of clinical applications for the different aspects of periodontal therapy. As such, these devices can successfully replace and/or serve as an adjunct to conventional instruments in a great variety of procedures including but not limited to soft tissue grafting, crown lengthening, tumor removal, and osseous surgery. However, no significant benefits could be expected with regard to long-term outcomes after the utilization of lasers when compared to traditional instrumentation [32]. On the other hand, Laser therapy for periodontal surgery can provide with clinical advantages including hemostatic effect and reduced bleeding, reduced need for suturing, shorter operative time, and bacterial decontamination. The comprehensive understanding of the characteristics and indications of each particular laser is of paramount importance since their effect will significantly vary depending on their properties.

References

1. Periodontology TAAO. Glossary of periodontal terms. 4th Edition. 2001.
2. Maiman T. Stimulated optical radiation in ruby. Nature. 1960;187:493–4.
3. Goldman L, Hornby P, Meyer R, Goldman B. Impact of the Laser on Dental Caries. Nature. 1964;203:417.
4. Stern RH, Sognnaes RF. Laser inhibition of dental caries suggested by first tests in vivo. J Am Dent Assoc. 1972;85(5):1087–90.
5. Myers TD. What lasers can do for dentistry and you. Dent Manage. 1989;29(4):26–8. 30
6. Cobb CM. Lasers in periodontics: a review of the literature. J Periodontol. 2006;77(4):545–64.
7. Passanezi E, Damante CA, de Rezende ML, Greghi SL. Lasers in periodontal therapy. Periodontol. 2015;67(1):268–91.
8. Aoki A, Mizutani K, Schwarz F, Sculean A, Yukna RA, Takasaki AA, Romanos GE, Taniguchi Y, Sasaki KM, Zeredo JL, Koshy G, Coluzzi DJ, White JM, Abiko Y, Ishikawa I, Izumi Y. Periodontal and peri-implant wound healing following laser therapy. Periodontol. 2015;68(1):217–69.
9. Aoki A, Mizutani K, Schwarz F, Sculean A, Yukna RA, Takasaki AA, et al. Periodontal and peri-implant wound healing following laser therapy. Periodontol. 2015;2000(68):217–69.
10. Takasaki AA, Aoki A, Mizutani K, Schwarz F, Sculean A, Wang C-Y, et al. Application of antimicrobial photodynamic therapy in periodontal and peri-implant diseases. Periodontol. 2009;2000(51):109–40.
11. Mizutani K, Aoki A, Coluzzi D, Yukna R, Wang C-Y, Pavlic V, et al. Lasers in minimally invasive periodontal and peri-implant therapy. Periodontol. 2016;2000(71):185–212.
12. Yukna RA, Carr RL, Evans GH. Histologic evaluation of an Nd:YAG laser-assisted new attachment procedure in humans. Int J Periodontics Restorative Dent. 2007;27:576–87.
13. Nevins M, Kim S-W, Camelo M, Sanz Martin I, Kim D, Nevins M. A prospective 9-month human clinical evaluation of laser-assisted new attachment procedure (LANAP) therapy. Int J Periodontics Restorative Dent. 2014;34:21–7.
14. Zhao Y, Yin Y, Tao L, Nie P, Tang Y, Zhu M. Er:YAG laser versus scaling and root planing as alternative or adjuvant for chronic periodontitis treatment: a systematic review. J Clin Periodontol. 2014;41:1069–79.
15. Sanz M, Teughels W, on behalf of group A of the European Workshop on Periodontology. Innovations in non-surgical periodontal therapy: consensus report of the sixth european workshop on periodontology. J Clin Periodontol. 2008;35:3–7.
16. Cobb CM. Commentary: is there clinical benefit from using a diode or Neodymium:Yttrium-Aluminum-Garnet laser in the treatment of periodontitis? J Periodontol. 2016;87:1117–31.
17. Raghavendra M, Koregol A, Bhola S. Photodynamic therapy: a targeted therapy in periodontics. Aust Dent J. 2009;54:S102–9.
18. Crespi R, Capparè P, Gherlone E, Romanos GE. Comparison of modified Widman and Coronally advanced flap surgery combined with Co2 laser root irradiation in periodontal therapy: a 15-year follow-up. Int J Periodontics Restorative Dent. 2011;31:640–51.
19. Dilsiz A, Canakci V, Aydin T. The combined use of Nd:YAG laser and enamel matrix proteins in the treatment of periodontal infrabony defects. J Periodontol. 2010;81:1411–8.
20. Behdin S, Monje A, Lin G-H, Edwards B, Othman A, Wang H-L. Effectiveness of laser application for periodontal surgical therapy: systematic review and meta-analysis. J Periodontol. 2015;86:1352–63.
21. Cochran DL, Cobb CM, Bashutski JD, Chun Y-HP, Lin Z, Mandelaris GA, et al. Emerging regenerative approaches for periodontal reconstruction: a consen-

sus report from the AAP regeneration workshop. J Periodontol. 2014;86:S153–6.
22. Atsawasuwan P, Greethong K, Nimmanon V. Treatment of gingival hyperpigmentation for esthetic purposes by Nd:YAG laser: report of 4 cases. J Periodontol. 2000;71:315–21.
23. Dilsiz A, Aydin T, Yavuz MS. Root surface biomodification with an Er:YAG laser for the treatment of gingival recession with subepithelial connective tissue grafts. Photomed Laser Surg. 2010;28:511–7.
24. Dilsiz A, Aydin T, Canakci V, Cicek Y. Root surface biomodification with Nd:YAG laser for the treatment of gingival recession with subepithelial connective tissue grafts. Photomed Laser Surg. 2010;28:337–43.
25. Fernandes-Dias SB, de Marco AC, Santamaria M, Kerbauy WD, Jardini MAN, Santamaria MP. Connective tissue graft associated or not with low laser therapy to treat gingival recession: randomized clinical trial. J Clin Periodontol. 2015;42:54–61.
26. Karam PSBH, Sant'Ana ACP, de Rezende MLR, Greghi SLA, Damante CA, Zangrando MSR. Root surface modifiers and subepithelial connective tissue graft for treatment of gingival recessions: a systematic review. J Periodontal Res. 2016;51:175–85.
27. Sculean A, Schwarz F, Berakdar M, Windisch P, Arweiler NB, Romanos GE. Healing of intrabony defects following surgical treatment with or without an Er:YAG laser. J Clin Periodontol. 2004;31:604–8.
28. Yoshino T, Aoki A, Oda S, Takasaki AA, Mizutani K, Sasaki KM, et al. Long-term histologic analysis of bone tissue alteration and healing following Er:YAG laser irradiation compared to electrosurgery. J Periodontol. 2008;80:82–92.
29. Nelson JS, Orenstein A, Liaw L-HL, Berns MW. Mid-infrared erbium:YAG laser ablation of bone: The effect of laser osteotomy on bone healing. Lasers Surg Med. 1989;9:362–74.
30. Doshi S, Jain S, Hegde R. Effect of low-level laser therapy in reducing dentinal hypersensitivity and pain following periodontal flap surgery. Photomed Laser Surg. 2014;32:700–6.
31. Yaghini J, Mogharehabed A, Safavi N, Mohamadi M, Ashtiju F. Evaluation of the effect of low level laser therapy toothbrush in treatment of dentin hypersensitivity. J Lasers Med Sci. 2015;6:85–91.
32. American Academy of Periodontology Statement. Efficacy of lasers in the non-surgical treatment of inflammatory periodontal disease. J Periodontol. 2011;82:513–4.

Laser-Assisted Therapy for Peri-implant Diseases

11

Jeff CW. Wang and Hom-Lay Wang

Contents

Abstract

Peri-implant disease is a new prevalent biological complication emerged from the popularity of implant therapy. Currently, there is no predictable treatment to manage advanced peri-implantitis lesions. Dental laser has a huge potential for the treatment of peri-implant disease, given that it provides a method to decontaminate implant surface without damaging its microstructures for re-osseointegration. In addition, biosimulation from low-energy laser attenuates the inflammatory status of the peri-implant defect to facilitate re-establishment of homeostasis. There are several wavelengths of dental laser available. Both Nd:YAG and Er:YAG lasers have shown promising results in vitro, and erbium lasers seem to be the most promising one due to its application on hard tissues. Although a few pilot randomized clinical trials did not show conclusive results, more well-designed controlled trials are warranted to optimize the application of laser-assisted therapy in identifying ideal indications and developing evidence-based protocol.

Keywords

Laser · Treatment · Peri-mucositis
Peri-implantitis

J. CW. Wang · H.-L. Wang (✉)
Department of Periodontics and Oral Medicine,
University of Michigan School of Dentistry,
Ann Arbor, MI, USA
e-mail: jeffwa@umich.edu; homlay@umich.edu

S. Stübinger et al. (eds.), *Lasers in Oral and Maxillofacial Surgery*,
https://doi.org/10.1007/978-3-030-29604-9_11

11.1 Introduction

The use of laser technology in dentistry has gained popularity since its first introduction half century ago. The indications and applications for laser therapy have also expanded, including stand-alone monotherapy or as an adjunctive aid. There are various laser devices with specific wavelengths and advantages that target different tissue types. Practitioners must learn the basic principles and characteristics of laser therapy in order to select the ideal laser device and settings for their practice or treatment procedures. For instance, peri-implant diseases are emerging serious complications and a major concern in modern dentistry that leads to tissue destruction, inflammation with pocketing, and disintegration of dental implants. Given that the traditional mechanical debridement did not provide predictable results, the utilization of laser therapy for the treatment of peri-implant diseases has therefore become the focus of recent clinical applications and researches. Although several in vitro and in vivo studies have shown favorable results with the use of laser therapy, preliminary clinical studies showed inconclusive results. Despite further well-controlled clinical studies are warranted to fully evaluate the efficacy of laser therapy, the benefits of hemostasis, enhanced healing, patient comfort, and possible positive outcomes have already been recognized by the clinicians. This chapter reviews the characteristics of laser therapy, especially for the treatment of peri-implant diseases. Existing nonsurgical and surgical treatment protocols are also compared together with their expected outcome for clinical implications.

11.2 Physics of Laser

Laser, which stands for light amplification by stimulated emission of radiation, is a medical device that delivers energy to a target. There are different media inside the laser that exert the energy, which can be gas, solid, or semiconductor. There are different mechanisms to excite the active medium to go through optical resonator for amplification, but it is the medium that determines the type of laser, which includes:

Gas: Carbon dioxide (CO_2) and argon

Solid: Neodymium-doped yttrium-aluminum-garnet (Nd:YAG)

- Erbium-doped yttrium aluminum garnet laser (Er:YAG)
- Erbium chromium-doped yttrium-scandium-gallium-garnet
- (Er, Cr:YSGG)

Semiconductor: Diodes

Generally, laser wavelengths are medium specific and cannot be changed. The most common range of wavelengths used in periodontics and implantology spans from 400 to 10,600 nm. This range includes both the invisible and visible electromagnetic spectra. The wavelength of a specific laser determines its unique characteristic and application. Studies have used different lasers for the treatment of peri-implant diseases, and thus the results should not be compared directly and data interpreted with caution.

11.2.1 Characteristics of Laser Therapy

The most common types of laser currently on the marker are listed in Table 11.1 describing some basic characteristics. Diode laser exerts the shortest wavelength (810–980 nm), and CO_2 has the longest ones (9600/10,600). Only CO_2 laser is a noncontact type of laser; the others are all contact type. When laser energy reached the tissue surface, the energy can be absorbed, or it can be reflected, scattered, or passed through the tissue without any effect (transmission).

Different substances or tissues have their efficiency in terms of resorption for various lasers (absorption of coefficient), and therefore therapeutic laser usually would target certain tissue; these include epithelium, water, bacteria, blood, pigmentation, bone, dentin, and enamel. The performance of a laser is determined by the degree of absorption from these chromophores. In these living tissues, the main components that influ-

Table 11.1 Characteristics of different laser types

Laser	Wavelength (nm)	Contact type	Penetration	Tissue-type ablation
CO_2	9600/10,600	Noncontact	Superficial	Soft only
Er:YAG	2940	Contact	Superficial	Hard + soft
Er, Cr:YSGG	2780	Contact	Superficial	Hard + soft
Nd:YAG	1064	Contact	Deep	Soft only
Diodes	810/940/980	Contact	Deep	Soft only

Table 11.2 Different effects of laser–tissue interactions

Photothermal effect	Thermomechanical effects	Biostimulation (photobiomodulation)
Light energy is converted into heat	Water molecules vaporized provoking "micro-explosions" that break the tissue	Low-level laser energy scattered from high-level energy that stimulatesphotochemical reactions
Evaporate soft tissues Kill bacteria Inactivate toxins Thermal denaturation Hemostasis	Hard tissue ablation	Reduce inflammation Promote wound healing Stimulate cells/tissues

ence the absorption are the presence of free water, proteins, pigments, and inorganic components (such as apatite). Simplified absorption spectra for each laser can be categorized into two groups: CO_2 and erbium (mainly water and hydroxyapatite) and Nd:YAG and CO_2 (pigmentation, hemoglobin, and melanin) (for full absorption coefficient curve, see [1]).

The penetration depth is an important characteristic for laser. It indicates the laser energy scattering deep into the tissue after penetration. Interestingly, the depth of the absorption is strongly associated with the absorption coefficient in water [2, 3]. The lower the absorption coefficient rate in water, the laser exerts deeper penetration. Therefore, the deep penetrating types of lasers are diode and Nd:YAG lasers, whereas the superficially absorbed types of lasers are CO_2 and erbium laser (high absorption in water). The absorption of energy by the water may also minimize collateral thermal effect to the adjacent tissues during irradiation.

When the laser energy reaches human tissue, there will be three main interactions occurring at the same time (see Table 11.2). It selectively vaporizes components of human tissue through photothermal effects. The energy of the laser is converted to heat absorbed by the tissue and directly evaporates itself ablating the soft tissue for cutting. There is also secondary thermal effect from the heated laser tip that can incise soft tissue, but it is a result of contact with the overheated tip rather than by the laser energy itself [4].

As for hard tissue ablation, it is thought to occur as a result of thermal-mechanical effects following photothermal interactions [5, 6]. The erbium laser seems to be the only laser that can effectively apply to hard tissue. During the hard tissue ablation process, water molecules within the hard tissue are vaporized after absorbing the energy and increasing pressure that provokes "micro-explosions." These water micro-explosions can cause mechanical breakdown of the hard tissues leaving a microstructured appearance with minimal thermal alteration [7–9]. The water micro-explosion is believed to play a major role in dental implant surface decontamination, especially over exposed implant surface within infrabony defects where undercut surface is expected under the threads. However, it is also important to preserve the microstructure of the dental implant after surface decontamination to allow re-osseointegration. Both Nd:YAG and Er:YAG lasers have shown promising results in vitro for implant surface decontamination [10, 11].

The most intriguing part of the laser–tissue interaction is the biostimulation or the photobiomodulation of the adjacent tissues. When high-level energy scatters into low-level energy, it may stimulate photochemical reactions within the cell and tissue without irreversible changes. It is also a concurrent and desired effect [12]. Although the detailed mechanism is still not clear, several clinical benefits are believed to be a result of bio-stimulation, including promoting wound healing [13–15], reduction of inflammation [16], and pain relief [13, 17]. Using laser to debride defect around the periodontal or peri-implant defect may also exert positive effect on regenerative therapy, which will be discussed in later sections.

Taken together, the effects of laser energy are diverse and synergized if used correctly. Laser therapy shows promising aid in wound healing, tissue ablation, bacterial reduction, epithelial ablation, connective tissue remodeling, bone metabolism, hemorrhage, and pain control.

11.2.2 Definition and Prevalence of Peri-implant Diseases

Peri-implant diseases constitute both peri-mucositis and peri-implantitis. The term *peri-implantitis* was first introduced almost 30 years ago [18] and then had the first definition in the 1990s [19] to describe an inflammatory progress that results in progressive bone loss around a dental implant. Contrary to peri-implantitis, peri-mucositis is a reversible inflammatory disease that does not cause bone loss beyond initial bone remodeling around the implant. It is similar to the definition of gingivitis and periodontitis around natural dentition. While the definition of peri-mucositis maintains the same, the definition of peri-implantitis kept evolving. Most recent consensus report from the American Academy of Periodontology [20] emphasizes that bone loss should be beyond the biological bone remodeling. However, the biological bone remodeling has yet to be determined and most likely varies among individuals, especially when peri-implant soft tissue thickness may play an important role in the initial bone remodeling process to determine the biological width around the dental implant [21]. Despite how much bone loss defines peri-implantitis, its rapid progressive bone loss associated with inflammation is well recognized as a serious concern following the popularity of dental implant therapy.

Peri-implantitis is an emerging new disease with a prevalence ranging from 7.1% up to 58% [22, 23] averaging 22% in a recent systematic review [24]. Although early stage mucositis may be controlled nonsurgically, established peri-implantitis lesions are still a challenge to manage due to the unpredictable results [25]. Before discussing about the treatment for peri-implant diseases and the role of laser therapy, it is prudent to understand the etiology of peri-implant diseases and recognize each contributing factor that needs to be addressed all together.

11.2.3 Main Etiologic Factors Associated with Peri-implant Diseases

The etiology of peri-implantitis is still an active quest for investigation. Although it was demonstrated that the main etiology to initiate peri-mucositis is the bacterial plaque [26–28], it is still unknown which individual will continue to develop bone loss around implants and constitutes peri-implantitis. Several other local and systemic host-related factors are emerging as important drivers and pathogenesis of the disease [20, 29, 30] (Table 11.3). Especially, the inflammatory response from the host immune system should also be considered as part of the main etiologic factor that determines the level of tissue destruction accumulated from various local stimuli. Each individual has their unique immune response that reacts differently to various local

Table 11.3 Potential local and systemic factors for peri-implantitis

Local factors	Systemic factors
1. Bacterial plaque	1. Genetic predisposition
2. Malpositioned implant	2. Past/active periodontal disease
3. Residual cement	3. Smoking
4. Poor prosthetic design	4. Uncontrolled diabetes
5. Peri-implant tissue quality	5. Osteoporosis?
6. Trauma from occlusion	6. Alcohol consumption?
7. Titanium particles?	7. Compromised conditions

factors. It is the same as the periodontal disease, as the response to the bacteria is a spectrum similar to normal distribution; there is about 10% of the population immune to bacterial plaque without developing periodontal disease [31]. Therefore, it is naive to believe that bacteria are the only cause of the peri-implant diseases. It is crucial to appreciate that peri-implant diseases are multifactorial and that all the contributing factors should be examined carefully as part of the diagnosis for treatment. Some critical iatrogenic factors, including malpositioning of the dental implants [32], residual cement [33, 34], poor prosthetic design, and occlusal trauma [35], should all be addressed as part of the treatment. Laser therapy cannot treat those factors, and sometimes implant will need to be removed if certain critical factor cannot be managed (e.g., malpositioned implant).

Therefore, before using the laser, the clinician must recognize if there are other factors that need to be addressed, including active periodontal disease, smoking, diabetes, or any systemic conditions that compromise the immune system [36, 37]. A prognosis system was developed considering whether all the other factors can be addressed or not. If all the factors can be addressed, the prognosis of the implant can be considered favorable; should there be some uncertainty, it will give questionable or unfavorable prognosis [38]. For the laser therapy, it can potentially both target bacteria decontamination over implant surface and biomodulate the host inflammatory response around the defect. The following paragraph will discuss the rationale and benefits of using laser as an adjunctive tool for treating the peri-implant diseases.

11.2.4 Why Can Laser Assist in the Treatment of Peri-implant Diseases

11.2.4.1 Implant Surface Detoxification with Laser Therapy

It was hypothesized that the main challenges in treating peri-implant diseases are from detoxification of the exposed contaminated dental implant surface. The conventional mechanical debridement with hand instrument may not be able to thoroughly scale the microstructure of the surface, whereas using rotary instruments may result in damaging the surface texture and compromising the re-osseointegration. Studies have evaluated the effectiveness of different methods for implant surface decontamination [39]. Among the available approaches for decontamination, laser therapy has been proven to reduce bacterial load [40–42] without damaging the implant surface (Nd:YAG and Er:YAG laser) [10, 11]. The notion that Nd:YAG can target pigmented pathogen (e.g., *Porphyromonas gingivalis*) may warrant further investigation as it may still present with relative abundance in peri-implantitis lesions [43]; however, its potential tendency in damaging implant surface even with lower energy power may require precaution [44]. Laser therapy not only can kill or devitalize the bacteria but also ablate or inactivate toxic substances, such as endotoxins [45, 46]. Therefore, together with the abovementioned micro-explosions, those characteristics of laser therapy make it a promising and effective way to detoxify implant surface.

However, given the limited clinical studies so far, it was difficult to assess if the goal of "surface decontamination" is achieved or not clinically and if it has an impact over the clinical outcome [47]. In animal models, there are several studies showing that with the Er:YAG laser treatment in preparation for bone grafting procedure, there is an increased regenerated bone-to-implant contact for a better regenerative outcome [48, 49]. Therefore, it may be more reasonable to assess the clinical attachment gain or radiographic bone fill over the specific defect site to indirectly assess the benefit of implant surface decontamination.

It is also important to note that proper laser therapy protocol is required to reach the bactericidal energy threshold for surface decontamination [42]. As most studies did not specify the setting of the laser and the detailed application time and methods, it may not have a strict protocol. Before more studies develop evidence-based application, it is prudent to recognize that a thorough implant surface decontamination takes time and should not be rushed.

11.2.4.2 Soft and Hard Tissue Wound Healing Following Laser Therapy

In addition to bactericidal effects, laser therapy has a distinct wound healing pattern following the treatment. The biostimulation effect from low-level energy laser is also an emerging area of interest, which may be an important characteristic of laser therapy to promote healing and tissue regeneration. Many earlier in vitro, in vivo, and clinical studies also have shown the benefits of laser to promote wound healing [13–15, 50] reduction of inflammation [16, 51, 52], as well as pain relief [13, 17, 53], which are all desirable biostimulatory effects [54].

At the cellular level, in vitro studies showed that low-level laser irradiation could attenuate the production of pro-inflammatory mediators (IL-1β and PGE_2) from both stimulated human gingival fibroblast and PDL cells [51, 52] as well as macrophages [55]. Diode laser at low dose can also activate human fibroblast transforming factor β1 signaling pathway and induce the expression human β-defensin 2 (HBD-2), both of which are potent factors to promote wound healing [56]. Additionally, low-level laser stimulates osteoblast proliferation, differentiation, release of several growth factors [57–59], and the formation of bone nodules in vitro [60]. Therefore, these cellular responses following laser biostimulation can attenuate inflammation and enhance both soft and hard tissue healing.

In the animal models, in vivo studies demonstrated that low-level laser therapy could induce dose-dependent reduction of tumor necrosis factor-alpha in acute inflammation [61]. Yamazaki et al. showed that low-level CO_2 laser induces expression of heat shock proteins in the collateral tissue exhibiting partial coagulation necrosis, but it promotes the repair process and tissue remodeling [62, 63]. Low-level laser therapy enhances fractured long bone healing in the animal model [64]. LED light irradiation promotes osteogenesis in periodontal intrabony defect with open flap debridement [65].

There are several interesting studies on laser enhancing implant osseointegration and healing of peri-implant tissues. Low-level laser therapy can stimulate faster osseointegration in the animal model [66] or even irradiate the recipient alveolar bone before implant placement to enhance the vitality of the osteocyte and promote faster bone formation around the dental implant for quick osseointegration [67, 68]. Omasa et al. utilized low-level laser to increase the stability of the mini implants placed in rat tibiae and found higher expression of the bone morphogenetic protein 2 from the surrounding cells as well [69]. Direct application of Er:YAG laser over contaminated implant surface can also induce more bone-to-implant contact with regenerative therapy [49], although such finding is not known to be a direct result of surface decontamination or biostimulation.

In a human split-mouth design study, using low-level laser therapy after gingivectomy incisions promotes better healing [70]; another human split-mouth study used diode laser to modulate modified Widman flap and found less edema of pain postoperatively [71]. More recently, Er:YAG laser has been used to conduct second-stage procedure to expose dental implant that resulted in significantly less postoperative pain score [53]. Another obvious clinical benefit for tissue management is hemostasis that is well recognized by the clinicians. However, strong hemostatic effect may compromise the wound healing, especially when hemostasis was generally achieved with carbonization, coagulation, and thermal denaturation of the adjacent tissue that clots the small blood vessels. Therefore, incision of the soft tissue with laser may not be the right application if severe bleeding is not expected. The carbonization of the incisional tissue would impair primary closure and delay wound healing [72–74]. Erbium lasers may not be the first choice in terms of hemostasis because it creates minimal thermal degeneration of the collateral tissue owing to its superficially penetrating characteristic [75]. However, given such characteristic, wound healing following erbium laser therapy may be more favorable. Sawabe et al. demonstrated faster and better gingival wound healing with Er:YAG laser compared with electrosurgery in rat animal models [74].

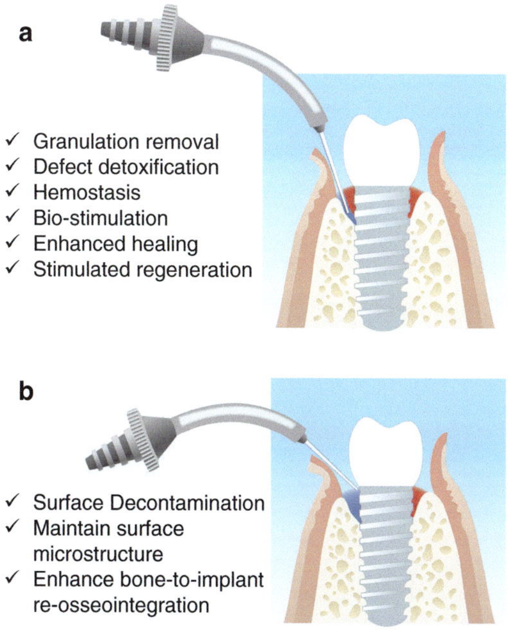

Fig. 11.1 The effect of laser therapy. (**a**) On peri-implant defect and (**b**) on implant surface

In summary, the effect of implant therapy is not only limited to implant surface decontamination but also enhances the soft and hard tissue healing around the inflamed peri-implant defect (Fig. 11.1).

11.2.5 How Can Laser Be Used in the Treatment of Peri-implant Diseases?

In general, nonsurgical treatment of peri-implantitis has shown limited clinical benefits [25, 76, 77], whereas surgical management of peri-implantitis may have more promising yet unpredictable outcomes [29, 78]. It was generally accepted that nonsurgical treatment should be able to manage peri-implant mucositis [28]. Laser can be used both nonsurgically and surgically. Most studies listed have combined laser as an adjunctive therapy with conventional debridement or anti-infective therapy. The types of lasers approved and reported for the treatment of peri-implantitis include CO_2, diodes, Er:YAG, and Er, Cr:YSGG. Two systemic reviews [79, 80] had evaluated the efficacy of various laser wavelengths in the treatment of peri-implantitis; however, very few RCTs with significant heterogeneity were identified, and meta-analysis of the pooled results revealed inconclusive benefits of laser usage. Here, we added recent studies and separated nonsurgical and surgical approaches into two groups to critically assess variables that may affect the results for clinical implications.

11.2.5.1 Nonsurgical Laser Therapy for Peri-implant Diseases

It is still an area of controversy that some investigators question whether nonsurgical application of laser is reliable or not due to the inconsistency where the laser actually applies and thus the study protocol may be heterogenous. However, some recent clinical trials demonstrate its efficacy and may stimulate more investigation considering it is a practical approach.

Regarding nonsurgical peri-implant laser therapy, attention must be paid to the inclusion criteria of peri-implant pocket depth. According to the classification proposed by Forum and Rosen [81], studies that included early peri-implantitis with probing depth (PD) of 4–6 mm had very limited clinical improvements [82, 83]. Other studies, which appear to have deeper PD, demonstrated a more significant additional peri-implant pocket reduction compared to the control group that favors the adjunctive use of laser [84–86] (Table 11.4). Therefore, the use of adjunctive laser on moderate to advanced peri-implantitis with deeper PD may expect to have a more favorable response if pocket reduction is the primary goal. In addition, reduction in bleed on probing (BOP) is also an important clinical outcome as all the peri-implantitis cases are defined with a requirement of bleeding and/or suppuration on probing as a sign of inflammation. Among the studies listed, there may be a clear trend that adjunctive laser application for nonsurgical application would have additional benefits in BOP reduction compared to control groups (~30–95% vs. ~15–40%; test vs. control), especially during short-term follow-up visits [87]. Another variable is the inclusion criteria for peri-implantitis bone

Table 11.4 Current literatures on nonsurgical laser treatment for peri-implantitis

Study (year)	Type of study	Type of laser	No. of pts (implants) criteria	Studylength	Test group/sites	Control group/sites	Critical summary of the results
Renvert et al. (2011), Persson et al. (2011)	RCT	Er:YAG	42 (90)PD ≥ 6 mmBL > 3 mm	6 months	Laser only 100 mJ/pulse, 10 Hz (12.7 J/cm^2) semicircular motion	Glycine powder polishing (15 s each site)	Similar outcomes between two groups PD and BOP reduction (0.9 vs. 0.8 mm and 31 vs. 25%)
Schär et al. (2013), Bassetti et al. (2014)	RCT	PDT	40 (40)PD: 4–6 mmBL ≤ 2 mm	6–12 months	Titanium curettes + glycine powder + 3% hydrogen peroxide		PD and BOP reduced similarly between two groups after 6 months (~0.36 vs. 0.49 mm; 30 vs. 15%)
					Adjunctive laser(100 nW, 10 s/pocket)repeat after 1 week	Local delivery of 1-mg minocycline microspheres	
Al-Falaki et al. (2014)	Case series	Er,Cr:YSGG	11 (28)PD > 4 mm	6 months	Adjunctive laser 1.5 W, 30 Hz, 50 mJ/pulseTwo rounds + titanium curette in between	N/A	Significant reduction in PD (~3.6 mm) and BOP (78%) after 6 months
Mettraux et al. (2015)	Case series	Diode	15 (23)PD ≥ 5 mm	2 years	Adjunctive laser 2.5 W, 50 Hz, 10 ms 30 s for three rounds + carbon & metal instrument	N/A	Significant improvements in deepest PD of each implant (7.7 → 3.8 mm)
Schwarz et al. (2015)	Prospectivecase series	Er:YAG	17 (21)PD ≥ 6 mm	6 months	Adjunctive laser 100 mJ/pulse (12.7 J/cm^2) and 10 Hz. 15–20° circular motion	N/A	Significant improvement in BOP (32%) and PD (0.9 mm)Complete resolution was obtained in 9/17 (52.9%) cases.
Arisan et al. (2015)	RCT	Diode	10 (48)PD: 4–6 mmBL < 3 mm	6 months	Adjunctive laser 3 J/cm^2; 400 mW/cm^2; 1.5 J for 1 min	Scaling and root planning (plastic curettes)	Similar results for minimal PD reduction;Adjunctive laser may yield more MBL
Lerario et al. (2016)	Controlledcase study	Diode	27 (125)PD > 4 mm	1 year	Adjunctive laser 1 W in pulsating mode, 50 Hz, 24.87 J/cm^2; 30 s for two rounds	Piezoelectric + ultrasonic magnetostrictive units (plastic tip) + titanium curettes + 0.5% chlorhexidine gel	Adjunctive laser significantly reduced PD (~2.7 vs. 1.1 mm) and BOP (95% vs. 40%) compare to control

loss. To the best of our knowledge, there is still no universally accepted threshold as individual physiologic marginal bone loss may vary [88]. Nonsurgical laser therapy may not work in case of severe peri-implant defect. Renvert et al. reported using laser as a monotherapy and found similar outcome with glycine powder polishing [89, 90]. Arisan et al. reported that adjunctive diode laser therapy may yield slightly more marginal bone loss compared to conventional scaling. However, the study primarily includes shallower pockets (4–5 mm), and the laser was applied for a longer period of time (1 min) compared to other studies, which may have a negative impact on peri-implant marginal bone [83]. Therefore, case selection remains critical.

In conclusion, nonsurgical laser therapy for peri-implantitis may not be predictable in complete resolution of the disease but has a tendency to give improvements, especially on bleeding on probing. Case selection may be the key factor to implement nonsurgical application. More studies are needed to optimize nonsurgical protocols. Repeated application for previously treated sites may also be a reinforcement approach for maintenance.

11.2.5.2 Surgical Laser Therapy for Peri-implantitis

In terms of surgical approaches (Table 11.5), to the best of our knowledge, there are only two randomized clinical trials published so far with two laser types (diode and Er:YAG). Papadopoulos et al. reported that adjunctive use of diode laser resulted in similar PD reduction compared with control group (~1.5 vs. 1.2 mm) at 6 months but achieved more CAL gain (~0.8 mm) compared to control group (~0.2 mm), which should also be a main clinical outcome to assess the efficacy of laser. On the contrary, Schwarz et al. [91] have reported the use of Er:YAG laser compared with "conventional therapy" (plastic curettes with cotton pellets and sterile saline) in preparation for regenerative therapy. It must be noted that implantoplasty over suprabony defect was part of the study protocol and thus the mean pocket depth reduction over all the implant surfaces may not be a good clinical outcome measurement. It was concluded that the control group seems to have better trends in pocket reduction and attachment gain after 6 months and remained similar results after 4 years [91, 92]. It was speculated that the titanium particles left in experimental group negatively impaired the clinical outcome and the degree of implantoplasty masked the beneficial effect from laser therapy by reporting the "mean" difference from all implant sites. Implant position may also be a contributing factor. Although complete resolution of the disease or defect was not always predictable, an improvement in resolving the defect is expected, and once established regenerated bone and peri-implant tissue can be maintained stable up to 7 years or longer [93]. Additionally, given the emerging evidence that titanium particles may have negative effect on peri-implant tissue [94], it may be prudent to use copious saline irrigation and cotton pellets swapping as a standard procedure following implantoplasty as it is still the most predictable procedure in managing peri-implant suprabony defects. Here we present a peri-implantitis case treated with laser-assisted surgical regenearitve therapy (Fig. 11.2).

Parma-Benfenati et al. published a case series utilizing a combined surface decontamination and detoxification approach and achieved complete radiographic bone fill in seven out of nine cases [95]. Most successful case reports published [11, 96–98] presented with moderate to advanced peri-implantitis with more prominent bony defect (mostly intrabony) and deeper initial periodontal pocket depth compared to RCTs. Complete resolution of the inflammation and regeneration of the bony defect seem more favorably achievable in these reports. However, more well-designed RCTs are needed to assess the predictability of laser-assisted surgical procedures and identify factors that determine the long-term prognosis and stability. In addition, human histology analyzing the re-established peri-implant support after laser therapy is also warranted. Given the histological study in rat and canine model from two different groups that demonstrated the adjunctive benefit of laser for surface decontamination to induce more bone-to-implant re-osseointegrated contact [49, 99], the positive histological outcome in human is likely to be promising.

Table 11.5 Current literatures on surgical laser treatment for peri-implantitis

Study(year)	Type of study	Type of laser	No. of pts(implants) criteria	Study length	Test group/sites	Control group/sites	Critical summary of the results
Schwarz et al. (2011, 2012, 2013)	RCT	Er:YAG	30 (35)17 (17) PD > 6 mm	6 months–4 years	Implantoplasty + laser100 mJ/pulse (11.4 J/cm^2, 10 Hz) semicircular motion+ GBR	Implantoplasty + Plastic curettes + cotton pellets + sterile saline + GBR	Similar reduction of BOP (72 vs. 85%) and PD (1.2 vs. 1.5 mm); Both showed peri-implant bone fill
Parma-Benfenati et al. (2015)	Case series	PDT	6 (9) PD > 6 mm	N/A	Ultrasonic, titanium curette, and tooth brush; air-powder abrasive; PDT (10 s); tetracycline; GBR	N/A	7/9 implants achieved complete bone fill
Papadopoulos et al. (2015)	RCT	Diode	16 (16) PD ≥ 6 mm	6 months	Adjunctive laser0.8 W at pulsating mode; 2 min for three times	Plastic curettes + cotton pellets + sterile saline	Both groups reduce BOP (73 vs. 67%) and PD (~1.5 vs. 1.2 mm) similarly but only test group had significant CAL gain whereas control group does not (~0.8 vs. 0.2 mm)
Badran et al. (2011)	Case report(combined)	Er:YAG	1 (1) PD: 5–9 mmBL~50%	6 months	Nonsurgical:ultrasonic scaling with laser, 120 mJ, 10 Hz60 s/site Surgical: laser + biphasic calcium phosphate	N/A	PD reduced (9 → 4 mm) without BOP and complete radiographic bone fill
Yamamoto et al. (2013)	Case report and animal study(surgical)	Er:YAG	1 (2)	4 years	50 mJ, 20 PPS+ GBR	N/A	Peri-implantitis was stabilized with radiographic bone gain. Osseointegration can occur over laser irradiated surface
Yoshino et al. (2015)	Case reports(surgical)	Er:YAG	2 (2)	2 years	Laser (40 mJ/10 pps) + GBR + PDGF + antibacterial therapy	N/A	Both cases achieved significant radiographic bone fill (7 and 3 mm vertical linear bone gain)

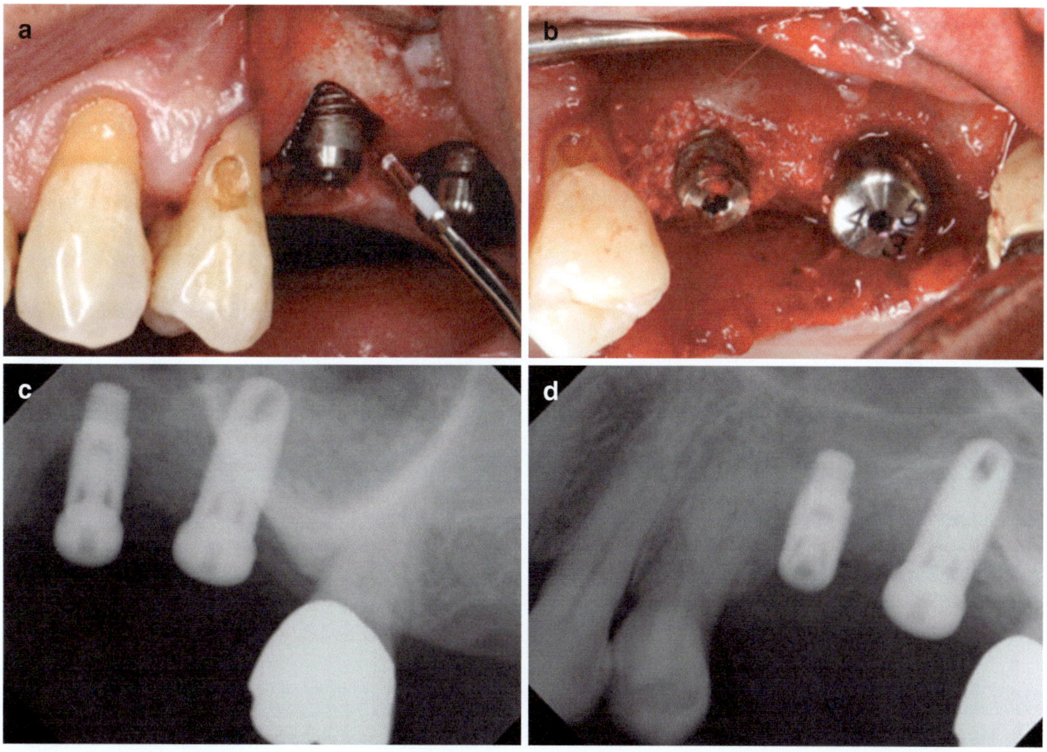

Fig. 11.2 Surgical laser therapy with bone grafting procedure for peri-implantitis. (**a**) Er:YAG laser application for infrabony defect region; (**b**) implantoplasty was performed for suprabony defect and bone grafting was placed within infrabony defect; (**c**) preoperative radiograph; (**d**) radiograph taken after the surgery

Of note, there is no standard treatment for peri-implantitis serving as a proper control group, variation in treatment outcome was present, and thus very few statistically significant results were reported. However, analyzing variables in each study revealed potential benefits from adjunctive use of laser and its promising role. Future studies should further examine the effect of laser implant surface decontamination and biostimulation through analyzing the microbial profile and inflammatory mediators in the peri-implant crevicular fluid. Clinical outcome should beware of other local factors, including titanium particles from implantoplasty, and evaluate the measurements only above the defect site where laser is applied. Future well-controlled RCTs are needed to establish evidence-based indications and protocol for the use of laser in the treatment of peri-implantitis.

11.3 Summary

Laser-assisted therapy for peri-implant diseases is a promising approach. In vitro and in vivo studies demonstrated that laser not only assists in implant surface detoxification but also promotes healing through biostimulation. Although a few pilot randomized clinical trials did not show conclusive results, more well-designed controlled trials are warranted to optimize the application of laser therapy to develop evidence-based protocol and ideal indications.

Acknowledgments The authors thank the assistant graphic designer Victoria Zakrzeski at the University of Michigan School of Dentistry for constructing the figure and the courtesy of postdoctoral resident Dr. Carlos Garaicoa, Graduate Periodontics, for sharing the case.

References

1. Coluzzi DJ. Fundamentals of lasers in dentistry: basic science, tissue interaction, and instrumentation. J Laser Dent. 2008;16:4–10.
2. Hale GMQM. Optical constants of water in the 200-nm to 200-lm wavelength region. Appl Opt. 1973;12:555–63.
3. Niemz MH. Laser-tissue interaction. Fundamentals and applications. Berlin Heidelberg: Springer-Verlag; 1996.
4. Schwarz F, Aoki A, Sculean A, Becker J. The impact of laser application on periodontal and peri-implant wound healing. Periodontol. 2009;51:79–108. https://doi.org/10.1111/j.1600-0757.2009.00301.x.
5. Seka WFJ, Fried D, Visuri SR, Walsh JT. Laser ablation of dental hard tissue: from explosive ablation to plasma-mediated ablation. Proc SPIE. 1996;2672(166):144–58.
6. Seka WRP, Featherstone JDB, Fried D. Laser ablation of dental hard tissue. J Laser Dent. 2007;15:61–72.
7. Nelson JS, Yow L, Liaw LH, Macleay L, Zavar RB, Orenstein A, et al. Ablation of bone and methacrylate by a prototype mid-infrared erbium:YAG laser. Lasers Surg Med. 1988;8(5):494–500.
8. Nuss RC, Fabian RL, Sarkar R, Puliafito CA. Infrared laser bone ablation. Lasers Surg Med. 1988;8(4):381–91.
9. Aoki A, Sasaki KM, Watanabe H, Ishikawa I. Lasers in nonsurgical periodontal therapy. Periodontol. 2004;36:59–97. https://doi.org/10.1111/j.1600-0757.2004.03679.x.
10. Goncalves F, Zanetti AL, Zanetti RV, Martelli FS, Avila-Campos MJ, Tomazinho LF, et al. Effectiveness of 980-mm diode and 1064-nm extra-long-pulse neodymium-doped yttrium aluminum garnet lasers in implant disinfection. Photomed Laser Surg. 2010;28(2):273–80. https://doi.org/10.1089/pho.2009.2496.
11. Yamamoto A, Tanabe T. Treatment of peri-implantitis around tiunite-surface implants using Er:YAG laser microexplosions. Int J Periodontics Restorative Dent. 2013;33(1):21–30.
12. Ohshiro T, Calderhead RG. Development of low reactive-level laser therapy and its present status. J Clin Laser Med Surg. 1991;9(4):267–75. https://doi.org/10.1089/clm.1991.9.267.
13. Enwemeka CS, Parker JC, Dowdy DS, Harkness EE, Sanford LE, Woodruff LD. The efficacy of low-power lasers in tissue repair and pain control: a meta-analysis study. Photomed Laser Surg. 2004;22(4):323–9. https://doi.org/10.1089/pho.2004.22.323.
14. Mester E, Spiry T, Szende B, Tota JG. Effect of laser rays on wound healing. Am J Surg. 1971;122(4):532–5.
15. Woodruff LD, Bounkeo JM, Brannon WM, Dawes KS, Barham CD, Waddell DL, et al. The efficacy of laser therapy in wound repair: a meta-analysis of the literature. Photomed Laser Surg. 2004;22(3):241–7. https://doi.org/10.1089/1549541041438623.
16. Albertini R, Aimbire FS, Correa FI, Ribeiro W, Cogo JC, Antunes E, et al. Effects of different protocol doses of low power gallium-aluminum-arsenate (Ga-Al-As) laser radiation (650 nm) on carrageenan induced rat paw oedema. J Photochem Photobiol B. 2004;74(2-3):101–7. https://doi.org/10.1016/j.jphotobiol.2004.03.002.
17. Bjordal JM, Johnson MI, Iversen V, Aimbire F, Lopes-Martins RA. Low-level laser therapy in acute pain: a systematic review of possible mechanisms of action and clinical effects in randomized placebo-controlled trials. Photomed Laser Surg. 2006;24(2):158–68. https://doi.org/10.1089/pho.2006.24.158.
18. Mombelli A, van Oosten MA, Schurch E Jr, Land NP. The microbiota associated with successful or failing osseointegrated titanium implants. Oral Microbiol Immunol. 1987;2(4):145–51.
19. Albrektsson T, Isidor F, editors. Consensus report of session IV. First European Workshop on Periodontology. London: Quintessence; 1994.
20. Peri-implant mucositis and peri-implantitis: a current understanding of their diagnoses and clinical implications. J Periodontol. 2013;84(4):436–43. https://doi.org/10.1902/jop.2013.134001.
21. Suarez-Lopez Del Amo F, Lin GH, Monje A, Galindo-Moreno P, Wang HL. Influence of soft tissue thickness on peri-implant marginal bone loss: a systematic review and meta-analysis. J Periodontol. 2016;87(6):690–9. https://doi.org/10.1902/jop.2016.150571.
22. Koldsland OC, Scheie AA, Aass AM. Prevalence of peri-implantitis related to severity of the disease with different degrees of bone loss. J Periodontol. 2010;81(2):231–8. https://doi.org/10.1902/jop.2009.090269.
23. Renvert S, Lindahl C, Rutger PG. The incidence of peri-implantitis for two different implant systems over a period of thirteen years. J Clin Periodontol. 2012;39(12):1191–7. https://doi.org/10.1111/jcpe.12017.
24. Derks J, Tomasi C. Peri-implant health and disease. A systematic review of current epidemiology. J Clin Periodontol. 2015;42(Suppl 16):S158–71. https://doi.org/10.1111/jcpe.12334.
25. Suarez-Lopez Del Amo F, Yu SH, Wang HL. Non-surgical therapy for peri-implant diseases: a systematic review. J Oral Maxillofac Res. 2016;7(3):e13. https://doi.org/10.5037/jomr.2016.7313.
26. Pontoriero R, Tonelli MP, Carnevale G, Mombelli A, Nyman SR, Lang NP. Experimentally induced peri-implant mucositis. A clinical study in humans. Clin Oral Implants Res. 1994;5(4):254–9.
27. Zitzmann NU, Berglundh T, Marinello CP, Lindhe J. Experimental peri-implant mucositis in man. J Clin Periodontol. 2001;28(6):517–23.
28. Salvi GE, Aglietta M, Eick S, Sculean A, Lang NP, Ramseier CA. Reversibility of experimental peri-implant mucositis compared with experimental gingivitis in humans. Clin Oral Implants Res. 2012;23(2):182–90. https://doi.org/10.1111/j.1600-0501.2011.02220.x.

29. Lindhe J, Meyle J, Group DoEWoP. Peri-implant diseases: consensus report of the sixth European Workshop on Periodontology. J Clin Periodontol. 2008;35(8 Suppl):282–5. https://doi.org/10.1111/j.1600-051X.2008.01283.x.
30. Padial-Molina M, Suarez F, Rios HF, Galindo-Moreno P, Wang HL. Guidelines for the diagnosis and treatment of peri-implant diseases. Int J Periodontics Restorative Dent. 2014;34(6):e102–11. https://doi.org/10.11607/prd.1994.
31. Loe H, Anerud A, Boysen H, Morrison E. Natural history of periodontal disease in man. Rapid, moderate and no loss of attachment in Sri Lankan laborers 14 to 46 years of age. J Clin Periodontol. 1986;13(5):431–45.
32. Monje A, Galindo-Moreno P, Tozum TF, Suarez-Lopez del Amo F, Wang HL. Into the paradigm of local factors as contributors for peri-implant disease: short communication. Int J Oral Maxillofac Implants. 2016;31(2):288–92. https://doi.org/10.11607/jomi.4265.
33. Linkevicius T, Puisys A, Vindasiute E, Linkeviciene L, Apse P. Does residual cement around implant-supported restorations cause peri-implant disease? A retrospective case analysis. Clin Oral Implants Res. 2013;24(11):1179–84. https://doi.org/10.1111/j.1600-0501.2012.02570.x.
34. Staubli N, Walter C, Schmidt JC, Weiger R, Zitzmann NU. Excess cement and the risk of peri-implant disease—a systematic review. Clin Oral Implants Res. 2016; https://doi.org/10.1111/clr.12954.
35. Fu JH, Hsu YT, Wang HL. Identifying occlusal overload and how to deal with it to avoid marginal bone loss around implants. Eur J Oral Implantol. 2012;5(Suppl):S91–103.
36. Renvert S, Polyzois I. Risk indicators for peri-implant mucositis: a systematic literature review. J Clin Periodontol. 2015;42(Suppl 16):S172–86. https://doi.org/10.1111/jcpe.12346.
37. Renvert S, Quirynen M. Risk indicators for peri-implantitis. A narrative review. Clin Oral Implants Res. 2015;26(Suppl 11):15–44. https://doi.org/10.1111/clr.12636.
38. Decker AM, Sheridan R, Lin GH, Sutthiboonyapan P, Carroll W, Wang HL. A prognosis system for peri-implant diseases. Implant Dent. 2015;24(4):416–21. https://doi.org/10.1097/ID.0000000000000276.
39. Claffey N, Clarke E, Polyzois I, Renvert S. Surgical treatment of peri-implantitis. J Clin Periodontol. 2008;35(8 Suppl):316–32. https://doi.org/10.1111/j.1600-051X.2008.01277.x.
40. Rooney J, Midda M, Leeming J. A laboratory investigation of the bactericidal effect of a NdYAG laser. Br Dent J. 1994;176(2):61–4. https://doi.org/10.1038/sj.bdj.4808364.
41. Ando Y, Aoki A, Watanabe H, Ishikawa I. Bactericidal effect of erbium YAG laser on periodontopathic bacteria. Lasers Surg Med. 1996;19(2):190–200. https://doi.org/10.1002/(SICI)1096-9101(1996)19:2<190::AID-LSM11>3.0.CO;2-B.
42. Coffelt DW, Cobb CM, MacNeill S, Rapley JW, Killoy WJ. Determination of energy density threshold for laser ablation of bacteria. An in vitro study. J Clin Periodontol. 1997;24(1):1–7.
43. Wang HL, Garaicoa-Pazmino C, Collins A, Ong HS, Chudri R, Giannobile WV. Protein biomarkers and microbial profiles in peri-implantitis. Clin Oral Implants Res. 2016;27(9):1129–36. https://doi.org/10.1111/clr.12708.
44. Kreisler M, Gotz H, Duschner H. Effect of Nd:YAG, Ho:YAG, Er:YAG, CO_2, and GaAIAs laser irradiation on surface properties of endosseous dental implants. Int J Oral Maxillofac Implants. 2002;17(2):202–11.
45. Folwaczny M, Aggstaller H, Mehl A, Hickel R. Removal of bacterial endotoxin from root surface with Er:YAG laser. Am J Dent. 2003;16(1):3–5.
46. Yamaguchi H, Kobayashi K, Osada R, Sakuraba E, Nomura T, Arai T, et al. Effects of irradiation of an erbium:YAG laser on root surfaces. J Periodontol. 1997;68(12):1151–5. https://doi.org/10.1902/jop.1997.68.12.1151.
47. Mailoa J, Lin GH, Chan HL, MacEachern M, Wang HL. Clinical outcomes of using lasers for peri-implantitis surface detoxification: a systematic review and meta-analysis. J Periodontol. 2014;85(9):1194–202. https://doi.org/10.1902/jop.2014.130620.
48. Takasaki AA, Aoki A, Mizutani K, Kikuchi S, Oda S, Ishikawa I. Er:YAG laser therapy for peri-implant infection: a histological study. Lasers Med Sci. 2007;22(3):143–57. https://doi.org/10.1007/s10103-006-0430-x.
49. Nevins M, Nevins ML, Yamamoto A, Yoshino T, Ono Y, Wang CW, et al. Use of Er:YAG laser to decontaminate infected dental implant surface in preparation for reestablishment of bone-to-implant contact. Int J Periodontics Restorative Dent. 2014;34(4):461–6. https://doi.org/10.11607/prd.2192.
50. Karu T. Laser biostimulation: a photobiological phenomenon. J Photochem Photobiol B. 1989;3(4):638–40.
51. Shimizu N, Yamaguchi M, Goseki T, Shibata Y, Takiguchi H, Iwasawa T, et al. Inhibition of prostaglandin E2 and interleukin 1-beta production by low-power laser irradiation in stretched human periodontal ligament cells. J Dent Res. 1995;74(7):1382–8. https://doi.org/10.1177/00220345950740071001.
52. Sakurai Y, Yamaguchi M, Abiko Y. Inhibitory effect of low-level laser irradiation on LPS-stimulated prostaglandin E2 production and cyclooxygenase-2 in human gingival fibroblasts. Eur J Oral Sci. 2000;108(1):29–34.
53. Matys J, Dominiak M. Assessment of pain when uncovering implants with Er:YAG laser or scalpel for second stage surgery. Adv Clin Exp Med. 2016;25(6):1179–84. https://doi.org/10.17219/acem/62456.
54. Aoki A, Mizutani K, Schwarz F, Sculean A, Yukna RA, Takasaki AA, et al. Periodontal and peri-implant wound healing following laser therapy. Periodontol. 2015;68(1):217–69. https://doi.org/10.1111/prd.12080.

55. Gavish L, Perez LS, Reissman P, Gertz SD. Irradiation with 780 nm diode laser attenuates inflammatory cytokines but upregulates nitric oxide in lipopolysaccharide-stimulated macrophages: implications for the prevention of aneurysm progression. Lasers Surg Med. 2008;40(5):371–8. https://doi.org/10.1002/lsm.20635.
56. Tang E, Khan I, Andreana S, Arany PR. Laser-activated transforming growth factor-beta1 induces human beta-defensin 2: implications for laser therapies for periodontitis and peri-implantitis. J Periodontal Res. 2016; https://doi.org/10.1111/jre.12399.
57. Stein E, Koehn J, Sutter W, Wendtlandt G, Wanschitz F, Thurnher D, et al. Initial effects of low-level laser therapy on growth and differentiation of human osteoblast-like cells. Wien Klin Wochenschr. 2008;120(3-4):112–7. https://doi.org/10.1007/s00508-008-0932-6.
58. Aleksic V, Aoki A, Iwasaki K, Takasaki AA, Wang CY, Abiko Y, et al. Low-level Er:YAG laser irradiation enhances osteoblast proliferation through activation of MAPK/ERK. Lasers Med Sci. 2010;25(4):559–69. https://doi.org/10.1007/s10103-010-0761-5.
59. Saygun I, Nizam N, Ural AU, Serdar MA, Avcu F, Tozum TF. Low-level laser irradiation affects the release of basic fibroblast growth factor (bFGF), insulin-like growth factor-I (IGF-I), and receptor of IGF-I (IGFBP3) from osteoblasts. Photomed Laser Surg. 2012;30(3):149–54. https://doi.org/10.1089/pho.2011.3079.
60. Ozawa Y, Shimizu N, Kariya G, Abiko Y. Low-energy laser irradiation stimulates bone nodule formation at early stages of cell culture in rat calvarial cells. Bone. 1998;22(4):347–54.
61. Aimbire F, Lopes-Martins RA, Castro-Faria-Neto HC, Albertini R, Chavantes MC, Pacheco MT, et al. Low-level laser therapy can reduce lipopolysaccharide-induced contractile force dysfunction and TNF-alpha levels in rat diaphragm muscle. Lasers Med Sci. 2006;21(4):238–44. https://doi.org/10.1007/s10103-006-0405-y.
62. Yamasaki A, Tamamura K, Sakurai Y, Okuyama N, Yusa J, Ito H. Remodeling of the rat gingiva induced by CO_2 laser coagulation mode. Lasers Surg Med. 2008;40(10):695–703. https://doi.org/10.1002/lsm.20712.
63. Yamasaki A, Ito H, Yusa J, Sakurai Y, Okuyama N, Ozawa R. Expression of heat shock proteins, Hsp70 and Hsp25, in the rat gingiva after irradiation with a CO_2 laser in coagulation mode. J Periodontal Res. 2010;45(3):323–30. https://doi.org/10.1111/j.1600-0765.2009.01239.x.
64. Rajaei Jafarabadi M, Rouhi G, Kaka G, Sadraie SH, Arum J. The effects of photobiomodulation and low-amplitude high-frequency vibration on bone healing process: a comparative study. Lasers Med Sci. 2016;31(9):1827–36. https://doi.org/10.1007/s10103-016-2058-9.
65. Tao CY, Lee N, Chang HC, Yang C, Yu XH, Chang PC. Evaluation of 660 nm LED light irradiation on the strategies for treating experimental periodontal intrabony defects. Lasers Med Sci. 2016;31(6):1113–21. https://doi.org/10.1007/s10103-016-1958-z.
66. Khadra M, Ronold HJ, Lyngstadaas SP, Ellingsen JE, Haanaes HR. Low-level laser therapy stimulates bone-implant interaction: an experimental study in rabbits. Clin Oral Implants Res. 2004;15(3):325–32. https://doi.org/10.1111/j.1600-0501.2004.00994.x.
67. Dortbudak O, Haas R, Mailath-Pokorny G. Effect of low-power laser irradiation on bony implant sites. Clin Oral Implants Res. 2002;13(3):288–92.
68. Naka T, Yokose S. Application of laser-induced bone therapy by carbon dioxide laser irradiation in implant therapy. Int J Dent. 2012;2012:409496. https://doi.org/10.1155/2012/409496.
69. Omasa S, Motoyoshi M, Arai Y, Ejima K, Shimizu N. Low-level laser therapy enhances the stability of orthodontic mini-implants via bone formation related to BMP-2 expression in a rat model. Photomed Laser Surg. 2012;30(5):255–61. https://doi.org/10.1089/pho.2011.3157.
70. Amorim JC, de Sousa GR, de Barros Silveira L, Prates RA, Pinotti M, Ribeiro MS. Clinical study of the gingiva healing after gingivectomy and low-level laser therapy. Photomed Laser Surg. 2006;24(5):588–94. https://doi.org/10.1089/pho.2006.24.588.
71. Sanz-Moliner JD, Nart J, Cohen RE, Ciancio SG. The effect of an 810-nm diode laser on postoperative pain and tissue response after modified Widman flap surgery: a pilot study in humans. J Periodontol. 2013;84(2):152–8. https://doi.org/10.1902/jop.2012.110660.
72. Arashiro DS, Rapley JW, Cobb CM, Killoy WJ. Histologic evaluation of porcine skin incisions produced by CO_2 laser, electrosurgery, and scalpel. Int J Periodontics Restorative Dent. 1996;16(5):479–91.
73. Sinha UK, Gallagher LA. Effects of steel scalpel, ultrasonic scalpel, CO_2 laser, and monopolar and bipolar electrosurgery on wound healing in guinea pig oral mucosa. Laryngoscope. 2003;113(2):228–36. https://doi.org/10.1097/00005537-200302000-00007.
74. Sawabe M, Aoki A, Komaki M, Iwasaki K, Ogita M, Izumi Y. Gingival tissue healing following Er:YAG laser ablation compared to electrosurgery in rats. Lasers Med Sci. 2015;30(2):875–83. https://doi.org/10.1007/s10103-013-1478-z.
75. Merigo E, Clini F, Fornaini C, Oppici A, Paties C, Zangrandi A, et al. Laser-assisted surgery with different wavelengths: a preliminary ex vivo study on thermal increase and histological evaluation. Lasers Med Sci. 2013;28(2):497–504. https://doi.org/10.1007/s10103-012-1081-8.
76. Renvert S, Roos-Jansaker AM, Claffey N. Non-surgical treatment of peri-implant mucositis and peri-implantitis: a literature review. J Clin Periodontol. 2008;35(8 Suppl):305–15. https://doi.org/10.1111/j.1600-051X.2008.01276.x.
77. Heitz-Mayfield LJ, Mombelli A. The therapy of peri-implantitis: a systematic review. Int J Oral Maxillofac Implants. 2014;29(Suppl):325–45. https://doi.org/10.11607/jomi.2014suppl.g5.3.

78. Chan HL, Lin GH, Suarez F, MacEachern M, Wang HL. Surgical management of peri-implantitis: a systematic review and meta-analysis of treatment outcomes. J Periodontol. 2014;85(8):1027–41. https://doi.org/10.1902/jop.2013.130563.
79. Kotsakis GA, Konstantinidis I, Karoussis IK, Ma X, Chu H. Systematic review and meta-analysis of the effect of various laser wavelengths in the treatment of peri-implantitis. J Periodontol. 2014;85(9):1203–13. https://doi.org/10.1902/jop.2014.130610.
80. Natto ZS, Aladmawy M, Levi PA Jr, Wang HL. Comparison of the efficacy of different types of lasers for the treatment of peri-implantitis: a systematic review. Int J Oral Maxillofac Implants. 2015;30(2):338–45. https://doi.org/10.11607/jomi.3846.
81. Froum SJ, Rosen PS. A proposed classification for peri-implantitis. Int J Periodontics Restorative Dent. 2012;32(5):533–40.
82. Schar D, Ramseier CA, Eick S, Arweiler NB, Sculean A, Salvi GE. Anti-infective therapy of peri-implantitis with adjunctive local drug delivery or photodynamic therapy: six-month outcomes of a prospective randomized clinical trial. Clin Oral Implants Res. 2013;24(1):104–10. https://doi.org/10.1111/j.1600-0501.2012.02494.x.
83. Arisan V, Karabuda ZC, Arici SV, Topcuoglu N, Kulekci G. A randomized clinical trial of an adjunct diode laser application for the nonsurgical treatment of peri-implantitis. Photomed Laser Surg. 2015;33(11):547–54. https://doi.org/10.1089/pho.2015.3956.
84. Al-Falaki R, Cronshaw M, Hughes FJ. Treatment outcome following use of the erbium, chromium:yttrium, scandium, gallium, garnet laser in the non-surgical management of peri-implantitis: a case series. Br Dent J. 2014;217(8):453–7. https://doi.org/10.1038/sj.bdj.2014.910.
85. Mettraux GR, Sculean A, Burgin WB, Salvi GE. Two-year clinical outcomes following non-surgical mechanical therapy of peri-implantitis with adjunctive diode laser application. Clin Oral Implants Res. 2016;27(7):845–9. https://doi.org/10.1111/clr.12689.
86. Lerario F, Roncati M, Gariffo A, Attorresi E, Lucchese A, Galanakis A, et al. Non-surgical periodontal treatment of peri-implant diseases with the adjunctive use of diode laser: preliminary clinical study. Lasers Med Sci. 2016;31(1):1–6. https://doi.org/10.1007/s10103-015-1785-7.
87. Abduljabbar T, Javed F, Kellesarian SV, Vohra F, Romanos GE. Effect of Nd:YAG laser-assisted non-surgical mechanical debridement on clinical and radiographic peri-implant inflammatory parameters in patients with peri-implant disease. J Photochem Photobiol B. 2017;168:16–9. https://doi.org/10.1016/j.jphotobiol.2017.01.015.
88. Monje A, Galindo-Moreno P, Canullo L, Greenwell H, Wang HL. Editorial: From early physiological marginal bone loss to peri-implant disease: on the unknown local contributing factors. Int J Periodontics Restorative Dent. 2015;35(6):764–5. https://doi.org/10.11607/prd.2597.
89. Renvert S, Lindahl C, Roos Jansaker AM, Persson GR. Treatment of peri-implantitis using an Er:YAG laser or an air-abrasive device: a randomized clinical trial. J Clin Periodontol. 2011;38(1):65–73. https://doi.org/10.1111/j.1600-051X.2010.01646.x.
90. Persson GR, Roos-Jansaker AM, Lindahl C, Renvert S. Microbiologic results after non-surgical erbium-doped:yttrium, aluminum, and garnet laser or air-abrasive treatment of peri-implantitis: a randomized clinical trial. J Periodontol. 2011;82(9):1267–78. https://doi.org/10.1902/jop.2011.100660.
91. Schwarz F, Sahm N, Iglhaut G, Becker J. Impact of the method of surface debridement and decontamination on the clinical outcome following combined surgical therapy of peri-implantitis: a randomized controlled clinical study. J Clin Periodontol. 2011;38(3):276–84. https://doi.org/10.1111/j.1600-051X.2010.01690.x.
92. Schwarz F, Hegewald A, John G, Sahm N, Becker J. Four-year follow-up of combined surgical therapy of advanced peri-implantitis evaluating two methods of surface decontamination. J Clin Periodontol. 2013;40(10):962–7. https://doi.org/10.1111/jcpe.12143.
93. Schwarz F, John G, Schmucker A, Sahm N, Becker J. Combined surgical therapy of advanced peri-implantitis evaluating two methods of surface decontamination: a 7-year follow-up observation. J Clin Periodontol. 2017;44(3):337–42. https://doi.org/10.1111/jcpe.12648.
94. Wilson TG Jr, Valderrama P, Burbano M, Blansett J, Levine R, Kessler H, et al. Foreign bodies associated with peri-implantitis human biopsies. J Periodontol. 2015;86(1):9–15. https://doi.org/10.1902/jop.2014.140363.
95. Parma-Benfenati S, Roncati M, Galletti P, Tinti C. Peri-implantitis treatment with a regenerative approach: clinical outcomes on reentry. Int J Periodontics Restorative Dent. 2015;35(5):625–36. https://doi.org/10.11607/prd.2374.
96. Badran Z, Bories C, Struillou X, Saffarzadeh A, Verner C, Soueidan A. Er:YAG laser in the clinical management of severe peri-implantitis: a case report. J Oral Implantol. 2011;37:212–7. https://doi.org/10.1563/AAID-JOI-D-09-00145.1.
97. Yoshino T, Yamamoto A, Ono Y. Innovative regeneration technology to solve peri-implantitis by Er:YAG laser based on the microbiologic diagnosis: a case series. Int J Periodontics Restorative Dent. 2015;35(1):67–73. https://doi.org/10.11607/prd.2116.
98. Suzuki JB. Salvaging implants with an Nd:YAG laser: a novel approach to a growing problem. Compend Contin Educ Dent. 2015;36(10):756–61.
99. Salmeron S, Rezende ML, Consolaro A, Sant'ana AC, Damante CA, Greghi SL, et al. Laser therapy as an effective method for implant surface decontamination: a histomorphometric study in rats. J Periodontol. 2013;84(5):641–9. https://doi.org/10.1902/jop.2012.120166.

Laser Applications and Autofluorescence

12

Paolo Vescovi, Ilaria Giovannacci, and Marco Meleti

Contents

Abstract

The diagnostic pathway for oral suspicious lesions usually starts with the clinical examination based on inspection and palpation of the oral mucosa. Such a phase is strongly related to the experience of the operator. Moreover, oral epithelial dysplasia and early oral carcinomas may already be present within areas of macroscopically intact oral mucosa. A great interest for techniques potentially improving the diagnostic accuracy has developed in several fields of surgical oncology in order to increase the specificity and sensitivity of the conventional diagnostic pathway. The development of noninvasive methods for real-time screening of neoplastic changes in oral cavity may be associated with the improvement of patients' quality of life and survival rate. The analysis of tissue autofluorescence (AF) for improving sensitivity and specificity in cancer diagnosis has been proposed for different organs, including colon, lung, cervix, and esophagus. Particularly, there are several

P. Vescovi · M. Meleti
Department of Dentistry (Oral Medicine, Oral Pathology, Oral Laser Surgery Unit), University of Parma, Parma, Italy
e-mail: paolo.vescovi@unipr.it; marco.meleti@unipr.it

I. Giovannacci (✉)
Department of Dentistry (Oral Medicine, Oral Pathology, Oral Laser Surgery Unit), University of Parma, Parma, Italy

Clinical and Experimental Medicine PhD program, Department of Dermatology, University of Modena and Reggio Emilia, Modena, Italy

S. Stübinger et al. (eds.), *Lasers in Oral and Maxillofacial Surgery*, https://doi.org/10.1007/978-3-030-29604-9_12

evidences supporting the effectiveness of this technique in head and neck cancer diagnosis. Autofluorescence shows high specificity and sensitivity for oral cancer and precancerous lesions: 72.4% and 63.79%, respectively. It can also provide valuable information for diagnosis, for planning of margin resection in surgical excision, and for monitoring the therapeutic response during follow-up. Direct visual fluorescence examination (DVFE) is based on the action of irradiation of specific wavelengths, between 375 and 440 nm, which excites some natural fluorochromes which show fluorescence in the range of the green color. The analysis of the lesions with AF tools must be performed in a dark environment to avoid the interference of white light wavelengths and to improve the quality of recorded images. Healthy oral mucosa emits fluorescence, detectable as green light. Cell and tissues within dysplastic and malignant lesions display modifications of the amount, distribution, and chemical–physical properties of the endogenous fluorophores. This results in an autofluorescence pattern variation that can be potentially used at diagnostic level. Loss of autofluorescence (LAF) seems to increase in correspondence to the progression of dysplasia, and altered tissue appears dark (brown to black). LAF in dysplasia and carcinoma seems to be connected to different mechanisms, such as altered metabolic activity of dysplastic keratinocytes, altered structure of subepithelial collagen, and absorbance of light by increased blood circulation due to inflammatory phenomena in dysplastic tissue and cancer. AF can be used for guiding incisional biopsy and in the excision to identify the resection margins.

Keywords

Autofluorescence (AF) · Fluorophores · Oral cancer diagnosis · Noninvasive tools for cancer diagnosis · Potentially malignant oral disorder surgical treatment · Biopsy of oral precancerous lesions

12.1 Noninvasive Methods in Diagnostics and Surgical Oncology

Oral cancer is a common malignant tumor. The 5-year survival rate of this neoplasm is low (approximately 50%), the delayed diagnosis being among the most important reasons. It is therefore important to emphasize the role of early diagnosis and treatment [1].

The diagnostic pathway for oral suspicious lesions usually starts with the clinical examination based on inspection and palpation of the oral mucosa. Such a phase is strongly related to the experience of the operator. Moreover, oral epithelial dysplasia and early oral carcinomas may already be present within areas of macroscopically intact oral mucosa.

A great interest for techniques potentially improving the diagnostic accuracy has developed in several fields of surgical oncology in order to increase the specificity and sensitivity of the conventional diagnostic pathway. The development of noninvasive methods for real-time screening of neoplastic changes in oral cavity may be associated with the improvement of patients' quality of life and survival rate.

Principles underlying the functioning of noninvasive visual diagnostic tools for oral cancer and dysplastic lesions are very different, being based on diverse specific cellular and tissue characteristics. Most common tools within such a context are chemiluminescence (CL), toluidine blue (TL), and chemiluminescence associated with toluidine blue (CLTB). Among these, the use of autofluorescence (AF) has recently attracted the interest of researchers.

The analysis of tissue autofluorescence for improving sensitivity and specificity in cancer diagnosis has been proposed for different organs, including colon, lung, cervix, and esophagus. Particularly, there are several evidences supporting the effectiveness of this technique in head and neck cancer diagnosis. Autofluorescence shows high specificity and sensitivity for oral cancer and precancerous lesions: 72.4% and 63.79%, respectively. It can also provide valuable information for diagnosis, for planning of margin resection in surgical excision, and for monitoring the therapeutic response during follow-up [2].

12.2 Autofluorescence: Background

The extent and nature of structural and biochemical changes taking place during the transformation from normal to precancerous state to oral cancer are poorly understood.

The *native cellular fluorescence* is the innate capacities of tissues to absorb and transmit light. It has been well recognized since many years that several subcellular components, called *fluorophores*, are capable of emitting light of specific wavelengths different from that of an exciting radiation.

Fluorophores can be classified into endogenous and exogenous. Endogenous fluorophores, either intracellular or extracellular, are present in several biologic tissues, being responsible for the phenomenon of autofluorescence (AF). Autofluorescence is a peculiar visual property of some tissues depending on the concentration and distribution of specific fluorophores.

In the literature, the use of this property in differentiating normal from neoplastic oral mucosa is widely reported [3].

The technique of AF detection is based on illumination of suspicious lesions with monochromatic light, followed by the recording of fluorescent spectra emitted by endogenous tissue fluorophores. The presence of disease results in alteration in concentration of fluorophores as well as in alteration of light scattering and absorption properties of tissue, nuclear size changes and distribution, collagen content, and epithelial thickness, which leads to spectral variations [4].

It has been hypothesized that fluorophores of oral human tissues are some proteins (e.g., structural proteins, collagen, elastin; coat proteins, keratin) and several coenzymes involved in cellular metabolism, including nicotinamide adenine dinucleotide (NADH) and flavin adenine dinucleotide (FAD). Such molecules are stimulated by wavelengths between blue and violet/ultraviolet light.

The reduced form of NADH and the oxidized form of FAD are important fluorophores that are good indicators of cellular metabolism. It has been shown that fluorescence intensity due to NADH increases with dysplastic progression, while that of FAD decreases. Maximum NADH fluorescence occurs at 340-nm excitation and 45-nm emission, and FAD occurs at 450-nm excitation and 515-nm emission [5].

Another source of AF originates in the submucosal collagen cross-links which have been demonstrated to decrease in the immediate vicinity of malignant or premalignant lesions.

Loss of collagen fluorescence is generally attributed to changes in its biochemistry, possibly due to the breakdown of the extracellular matrix by dysplastic cells.

Collagen cross-links and basal lamina of tissue affected by cancer or epithelial dysplasia are destroyed, and glucose is highly consumed in malignant tissue even in an aerobic environment. On the contrary, the concentration of FAD decreases in epithelial dysplastic tissues [6].

One hypothesis is that matrix metalloproteinase (MMP) expression in stromal cells and the consequent remodeling of the extracellular matrix are induced by altered signaling from dysplastic epithelial cells. Collagen yields maximum fluorescence at 340-nm excitation and 420-nm emission and has significant fluorescence when excited between 410 and 470 nm [5].

12.3 Autofluorescence: A Diagnostic Support in Oral Cancer and Precancerous Lesions

Oral squamous cell carcinoma (OSCC) has an incidence of more than 500,000 cases per year worldwide.

The most important prognostic factor in influencing the disease-specific survival rate is the tumor stage at diagnosis.

The 5-year relative survival rate is 64.3%. However, survival rates for OSCC are highly stage-dependent, with 83.7% of people alive 5 years after diagnosis when a localized cancer is diagnosed and 64.2% and 38.5% of people alive 5 years after diagnosis when regional and distant metastases are diagnosed, respectively. Approximately 70% of all new cases are diagnosed at a late stage, underscoring the importance of early detection and prevention [7].

The diagnostic pathway for oral suspicious lesions usually starts with the conventional objective examination (COE) based on inspection and palpation of the oral mucosa with the support of an incandescent light available on the dental chair. It is well known that COE mainly depends on a subjective interpretation, which is a consequence of the experience of the operator.

Oral epithelial dysplasia (OED) is often observed in the tissue surrounding oral squamous cell carcinoma (OSCC), and it is reportedly associated with a malignant transformation rate of 2.2–38.1% [8].

Moreover, epithelial dysplasia and early oral cancer can be located within the context of oral potentially malignant disorders such as leukoplakia, erythroplakia, submucous fibrosis, and oral lichen planus as well in areas of apparently healthy mucosa.

The gold standard for the diagnosis of oral dysplastic and neoplastic malignant lesions is the histological examination. Incisional or excisional biopsy techniques are the most reliable methods to collect a surgical specimen suitable for microscopic evaluation. However, despite the little invasivity of such techniques, they still have some disadvantages in terms of morbidity and possible artifacts induced by the method of collection.

Direct visual fluorescence examination (DVFE) is based on the action of irradiation of specific wavelengths, between 375 and 440 nm, which excites some natural fluorochromes which show fluorescence in the range of the green color. The analysis of the lesions with AF tools must be performed in a dark environment to avoid the interference of white light wavelengths and to improve the quality of recorded images (Fig. 12.1). Healthy oral mucosa emits fluorescence, detectable as green light (Figs. 12.2, 12.3, 12.4, and 12.5). Cell and tissues within dysplastic and malignant lesions display modifications of the amount and distribution and chemical–physical properties of the endogenous fluorophores.

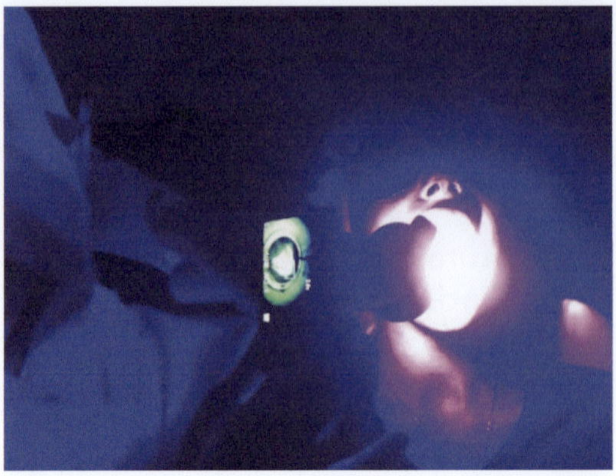

Fig. 12.1 The analysis of the lesions with AF tools must be performed in a dark environment to avoid the interference of white light wavelengths

This results in an autofluorescence pattern variation that can be potentially used at diagnostic level. Loss of autofluorescence (LAF) seems to increase in correspondence to the progression of dysplasia, and altered tissue appears dark (brown to black) (Figs. 12.6 and 12.7). LAF in dysplasia and carcinoma seems to be connected to different mechanisms, such as altered metabolic activity of dysplastic keratinocytes, altered structure of subepithelial collagen, and absorbance of light by increased blood circulation due to inflammatory phenomena in dysplastic tissue and cancer [2].

According to some clinical experiences reported in the literature, red lesions are related to hypofluorescence, whereas white lesions are mostly related to hyperfluorescence, most probably because of keratin increase. There is a significant association of OED and carcinoma and autofluorescence alteration considering both hypo- and hyperfluorescence.

OED and carcinoma are particularly associated with hypofluorescence, excluding verrucous car-

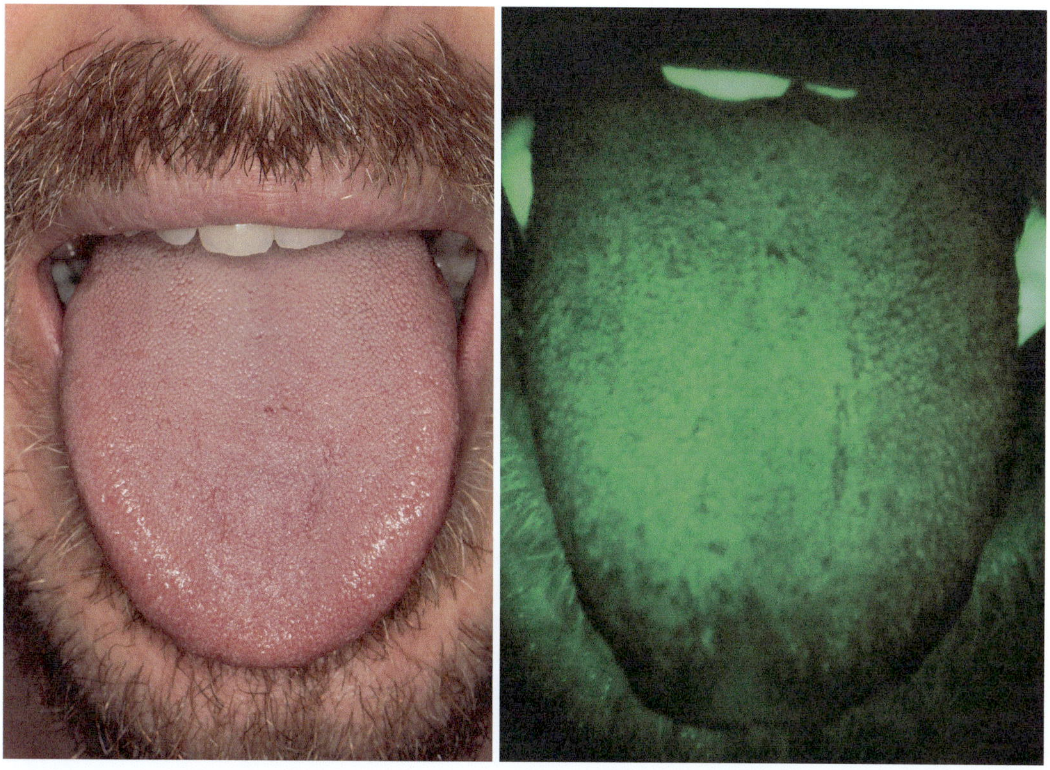

Figs. 12.2 and 12.3 Dorsum of the tongue under visible light and in AF: healthy oral mucosa, under 410–460-nm excitation, emits fluorescence detectable as a green light

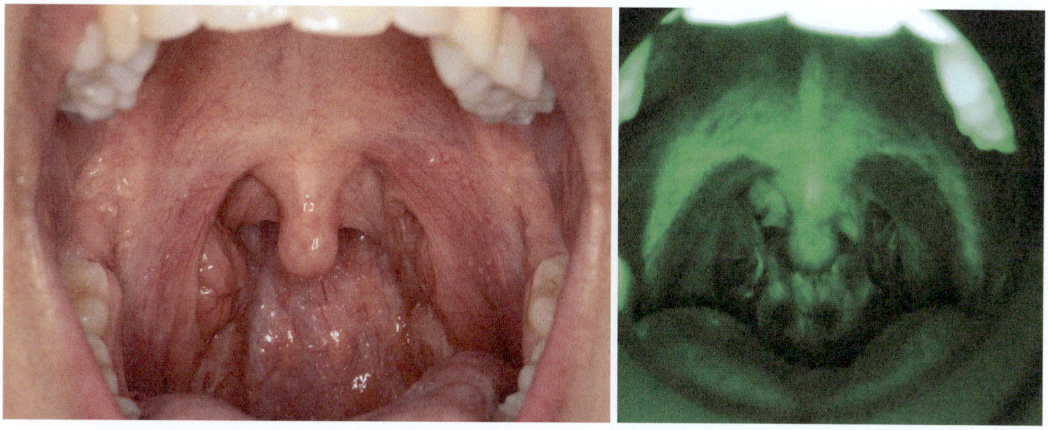

Figs. 12.4 and 12.5 Soft palate under visible light and in AF: healthy oral mucosa, under 410–460-nm excitation, emits fluorescence detectable as a green light

cinomas, which appear hyperfluorescent because of intense keratinization.

AF analysis could be a valid adjunctive technique if associated with the clinician experience and knowledge. It may be used to spot lesions at risk, to identify suitable sites for incisional biopsies, and to define excision margins of the lesions.

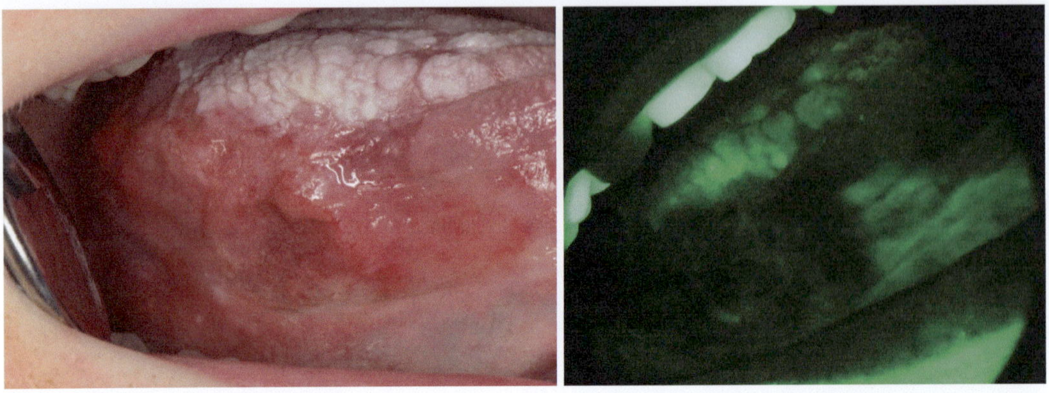

Figs. 12.6 and 12.7 Border of the tongue under visible light and in AF: oral squamous cell carcinoma exhibits a dark area of loss of autofluorescence (LAF)

12.4 Clinical Applications of Autofluorescence in Oral Surgery

AF can be used for guiding incisional biopsy and in the excision to identify the resection margins.

12.4.1 Autofluorescence-Guided Biopsy

For patients seeking care for suspicious lesions, immediate performance of a biopsy or referral to a specialist is an important recommendation in clinical practice.

Potentially malignant oral disorders are a group of clinically suspicious conditions, a small percentage of which will undergo malignant transformation. Dysplasia is the most well-established marker to distinguish high-risk lesions from low-risk lesions, and performing a biopsy to establish dysplasia is the diagnostic gold standard. *Dysplasia* is defined as the presence of specific epithelial architectural and cytologic changes, and it can be graded as mild, moderate, or severe based on the depth and severity of the cellular changes. It is frequently assumed that oral carcinogenesis involves oral premalignant disorders that undergo a gradual progression evolving through stages of mild dysplasia, moderate dysplasia, severe dysplasia, carcinoma in situ, and finally carcinoma after cellular invasion through the basement membrane [9]. However, oral premalignant disorders with dysplasia are considered non-obligate precursors of OSCC, indicating that not all dysplastic lesions will progress to invasive cancer [10].

COE is generally effective for lesion identification, but not always for the biopsy planning. Once the decision has been made to perform a biopsy lesion, clinicians must select a bioptic site, which should represent the area of the lesion most likely to contain dysplasia or carcinoma [11].

AF can be useful for simple incisional biopsies for homogeneous lesions or multiple biopsies for multifocal, large, or nonhomogeneous lesions. In particular, for the last type of lesions, it is difficult to indicate representative biopsy area.

In a surface with a diffuse and homogeneous green light aspect, some area of hypofluorescence (or in certain cases of hyperfluorescence) can be suspected, and the biopsy can be performed at these sites [12] (Figs. 12.8, 12.9, 12.10, 12.11, 12.12, and 12.13).

According to the literature, tissue AF imaging revealed a heterogeneous pattern of loss and increase of fluorescence in patients with actinic

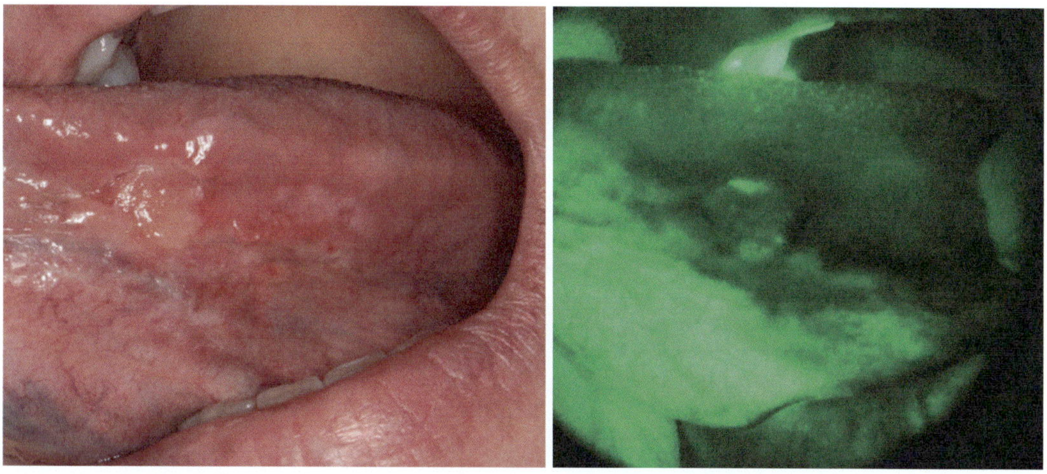

Figs. 12.8 and 12.9 Border of the tongue under visible light and in AF: erythroplasic nonhomogeneous lesion with area of loss of autofluorescence (LAF)

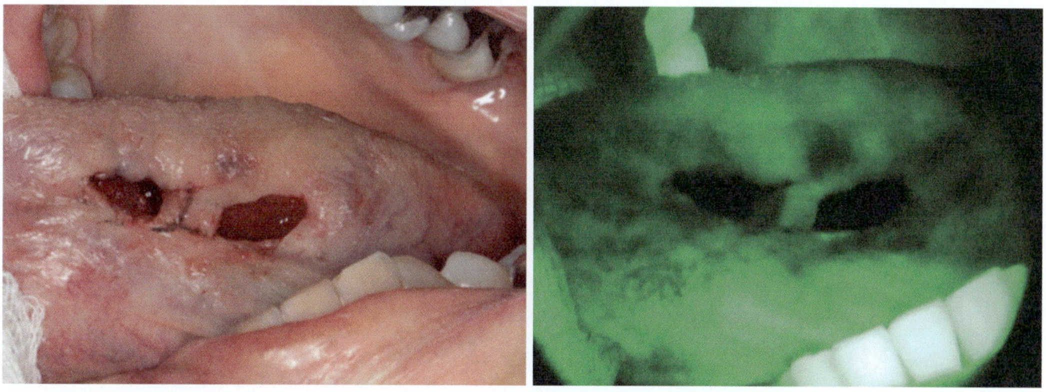

Figs. 12.10 and 12.11 Two biopsies performed in the hypofluorescent areas

cheilitis (AC). Epithelial dysplasia was found in 93% of the cases, and most of the areas graded as moderate or severe were chosen for incisional biopsy with the aid of AF.

The advantages of AF in incisional biopsies include high sensitivity for dysplasia and cancer, capability to assess large areas of the oral mucosa at the point of care, nonrequirement of consumables, and noninvasiveness (Figs. 12.14, 12.15, 12.16, 12.17, and 12.18).

Unfortunately, the application of AF can be limited by false-positive results: inflammatory benign lesions, infectious stomatitis, and vascular diseases often exhibit a loss of fluorescence (Figs. 12.19 and 12.20). Keratin is autofluorescent, and hyperkeratinized high-risk diseases such as proliferative verrucous leukoplakia may not show LOF even in the presence of dysplasia or cancer (Figs. 12.21 and 12.22). AF may have clinical utility for risk assessment during longitudinal monitoring of patients with known high-risk potentially malignant oral disorders (such as proliferative verrucous leukoplakia, oral lichenoid lesions, and oral lichen planus) or

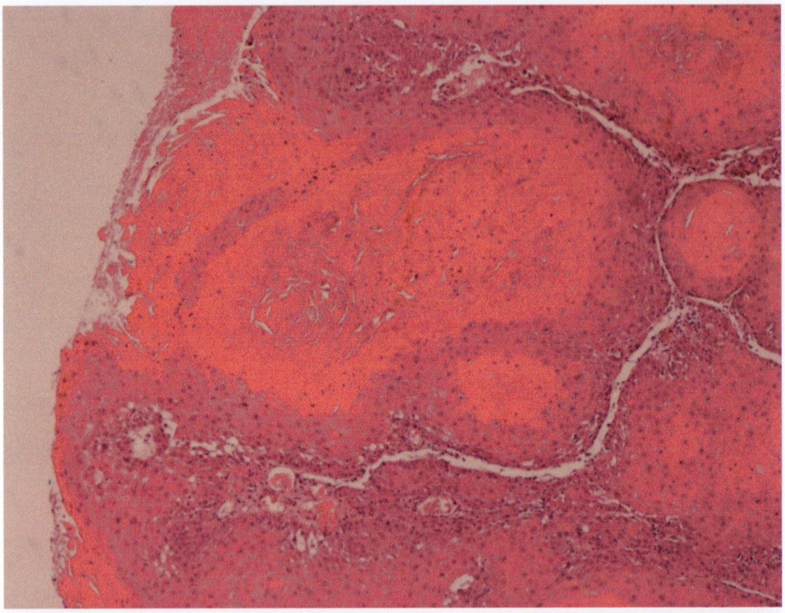

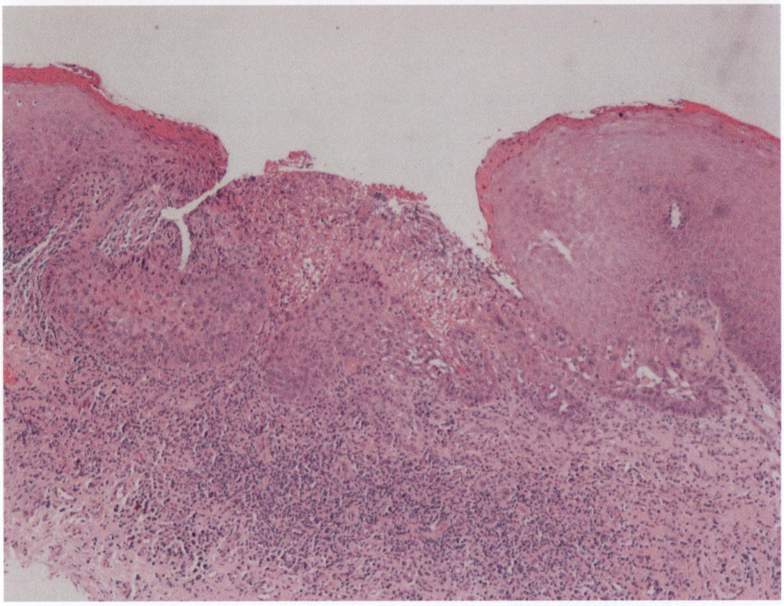

Figs. 12.12 and 12.13 Histopathological results: invasive (Fig. 12.12) and microinvasive (Fig. 12.13) oral squamous cell carcinoma (OSCC)

previous history of cancer of the upper aerodigestive tract [13].

12.4.2 Autofluorescence-Guided Excision

Excisional biopsy can be performed for smaller lesions and could prevent sampling bias, but the risk of incomplete excision of malignant lesions exists, and the procedure may be not indicated in case of benign lesions.

Because the statistically significant reported risk factors for malignant transformation of leukoplakia include the presence of epithelial dysplasia, we support the opinion that surgical resection with adequately radical margins including the area of epithelial dysplasia would be effective in preventing malignant transformation.

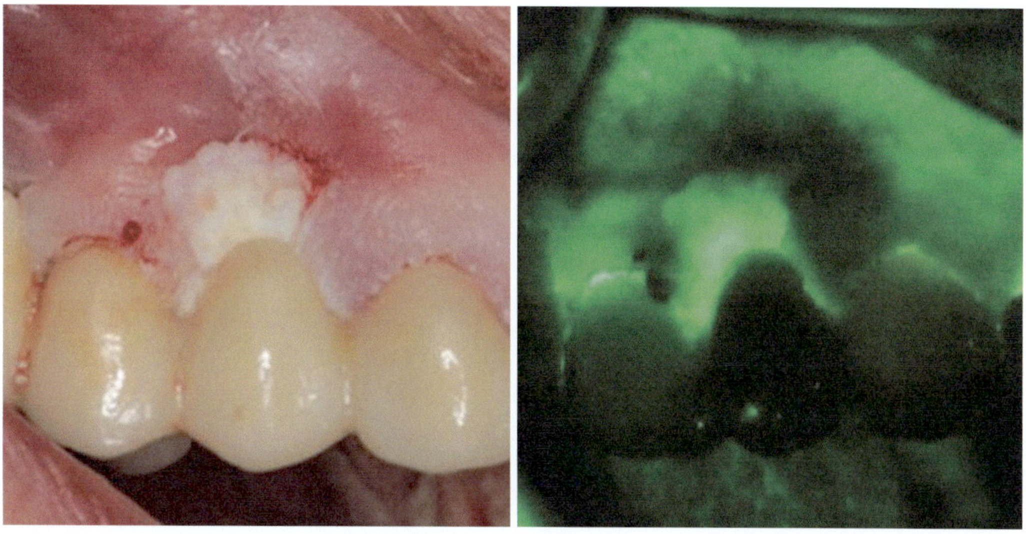

Figs. 12.14 and 12.15 Gingiva under visible light and in AF: hyperfluorescent surface surrounded by hypofluorescent area

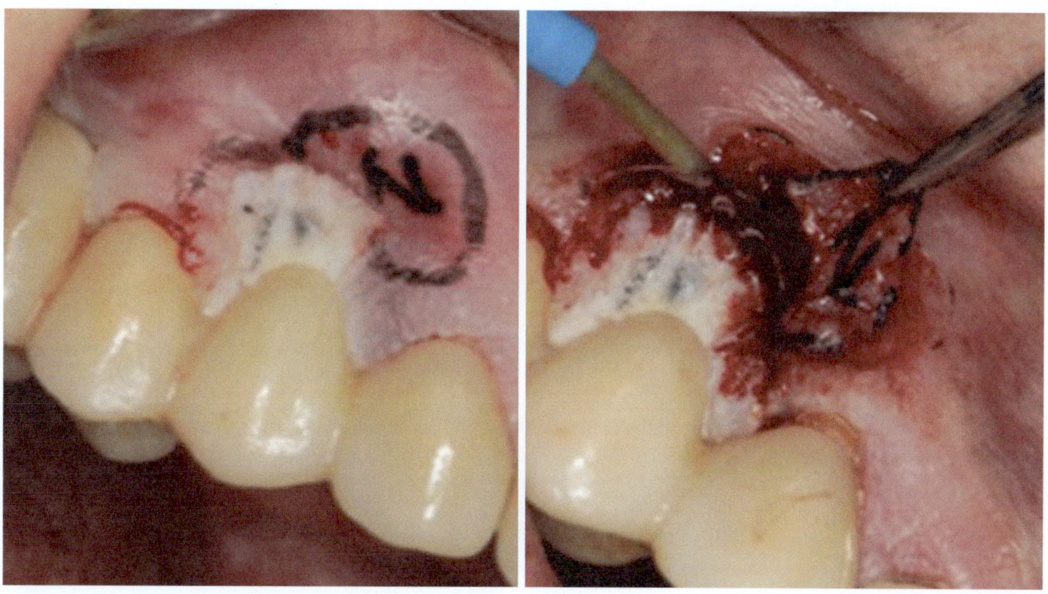

Fig. 12.16 Biopsy performed in two different areas

Residual epithelial dysplasia after surgical treatment of oral cancer is an important risk factor for poor prognosis, and precise detection of affected areas with epithelial dysplasia prior to surgical resection of malignant lesions is important to prevent local recurrence [14].

AF can be used to delineate margins during surgical resection of OSCC to reduce recurrence rates. LOF frequently extends beyond the visible borders of a lesion, and such extension often shows dysplasia and loss of heterozygosity (Figs. 12.23, 12.24, 12.25, and 12.26).

Recent experiences reported in the literature indicate that the molecular profile of oral potentially malignant disorders changes with divergence away from the center of the lesion and that

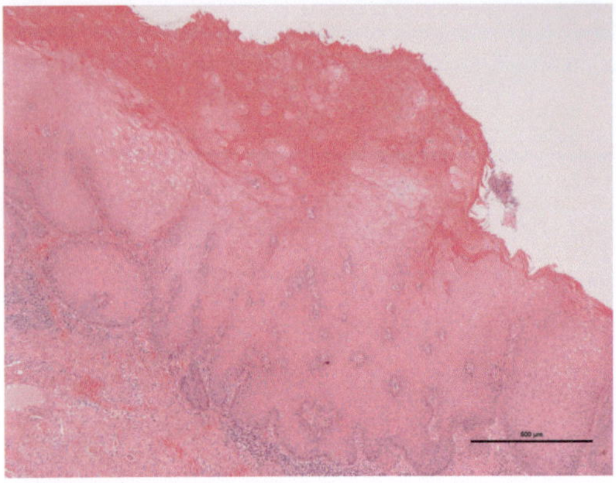

Fig. 12.17 Hyperfluorescent tissue revealed verrucous carcinoma

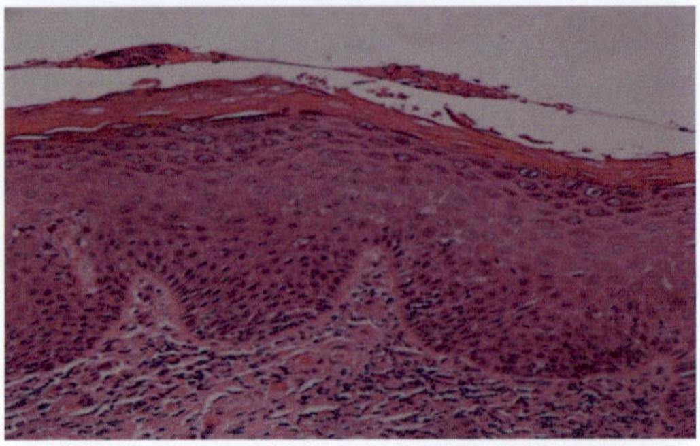

Fig. 12.18 Hypofluorescent area showed mild dysplasia

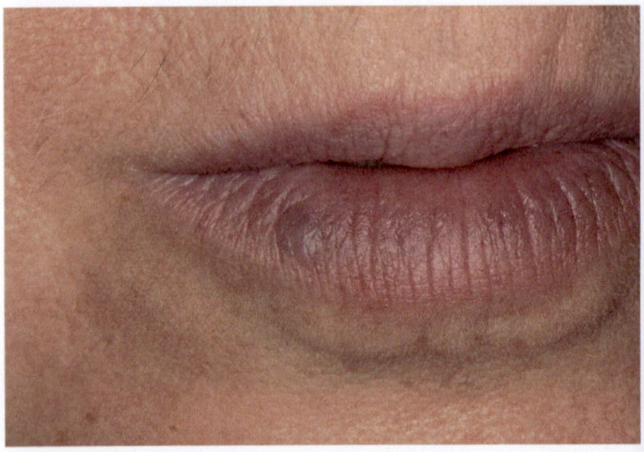

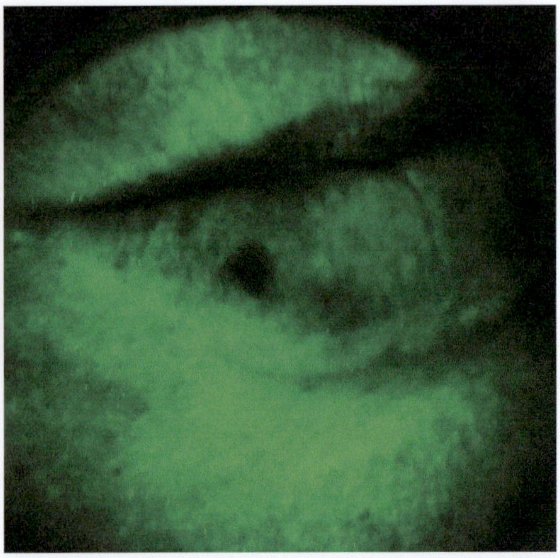

Figs. 12.19 and 12.20 False positive: vascular benign lesion of the lip shows area of a loss of autofluorescence (LAF) for the presence of blood and hemoglobin

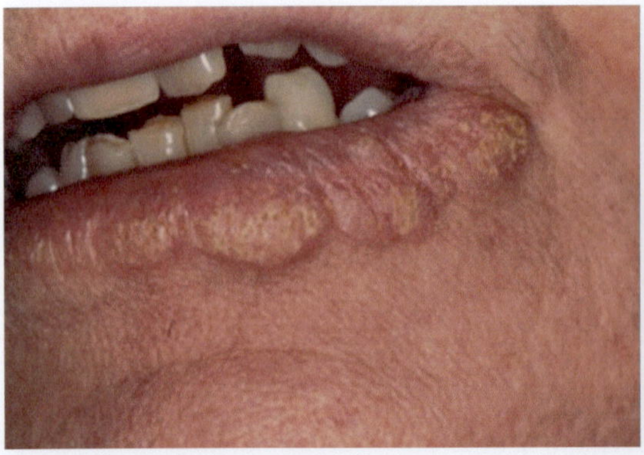

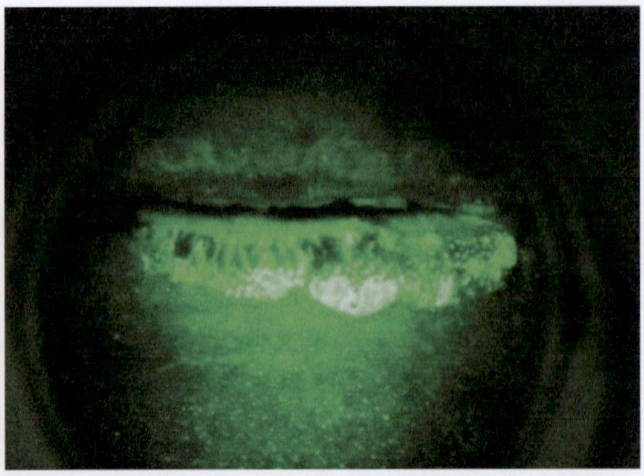

Figs. 12.21 and 12.22 False negative: squamous cell carcinoma of the lip shows intense hyperfluorescence for the presence of intense keratinization

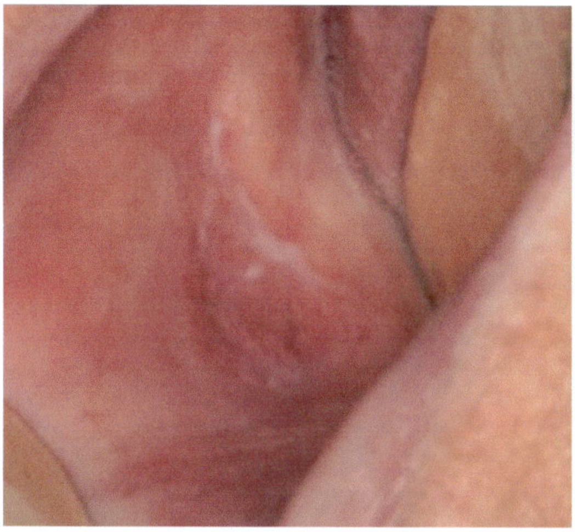

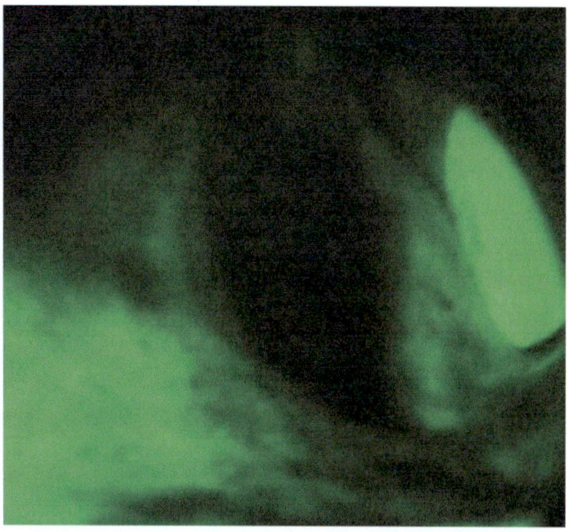

Figs. 12.23 and 12.24 Dishomogeneous oral lichenoid lesion of the cheek under visible light and in AF: intense dark area (loss of autofluorescence, LAF) much wider than the visible lesion in conventional objective examination (COE)

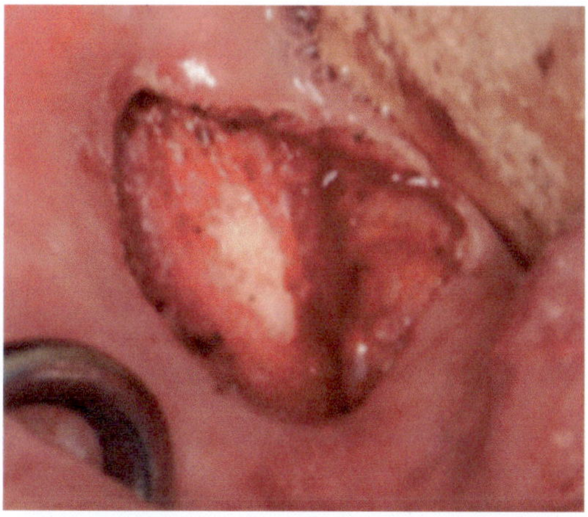

Fig. 12.25 Surgical excision extended to margins of hypofluorescent area

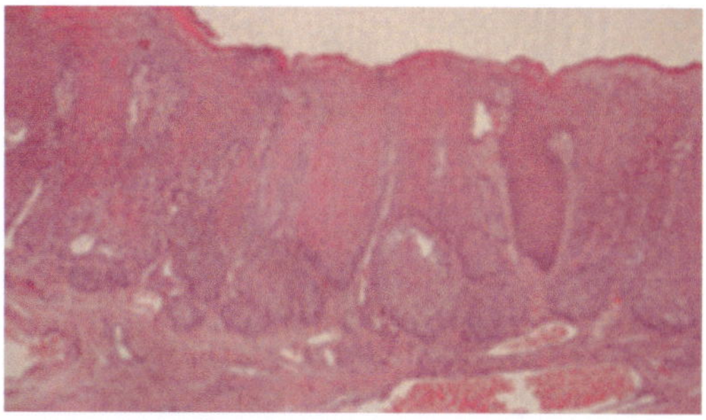

Fig. 12.26 Histopathological examination revealed micro-invasive oral squamous cell carcinoma (OSCC)

autofluorescence determined margins are superior to the white light margin in achieving a clear molecular margin when excising an OPMD [15].

Some leukoplakias show clinically invisible extensions during histopathological examination and AF. Most of leukoplakias are not surrounded by green light but by dark areas, indicating LOF with a mean size of 66%, exceeding the clinically visible margins of the disease. This technique enables clinicians to measure the extent of lesions beyond their visible margins [16].

Surgical operations for advanced stages of oral cancer are invasive with poor prognosis. On the contrary, a minimal and faster intervention under local anesthesia is useful both for compliance of the patients and for the success of the treatment. Early detection of suspicious lesions through AF and less invasive surgery performed with different lasers (Er:YAG, CO2, diode, Nd:YAG) guided by AF for healthy margin detection may determine a complete mucosal healing containing the risk of spread of the disease and reduce the risk of cancerization [17–20].

12.5 Conclusions

The usefulness of autofluorescence for oral tissue examination, especially within an oral medicine secondary care facility, before performing a biopsy and in monitoring oral lesions is confirmed by several studies [21]. In patients with clinically evident, potentially malignant, or seemingly malignant lesions, clinicians should perform a biopsy of the lesion. Autofluorescence represents an important support to conventional objective examination and palpation. For general dental practitioners, devices using AF are potentially useful for screening purposes. Furthermore, referral to a specialist for a biopsy (clinicians with training in oral and maxillofacial surgery, oral and maxillofacial pathology, oral medicine, and otolaryngology–head and neck surgery) is indicated when clinicians are not trained adequately to perform a biopsy of precancerous or cancerous lesions.

References

1. Warnakulasuriya S. Global epidemiology of oral and oropharyngeal cancer. Oral Oncol. 2009;45:309–16.
2. Giovannacci I, Vescovi P, Manfredi M, Meleti M. Non-invasive visual tools for diagnosis of oral cancer and dysplasia: a systematic review. Med Oral Patol Oral Cir Bucal. 2016;21(3):e305–15.
3. Nazeer SS, Asish R, Venugopal C, Anita B, Gupta AK, Jayasree RS. Noninvasive assessment of the risk of tobacco abuse in oral mucosa using fluorescence spectroscopy: a clinical approach. J Biomed Opt. 2014;19(5):057013.
4. Jayanthi JL, Mallia RJ, Shiny ST, Baiju KV, Mathews A, Kumar R, et al. Discriminant analysis of autofluorescence spectra for classification of oral lesions in vivo. Lasers Surg Med. 2009;41(5):345–52.
5. Lane PM, Gilhuly T, Whitehead P, Zeng H, Poh CF, Ng S, et al. Simple device for the direct visualization of oral-cavity tissue fluorescence. J Biomed Opt. 2006;11(2):024006.
6. Monici M. Cell and tissue autofluorescence research and diagnostic applications. Biotechnol Annu Rev. 2005;11:227–56.
7. Lingen MW, Abt E, Agrawal N, et al. Evidence-based clinical practice guideline for the evaluation of potentially malignant disorders in the oral cavity. J Am Dent Assoc. 2017;148:712–27.
8. Yamamoto N, Kawaguchi K, Fujihara H, Hasebe M, et al. Detection accuracy for epithelial dysplasia using an objective autofluorescence visualization method based on the luminance ratio. Int J Oral Sci. 2017;9:e2. https://doi.org/10.1038/ijos.2017.37. Online publication 10 Nov 2017.
9. Warnakulasuriya S, Johnson NW, Van Der Waal I. Nomenclature and classification of potentially malignant disorders of the oral mucosa. J Oral Pathol Med. 2007;36:575–80.
10. Patel KJ, De Silva HL, Tong DC, Love RM. Concordance between clinical and histopathologic diagnoses of oral mucosal lesions. J Oral Maxillofac Surg. 2011;69:125–33.
11. Epstein JB, Güneri P, Boyacioglu H, Abt E. The limitations of the clinical oral examination in detecting dysplastic oral lesions and oral squamous cell carcinoma. J Am Dent Assoc. 2012;143:1332–42.
12. Rana M, Zapf A, Kuehle M, Gellrich NC, Eckardt AM. Clinical evaluation of an autofluorescence diagnostic device for oral cancer detection: a prospective randomized diagnostic study. Eur J Cancer Prev. 2012;21(5):460–6.
13. Takahama Junior A, Kurachi C, Cosci A, Pereira Faustino IS, Camisasca DR, da Costa Fontes KB, Pires FR, Azevedo RS. Usefulness of tissue autofluorescence imaging in actinic cheilitis diagnosis. J Biomed Opt. 2013;18(7):76023. https://doi.org/10.1117/1.JBO.18.7.076023.
14. Yang EC, Tan MT, Schwarz RA, Richards-Kortum RR, Gillenwater AM, Vigneswaran N. Noninvasive diagnostic adjuncts for the evaluation of potentially premalignant oral epithelial lesions: current limitations and future directions. Oral Surg Oral Med Oral Pathol Oral Radiol. 2018. pii: S2212-4403(18)30092-0.; https://doi.org/10.1016/j.oooo.2018.02.020.
15. Farah CS, Kordbacheh F, John K, Bennett N, Fox SA. Molecular classification of autofluorescence excision margins in oral potentially malignant disorders. Oral Dis. 2017;24:732. https://doi.org/10.1111/odi.12818. [Epub ahead of print].
16. Elvers D, Braunschweig T, Hilgers RD, Ghassemi A, Möhlhenrich SC, Hölzle F, Gerressen M, Modabber A. Margins of oral leukoplakia: autofluorescence and histopathology. Br J Oral Maxillofac Surg. 2015 Feb;53(2):164–9.
17. Monteiro L, Barbieri C, Warnakulasuriya S, Martins M, Salazar F, Pacheco JJ, Vescovi P, Meleti M. Type of surgical treatment and recurrence of oral leukoplakia: a retrospective clinical study. Med Oral Patol Oral Cir Bucal. 2017;22(5):e520–6.
18. Nammour S, Zeinoun T, Namour A, Vanheusden A, Vescovi P. Evaluation of different laser-supported surgical protocols for the treatment of oral leukoplakia: a long-term follow-up. Photomed Laser Surg. 2017;35(11):629–38.

19. Del Corso G, Gissi DB, Tarsitano A, Costabile E, Marchetti C, Montebugnoli L, Foschini MP. Laser evaporation versus laser excision of oral leukoplakia: a retrospective study with long-term follow-up. J Craniomaxillofac Surg. 2015;43(6):763–8. https://doi.org/10.1016/j.jcms.2015.04.009. Epub 2015 Apr 17.
20. Huang Z, Wang Y, Liang Q, Zhang L, Zhang D, Chen W. The application of a carbon dioxide laser in the treatment of superficial oral mucosal lesions. J Craniofac Surg. 2015;26(3):e277–9.
21. Paderni C, Compilato D, Carinci F, Nardi G, Rodolico V, Lo Muzio L, Spinelli G, Mazzotta M, Campisi G. Direct visualization of oral-cavity tissue fluorescence as novel aid for early oral cancer diagnosis and potentially malignant disorders monitoring. Int J Immunopathol Pharmacol. 2011;24(2 Suppl):121–8.

13 Cartilage Reshaping

Jeffrey T. Gu and Brian J. F. Wong

Contents

Abstract

In this chapter, we introduce the working theory of cartilage reshaping and highlight landmark papers in the development and refinement of this technique. We discuss the tissue and mechanical properties of cartilage and define how optical techniques may be utilized to manipulate these properties. The goal of cartilage reshaping is to ultimately reduce the need for more invasive traditional approaches with scalpel and suture, in favor of much less invasive techniques. Therefore, we discuss the challenges associated with its development and delineate its translation toward clinical applications.

Keywords

Cartilage reshaping · Optical techniques
Airway reshaping · Rhinoplasty · Otoplasty

J. T. Gu · B. J. F. Wong (✉)
Department of Otolaryngology-Head & Neck Surgery, UC Irvine School of Medicine, Irvine, CA, USA
e-mail: jtgu@uci.edu; bjwong@uci.edu

S. Stübinger et al. (eds.), *Lasers in Oral and Maxillofacial Surgery*,
https://doi.org/10.1007/978-3-030-29604-9_13

13.1 Introduction

Classical approaches to altering the shape of cartilage in the head, neck, and upper airway have focused on creating incisions in the cartilage to weaken it focally or using sutures to balance the forces which resist sustained deformation. Surgery as a whole is steeped in the use of these conventional approaches which require gaining access to individual cartilage specimens through incisions within the nose or neck.

Cartilage itself is a complex tissue which is triphasic in structure, having its mechanical state determined by the interplay of viscoelastic, hydrodynamic, and electrostatic forces. This specific behavior is well beyond the scope of this discussion here but has been examined in detail by Mow and Lai, among others [1–4]. Importantly, cartilage may be thought of as a charged polymer hydrogel, and if one examines cartilage from the vantage of a materials scientist, one can think of alternate ways of creating shape change, without the need potentially for either destructive techniques involving scalpels or techniques involving sutures. Early in the 1950s, Lewis Thomas, in fact, had examined the potential use of enzymes to locally disrupt the bonds between the glycosaminoglycans in the cartilage of rabbit ears and was able to demonstrate transient changes in tissue geometry [5–9]. While promising, the effect was noted to be completely reversible, which negated any further exploration of this approach toward clinical implementation.

In contemporary times, Emil Sobol of the Russian Academy of Sciences in Troitsk, while on sabbatical in Crete, had the opportunity to work with Emmanuel Helidonis, who is an otolaryngologist. Helidonis had an extensive medical laser facility, and Sobol spent his time identifying areas where advanced laser technology might optimize surgery. As an alternative to morselization, Sobol proposed that cartilage could be heated and then undergo a phase transformation that would lead to an alteration of shape. In this implementation, cartilage which is itself curved or misshapen is first mechanically deformed, and then laser energy is directed at areas where internal stress is concentrated. Focally within these regions of interest, temperature elevation leads to a local alteration in tissue mechanical properties and an acceleration of stress relaxation.

The net effect is shape change, which in this case early on was focused on changing the shape of the nasal septal cartilage. Regardless, the use of photothermal techniques to reshape cartilage is still investigational, though much basic research has focused on this application. The use of lasers to reshape cartilage has been studied in great detail, though the precise mechanism still remains elusive. The hope and goal of this technique is that traditional cut-and-suture approaches to altering cartilage shape could be replaced by methods which are minimally invasive, potentially transcutaneous, or delivered via fiber optics and small-bore needles.

Likewise, in parallel with research performed in laser reshaping, other techniques that alter the shape of facial cartilages have been developed. These include the application of radiofrequency energy as well as the creation of in situ redox reactions in the tissue. All of these approaches do share in common a fundamental difference from classic surgical technique in that these view cartilage as a plastic material.

The remainder of this chapter reviews the basic science behind facial cartilage reshaping using laser and related technologies and provides a comprehensive review of the literature.

13.2 Basic Science of Cartilage Reshaping

13.2.1 Laser Shaping of Cartilage

In living organisms, cartilage serves to support and fasten soft tissues and to absorb shock for skeletal bones. Cartilage is a dense connective tissue composed of 65–80% of water containing a small proportion of chondrocytes within an extracellular matrix (ECM). The ECM is a hydrated gel containing proteoglycans (5–15%) and collagen fibers (20–25%). The proteoglycan matrix possesses negatively charged ion groups (SO^{3-} and COO^{-} moieties). Therefore, cartilage can be thought of as a charged hydrogel where free space is filled with water in either partially bound or free states. Polarized water molecules bind weakly to the negatively charged groups attached to both proteoglycan and collagen molecules. Free water within the cartilage matrix contains dissolved minerals such as Na^+ and Ca^{2+} ions, which are attracted to the negatively charged components of proteoglycan molecules (Fig. 13.1). These ions are therefore trapped in the matrix when free water is forced out of it during deformation or evaporation. A gradient in distribution of negatively charged groups in the tissue accounts for the intramolecular internal stresses of the tissue. Since the ECM is nonvascular, maintenance of its mechanical structure and nutrition for chondrocytes depends on the diffusion of fluids [11]. The mechanical properties of cartilage shape retention are accounted for by the development of areas of high internal stress upon mechanical deformation and the property of shape memorization whereby shape recovery is possible after deformation.

In 1993, Emil Sobol et al. were the first to describe the use of lasers in altering cartilage shape [11]. Sobol hypothesized that local laser heating may lead to increased plasticity by relaxing the internal stresses, thereby leading to shape change with fluence rate profiles below the ablation threshold. Under ordinary conditions, mechanical resistance to sustained cartilage deformation is largely due to the intermolecular forces between water and proteoglycan models. Under moderate laser heating, Sobol hypothesized that there is a momentary relaxation in internal stress when water transitions from a state in which it is bound to proteoglycans to a liberated free state. If this bound-to-free phase transition of water can occur without damaging surrounding protein or carbohydrate molecules, then a stable modified cartilage configuration may be achieved.

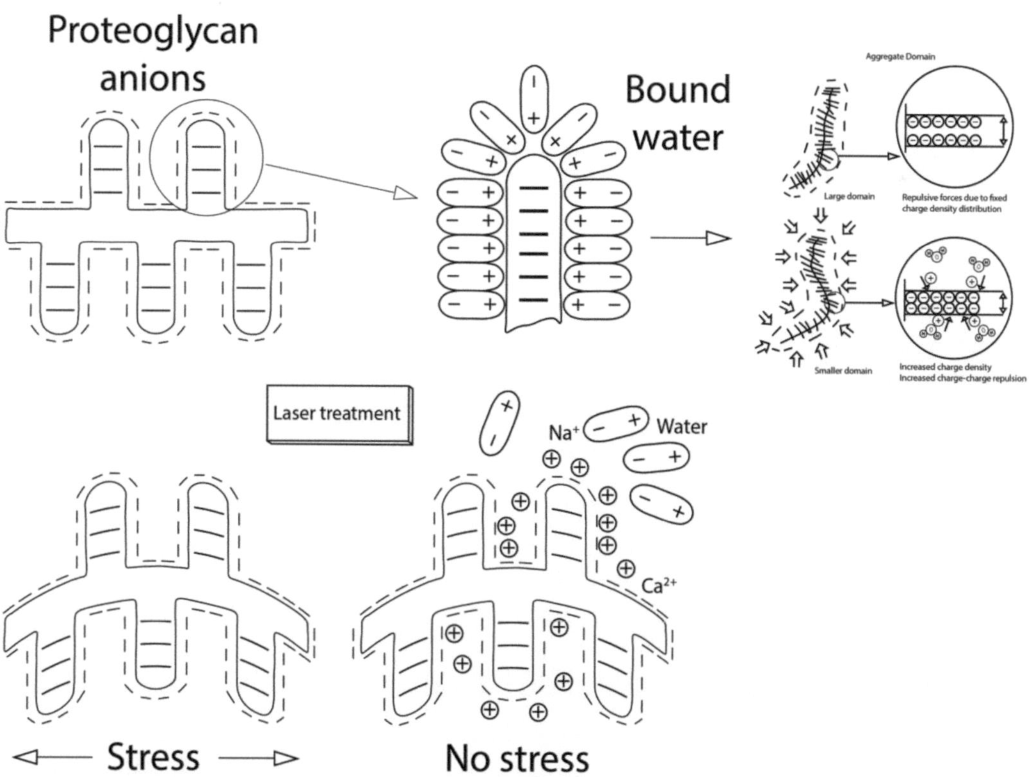

Fig. 13.1 Mechanisms of stress relaxation in cartilage (After Sobol et al. Laser Reshaping of Cartilage. Biotechnology and Genetic Engineering Reviews 2000 [10])

Sobol et al. demonstrated laser shape change on samples of cartilage from 0.2 to 1.5 mm in thickness using a CO_2 laser with 1–10 W in average power output. Cartilage samples were mechanically fixed in a new shape and exposed to either repetitively pulsed (pulse duration of 0.2 s, pulse repetition rate of 1 Hz) or continuous wave treatment regimens. Cartilage samples treated in this manner retained their shape for several months and could be implanted into animal models or kept in storage for later use, though banking of autologous cartilage is by no means common practice in North America.

13.2.2 Ex Vivo Cartilage Reshaping

After Sobol's initial studies on the use of lasers for reshaping cartilage, more detailed studies followed to characterize the effects of laser irradiation on tissue structure and viability and to attempt to identify optimal dosimetry. In subsequent studies, a holmium:YAG (Ho:YAG) laser (2.12-μm wavelength) was used to reshape a 1-mm-thick cartilage specimen without overheating or gross destruction of tissue near the surface [10]. Confocal microscopy and histology determined that thermal injury was deeper using Ho:YAG (up to more than 1800 μm) than with an Er:YAG laser (2.94 μm) (up to 70 μm) as expected, suggesting that Ho:YAG lasers should be used judiciously with pulse energies as low as possible to reduce collateral tissue damage [12].

Atomic force microscopy images of the fine structure of cartilage following CO_2 laser irradiation showed the formation of micro-channels of 100–400 nm in cross section, lending some credence to a proposed mechanism for laser-induced stress relaxation of cartilage being based on short-time polymerization and subsequent reformation of proteoglycan units. These micro-channels may facilitate transport of traces of proteoglycan units possessing a length of ~300–400 nm and a width of ~80 nm. These results were also consistent with changes in light-scattering behavior in cartilage after laser-induced stress relaxation, whereby it is thought that the number of scattering centers first increases due to the short-time liberation of proteoglycan units and then decreases after the new proteoglycan configuration has been formed. Furthermore, sodium carbonate crystals were observed, suggesting that prolonged laser heating of cartilage induces denaturation of proteoglycans and can lead to local mineralization of the cartilaginous matrix [13].

13.2.2.1 Dosimetry Studies

In 2000, Helidonis et al. performed histologic and morphological analysis on CO_2 laser-irradiated rabbit auricular cartilage to assess shape retention and viability [14]. Straight cartilage samples were removed from the ears of 21 rabbits, and the cartilage was reshaped using CO_2 laser at an output power of 3 W, a spot diameter of 2 mm, and exposure time of 0.5 s. Remodeled cartilage, along with control cartilage, was then implanted into the rabbits' backs and retrieved 6–12 months later, after which histology and morphological analyses revealed shape retention and viability of chondrocytes.

Subsequently, investigations were conducted to optimize parameters for cartilage reshaping and to define the therapeutic window within which cartilage is reshaped but not thermally damaged (Fig. 13.2). To this end, Wong et al. designed a computer-controlled instrument to evaluate the effect of laser dosimetry on shape change during laser-mediated cartilage reshap-

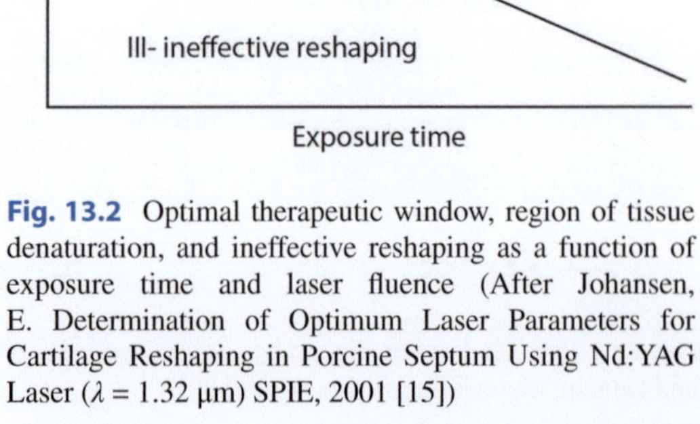

Fig. 13.2 Optimal therapeutic window, region of tissue denaturation, and ineffective reshaping as a function of exposure time and laser fluence (After Johansen, E. Determination of Optimum Laser Parameters for Cartilage Reshaping in Porcine Septum Using Nd:YAG Laser ($\lambda = 1.32$ μm) SPIE, 2001 [15])

ing using an Nd:YAG laser at a wavelength of 1.32 μm [15]. Real-time measurements of tissue optical properties and surface temperatures were obtained, and to determine optimal reshaping, the radius of curvature of the specimen was compared to that of the reshaping jig. Optimal reshaping was observed at 6 W with an irradiation time of 16 s or alternatively at 10 W with an irradiation time of 8 s.

Subsequent investigations focused on characterizing the safety of LCR by determining shape change and tissue viability as a function of laser dosimetry [16]. Similarly, Dobrikov et al. used changes in backscattered He-Ne light intensity to characterize the temperature range in which stress relaxation occurs [17]. Wong et al. utilized the same Nd:YAG laser at 1.32 μm as in previous studies but with a spot diameter of 5.4 mm instead of 5 mm; exposure times of 4, 6, 8, 10, 12, and 16 s; and powers of 4, 6, and 8 W. Cartilage surface temperature measured using infrared thermography and a live/dead viability assay combined with fluorescent confocal microscopy was used to determine the amount of thermal damage generated in irradiated specimens. Confocal microscopy identified dead cells spanning the entire cross-sectional thickness of cartilage specimen within the laser spot at laser power density and exposure times above 4 W and 6 s, with damage proportional to increases in time and irradiance. These results suggested that thermal tissue damage is concurrent with shape change and that significant cell death occurs at laser dosimetry parameters necessary to produce clinically relevant shape changes.

13.2.3 Cartilage Properties

Mow and Lai proposed a triphasic model of articular cartilage as an extension of their earlier biphasic theory [2, 3, 18]. The triphasic model consists of the following three phases: (1) an intrinsically incompressible porous permeable charged solid phase, (2) an intrinsically incompressible interstitial fluid phase, and (3) an ion phase with two monovalent ions (anion and cation). In this theory, the motive forces for water and ions are described by the gradient of chemical or electrochemical potentials. These driving forces are balanced by the frictional forces between the phases as one phase flows through the other. Stress and strain in cartilage is determined by a balance of tissue elastic properties, fluid flow or shift, and electrostatic charge. This model was later extended to incorporate multiple polyvalent ions by Gu et al. [19]

13.2.3.1 Optical Properties of Cartilage

In order to optimize laser cartilage reshaping (LACR), it was important to determine the optical properties of cartilage to facilitate computational modeling. It is well established in the literature that different types of cartilage have different structures and compositions. Sobol's group in 1993 demonstrated that light scattering may identify a phase transformation in cartilage after laser irradiation [20]. Bagratashvili et al. demonstrated that human, pig, and bovine cartilages have similar transmission and reflection spectra, which opened the door for the development of animal models for in vivo studies [21]. Wong et al. through a series of studies that measured integrated backscattered light intensity of He:Ne laser light (λ = 632.8 nm) during laser irradiation by Nd:YAG laser (λ = 1.32 μm) observed an increase, plateau, and then decrease in diffuse reflectance during heating [22–24].

The above developments allowed for later studies by Youn et al. to further characterize optical and thermal properties of nasal septal cartilage using double integrating sphere experiments and thermocouple techniques [25]. Wong et al. demonstrated in 2001 that the tissue optical, mechanical, and biologic properties of septal cartilage varied spatially within each individual sample, as well as between animals within the same species [26]. These measurements would establish baseline values for tissue metabolism, cell density, and the basic biomechanical behavior of porcine and rabbit septal cartilage.

13.2.3.2 Thermal and Mechanical Properties of Cartilage

Stress Relaxation

From a materials science point of view, cartilage may be thought of as a charged polymer hydrogel, with a triphasic structure formed by the interplay of viscoelastic, hydrodynamic, and electrostatic forces. Early hypotheses by Sobol et al. on the mechanism of stress relaxation that occurs upon heating cartilage proposed that this phenomenon relied on a phase transformation dominated by the movement of the water through the matrix [27]. The underlying principle of this hypothesis is that water exists in two forms to form the structure of cartilage: bound, or non-exchangeable, and free, or exchangeable. Upon heating and deformation, a phase change between the two states of water within cartilage allows for stress relaxation to occur within the areas of highest stress, thereby allowing for shape change. The first of many studies to explore this hypothesis examined the thermodynamic characteristics of this "bound-to-free" phase transformation of water [28].

An important observation was made by Sobol et al. in 1997, where it was noted that light scattering increases with stress relaxation and at a temperature exceeding 70 °C [29]. Changes in light scattering were thought to represent the bound-to-free water phase transition, beginning with the formation of nucleus centers or local regions of anomalous refractive index created when water bound to large proteoglycan molecules becomes liberated. When examining the mechanical properties of cartilage following this phase transition, it was observed that stress indeed decreases with some time delay after tissue temperature reaches 70 °C, which was initially hypothesized to represent the internal friction coefficient of cartilage. These observations were used to develop theoretical models which incorporated thermal and mass transfer in a tissue to study the effect of laser irradiation, water evaporation from the surface, and the temperature dependence of the diffusion coefficient [30]. From this model, it was shown that surface temperature reaches a plateau quicker than the maximal temperature, laser-induced mass transfer in cartilage is heterogeneous along the depth, and depth of the denatured area depends on laser fluence, wavelength, exposure time, and thickness of cartilage.

Wong et al. investigated the pattern of backscattered light intensity and internal stress and found that both tend to increase, plateau, and then decrease in similar ways during laser irradiation [31]. The plateau region occurred when the cartilage surface temperature approached 65 °C. These observations clarified the potential of using backscattered light intensity to control the process of laser-assisted cartilage reshaping, which would allow for greater precision of heating, and minimize nonspecific thermal injury due to uncontrolled heating. Bagratashvili et al. examined the phase change through multiple modalities including optical coherence tomography [32]. They describe a bleaching effect similar to the increase in backscattered light described by earlier studies. This bleaching effect was due to structural alterations in irradiated cartilage caused by the removal of water; since water and cartilage matrix have different refractive indices, removal of water leads to increases in scattering signal.

Temperature Dependence of LCR

Although early reports show this transition to occur above 70 °C, later studies have described a range of critical temperatures T_c from 60 °C to 70 °C [31, 33]. To refine this range, Wong et al. studied temperature-dependent changes in thermal properties using modulated differential scanning calorimetry (MDSC), a very precise technique to measure temperature and heat flow associated with transitions in materials as a function of temperature and time [34]. It was observed that slow heating results in a lower critical transition temperature of around 55 °C, in contrast to the rapid heating associated with laser irradiation, with a critical transition temperature of around 65 °C. At around 70 °C, it was noted that heat flow into the specimen reaches a maximum and subsequently decreases, which is in agreement with previous results regarding temperature-dependent changes in optical and mechanical properties of cartilage. Further studies by Sobol et al. demonstrated that light scattering may be useful for measuring denaturation thresholds and kinetics for biological tissues, with denaturation thresholds showing an inverse correlation with the absorption spectrum of the tissue [35].

Mechanical Properties

The elastic modulus describes the intrinsic stress-strain relationships in a material independent of geometry and is the best characterization of the mechanical behavior of cartilage. Investigations into the elastic modulus of cartilage samples contributed to the understanding of shape change in cartilage during laser irradiation and the optimization of this process. Gaon et al. determined the elastic moduli of porcine cartilage before and after Nd:YAG laser irradiation ($\lambda = 1.32$ μm, 21.22 W/cm^2) and found the elastic moduli to be much lower following irradiation [36]. This result confirms that cartilage becomes more flexible after undergoing stress relaxation due to photothermal heating. Gaon et al. also examined the changes in elastic moduli after total thermal denaturation of cartilage samples, which also resulted in a lower elastic modulus. However, the mechanical changes in elastic modulus after laser irradiation were reversible, whereas those following total thermal denaturation were not. Chao et al. conducted similar investigations on the elastic modulus of rabbit nasal septal cartilage and confirmed that this pattern of reversible decreases in elastic modulus is seen in the porcine model and is also seen in the rabbit model [37].

Thermal Properties

It has been hypothesized that cartilage reshaping occurs due to a heat-induced transition that leads to the rearrangement of molecular bonds in the cartilage matrix macromolecules. Chae et al. studied the thermomechanical behavior of cartilage using dynamic mechanical analysis (DMA) and time-temperature superposition (TTS)—techniques used in the rheological sciences to characterize viscoelastic material properties, such as storage and loss modulus, and damping properties [38]. They identified a temperature transition range between 50 °C and 67 °C—consistent with previous results. By using TTS, Chae et al. were able to estimate the activation energy associated with the mechanical relaxation of cartilage as approximately 148 kJ/mole. This estimated activation energy for stress relaxation exceeds that of the evaporation of free water (41–44 kJ/mole), as well as the activation energy of water diffusion (30.6 kJ/mole). Additionally, it was found that a relatively larger activation energy was required for relatively lower concentration of water. This may be due to an increased amount of energy needed to facilitate water movement through the dense ECM and liberate bound water from the proteoglycan side groups.

In order to estimate the thermal influence on the physical shape of a cartilage sample, Wright et al. rapidly immersed porcine nasal septal cartilage in saline water baths and measured resulting bend angles [39]. This was performed to emulate uniform or bulk volumetric heating of thin cartilage specimens held in deformation. The largest bend angle was seen at 74 °C with an immersion time of 320 s. In a following study, Wright et al. examined the dependence of cartilage shape change on both temperature and laser dosimetry using laser irradiation in addition to saline bath immersion [40]. From this investigation, the critical transition temperature region was determined by the sharp increase in bend angle at consecutive times of immersion at the same temperature (59–68 °C and 62–68 °C for porcine and rabbit cartilage, respectively). As for laser irradiation, similar transition zones for dosimetry occurred below 20.4 W/cm^2 for both species.

In a later study by Chae et al., temperature modulate differential scanning calorimetry (TMDSC) is a technique that is used to differentiate between thermodynamic and kinetic components of heat flow [41]. From this analytic technique, two enthalpic events were identified in samples with low water loss, with the first event occurring between 50 °C and 52 °C. When water loss exceeded about 35–40%, only one endothermic event was observed. Thus, the water content of the sample has a profound effect on the temperature range of phase transformation. Laser heating of cartilage creates a localized region of dehydration within cartilage samples within the area of light distribution. This variation in water content could lead to changes in temperature thresholds for stress relaxation and thus phase transformation.

Modeling of Cartilage Reshaping

During laser irradiation of biological tissue, many important physical processes occur that determine temperature elevation and thermal damage rates. Of note are the propagation of light within a scattering media; transformation of laser light into photochemical, acoustic, or thermal energy; tissue-tissue and tissue-environment heat and mass transfer; and the occurrence of low-energy phase transformations. In order to optimize the reshaping process, it is essential to characterize the temperature-dependent stress relaxation and physical properties of cartilage, namely, elastic modulus, thermal diffusivity, and optical scattering. These processes have been used by Diaz et al. to create a finite element model (FEM) to predict the temperature distribution in a slab of porcine nasal cartilage during laser irradiation [42, 43]. These models can be used to make predictions of the onset, extent, and severity of thermal injury—information which may be used to develop dosimetry guidelines for medical applications of lasers.

In order to guide and optimize laser cartilage reshaping for clinical use in septal cartilage reshaping, Protsenko et al. used FEM to model the forces applied during cartilage straightening deformation before and after laser irradiation as a function of the number, pattern, and location of laser target sites [44]. From the FEM model, it was observed that straightening deformation produced a nonhomogeneous stress field with regions of tension and compression. With an increase in number of laser irradiation sites and delivered laser energy, it was noted that reaction force decreased. The model showed that in order to reduce reaction force by 95%, approximately 50% of thermal damage to septal cartilage would also occur.

13.2.3.3 Biophysical Properties and Cartilage Behavior

Cartilage is a charged, hydrated, protein-based polymer that is at risk for denaturation upon heating. It is well known that laser heating may result in thermal decomposition of biopolymers as intermolecular bonds break as temperature rises. The safe practice of LCR necessitates investigation into thresholds of denaturation to minimize the risk of uncontrolled thermal injury. Tissue changes due to laser irradiation may be monitored by examining the number and size of light-scattering centers in the tissue, which has been discussed in previous sections for the application of monitoring the phase transformation of water in cartilage during laser-induced stress relaxation.

Sobol et al. used data on the time dependence of light scattering in tissue to estimate the approximate values of kinetic parameters for denaturation as a function of laser wavelength and radiant exposure [45]. An inverse correlation between denaturation thresholds and the absorption spectrum of the tissue was observed for many wavelengths. This was observed except at wavelengths near 3 and 6 μm, where denaturation threshold is instead governed by heating kinetics of tissue, as the initial absorption coefficient is very high. In a following study, Sobol et al. examined the alterations in the absorption of tissue water by laser heating with a short, single laser pulse with negligible movement and evaporation of water [46]. For temperatures less than 50 °C, it was observed that the absorption coefficient for cartilage remained approximately constant. However, for temperatures above this critical threshold temperature, the absorption of coefficient decreases at a nearly constant rate. Therefore, the critical threshold temperature is the characteristic temperature for a change in the molecular structure of the tissue, and the changes observed are due to a decrease of intermolecular interaction energy, such as by the disaggregation of water molecules.

In another series of studies, Ignat'eva et al. investigated the thermal stability of collagen in cartilage and factors that may alter the degree of denaturation upon heating [47, 48]. Cartilage is composed primarily of type II collagen fibers embedded in a mesh-like network of proteoglycan fibers. In their 2004 results, Ignat'eva et al. generated the curve of endothermic melting of collagen and observed three peaks with maximums at 60, 65, and 70 °C. These peaks correspond to melting of three fractions of collagen: tropocollagen, fibril surface collagen, and fibrillary collagen, respectively. Analysis of thermal and thermomechanical behavior of the samples revealed that the initial melting point of the first fraction corresponded to the phase of softening of the preparations (40–50 °C), whereas the initial melting point of the third fraction (65 °C) corresponded to abrupt changes in sample shape. In their subsequent study, Ignat'eva et al. determined that hyaline cartilage, such as that of the nasal septum, is thermally stable and remains incompletely denatured up to 100 °C. However, partial destruction of glycosaminoglycans in hyaline cartilage leads to an increase in degree of denaturation of collagen II upon heating. Proteoglycan aggregates therefore may play a key role in creating topological hindrances for moving polypeptide chains, reducing the configurational entropy of collagen macromolecules during denaturation. Later, Hajiioannou et al. determined the distinct role of the collagen network in cartilage shape and tensile strength preservation by enzymatically incubating cartilage strips and subsequently using laser irradiation for reshaping [49]. Collagen degradation was observed to be a substantial factor leading to the release of cartilage tensile stresses.

Polarization-sensitive optical coherence tomography (PS-OCT) has been used to characterize the polarization state of backscattered light as a function of optical path length in birefringent biological tissues. Birefringence in cartilage is due to asymmetrical collagen fibril structure, and changes in birefringence may signal disruption of cartilaginous structure due to laser irradiation. Youn et al. investigated the use of PS-OCT to measure thermodynamically induced changes of phase retardation in cartilage during LACR. It was observed that the retardation of light in the cartilage sample was changed due to laser irradiation, with two possible causes: dehydration and thermal denaturation (Fig. 13.3). The two conditions were then tested via either dehydration in glycerol or thermal denaturation in heated physiological saline. The results suggested that the observed retardation changes in cartilage were primarily due to dehydration.

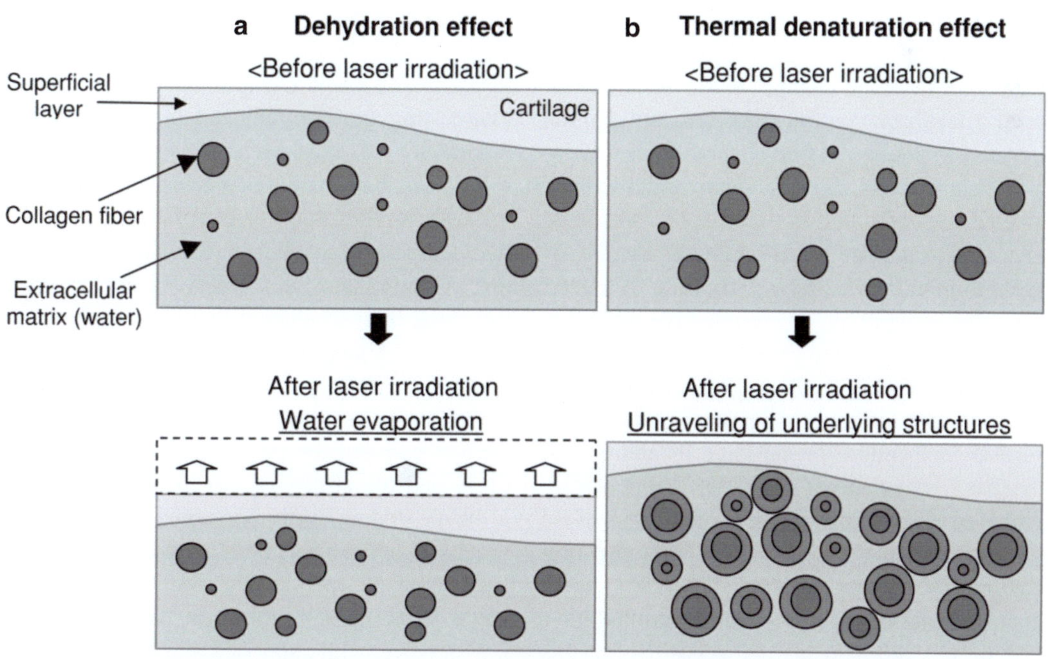

Fig. 13.3 Dehydration (**a**) and thermal denaturation effects (**b**) before and after laser irradiation (Youn et al. 2005 [48] © Institute of Physics and Engineering in Medicine. Reproduced by permission of IOP Publishing. All rights reserved)

Numerous methods have been used to evaluate phase transition during stress relaxation of cartilage samples undergoing LAR. Ultrasound monitoring can be used, as it has been demonstrated that the speed of the ultrasonic pulse is indicative of permanent stress relaxation [50]. By using a double integrating sphere system to measure diffuse transmittance, diffuse reflectance, and collimated transmittance of cartilage and polyacrylamide hydrogel samples as a function of temperature under 1560-nm laser irradiation, it was found that raising the temperature of cartilage samples to 80 °C caused the absorption coefficient to decrease by about 25% [51]. Other studies have shown that the effect of structural anisotropy of costal cartilage reveals itself in the increasing scattering of IR radiation passing crosswise the collagen orientation when tissue water content is decreased [52].

13.2.4 Control Systems in Laser Cartilage Reshaping

Since prolonged laser heating of cartilage leads to temperatures incompatible with chondrocyte survival, it is critical to develop a feedback system to control this process while still providing for adequate shape change. Wong et al. developed a feedback-controlled process utilizing an integrating sphere and silicon photodiode to measure backscattered light intensity. Additionally, a feedback-controlled cryogen spray was used to maintain surface temperatures below 50 °C [53]. Similar results were presented in a later study by Wong et al., where effective reshaping was also demonstrated [54]. Bagratashvili et al. have proposed a feedback mechanism integrating measurements of heat conductive or radiometric surface temperature of cartilage in addition to detecting backscattered light [55]. Burden et al. proposed using a thermopile to measure surface temperature, in addition to a silicon photoreceiver to detect backscattered light [56]. Sobol et al. have tested their feedback-controlled laser system on 380 patients with positive results obtained for 95% of patients with 2-year follow-up [57]. The following sections will discuss the clinical use of feedback-controlled laser systems for cartilage reshaping.

13.3 Clinical Applications

13.3.1 In Vivo LCR

Cartilage reshaping has myriad clinical applications throughout head and neck surgery and has been an ongoing area of investigation for many decades. Classical approaches to altering the shape of cartilage in the head, neck, and upper airway have focused on manipulating the interlocking stresses and forces through partial thickness incisions or through sutures [58]. In the 1950s, Thomas showed that intravenous injections of the enzyme papain lead to reversible shape change in rabbit ears, an effect further potentiated by cortisone [59]. In the 1960s, De Palma then described that saline immersion of rabbit auricular cartilage would increase pliability and allow for shape change after at least 8 days of autotransplantation to the anterior abdominal wall [60]. Around that time, Rubin demonstrated the neutralization of interlocking stress forces through the use of morselization [61].

Although the above techniques were able to produce a shape change, this effect was not long-lasting or was achieved through invasive maneuvers. Laser cartilage reshaping provides a solution to both of these problems. The refinement and optimization of laser cartilage reshaping necessary for clinical use would involve investigations into the viability of chondrocytes following laser irradiation and understanding of the effect of laser dosimetry on tissue thermal injury.

Following the many in vitro and ex vivo studies that clarified the material properties of cartilage and the effects of laser irradiation, early in vivo studies were performed by multiple groups. Shapshay et al. induced tracheal wall collapse in beagles and irradiated tracheal cartilage under deformation with 1.44-μm Nd:YAG laser at 2 W of power with a spot of 3 mm on the mucosal side of the cartilage surface along the line where internal stresses were expected to be maximum

[62]. After 6 weeks, endoscopic examination displayed corrected tracheal wall with adequate airway, and histopathologically the overlying mucosa was fully regenerated, and a number of viable chondrocytes with normal appearance were observed within the local cartilage.

Omelchenko et al. reported similar findings in an in vivo investigation of porcine auricular cartilage reshaping [63]. Shape change was produced through irradiation by Ho:YAG laser of 2.1 μm with an energy from 0.1 to 1.0 J, pulse duration of 300 μs, and repetition rate of 5 Hz. They describe a set of zones corresponding to changes in cartilage structure expanding radially from the irradiated areas (Fig. 13.4). In the central zones 1 and 2, the cartilage matrix is nearly completely destroyed, with few viable chondrocytes. In the more peripheral zone 3, the matrix is not destroyed, but cell dystrophy is observed, and most peripherally, in zone 4, the matrix and chondrocytes are unchanged. At 2–4 months following laser irradiation, treated cartilage was observed to maintain shape change.

In multiple later studies, dosimetry, shape change, and chondrocyte viability were examined in vivo. Lowe et al. examined porcine ears following exposure to Ho:YAG laser irradiation at 2.1 μm with a pulse energy of 2 J/cm^2 at 20 Hz with a spot diameter of 1.1 mm for 7 s [64]. For this set of parameters, shape change was retained

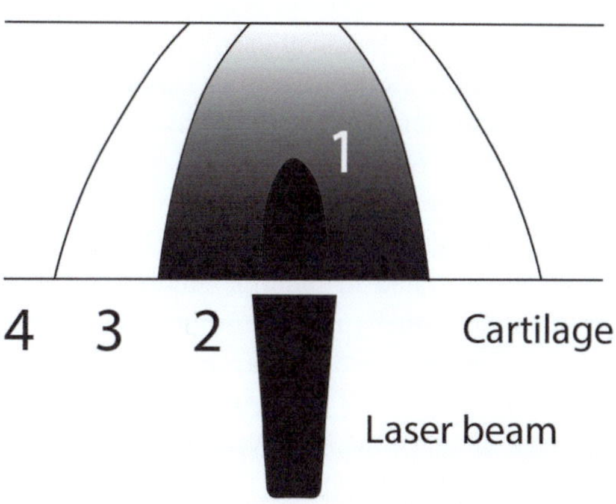

Fig. 13.4 The structural alteration zones induced by laser radiation in cartilage (in vitro experiment) (After Sviridov A. In vivo study and histological examination of laser reshaping of cartilage (1999, SPIE) [63])

for at least 14 days. Samples treated for less than 4 s returned to their original shape after 24 h, and those exposed for 9 s showed evidence of tissue necrosis. In all laser-irradiated areas, there was a loss of viable chondrocytes; however, in areas away from the center of irradiation, there was a marked proliferation of cartilage with a noticeable absence of any inflammation. Wong et al. examined an in vivo model of rabbit nasal septal cartilage reshaping using an Nd:YAG laser at 1.32 μm, 25 W/cm^2, and determined that shape change took place at the thermal range of 60–70 °C [65]. Creusy et al. examined multiple treatments in rabbit auricular cartilage using 1.54-μm Er:glass laser at 3 ms, 7 pulses, 12 J/cm^2, 2 Hz applied on 10 contiguous parallel rows along the ear, and examined biopsies from irradiated areas at 1, 3, and 6 weeks [66]. Shape change was observed in all treated ears. At 3 weeks, a chondroblastic proliferation was noted in areas of contracted cartilage, and at 6 weeks, the presence of new chondrocytes was observed.

13.3.1.1 Effects of LCR on Chondrocyte Viability

In general, chondrocytes are more sensitive to damage by laser irradiation than their surrounding ECM. The effect of laser irradiation on chondrocytes may be observed as either cytoplasmic focal vacuolation or nuclear condensation, representing reversible cell injury and cell death, respectively. Sviridov et al. showed in 1998 that there are conditions, such as laser fluence of 1.7 J/cm^2 and exposure time of 4 s, which allow for reshaping without nuclear condensation and only minor cell vacuolation. Lower values for these parameters produced less cell damage but were unfortunately not able to produce shape change [63].

The characterization of laser irradiation on cellular components of cartilage began with studies by Pullin, who investigated such effects from Ho:YAG irradiation in equine articular cartilage [67]. This study piggybacked off recent results showing potential applications for accelerating the healing process using laser irradiation and involved histological and biochemical assessments. Biochemical analyses included examination of GAG synthesis and cell proliferation at baseline and 24 weeks after irradiation between injured areas and an internal control. Their results demonstrated a clustering effect on chondrocytes at the exposure boundary, which may represent destructive changes or actual upregulation of chondrocyte metabolism. Additionally, they observed an inhibition of GAG synthesis in laser-treated perilesional tissue. However, no changes were noted on cell proliferation in irradiated areas, except in areas of lesional tissue, where increased proliferation was noted. This phenomenon may be caused by changes in the water diffusion kinetics in cartilage and the relaxation of the ECM.

Subsequent studies by Wong investigated proteoglycan synthesis in porcine nasal cartilage following Nd:YAG laser reshaping [68]. Cellular viability was evaluated by measuring the incorporation of Na_2 [32]SO_4 into proteoglycan macromolecules in whole-tissue culture. Wong et al. determined that average proteoglycan synthesis rates decreased with successive laser exposures but did not result in complete elimination of viable chondrocytes. The reduction in proteoglycan synthesis correlated with the time-temperature-dependent heating profile created during laser irradiation, which provided greater support to the need for careful monitoring of laser dosimetry to preserve chondrocyte viability.

In a later study, Wong et al. used flow cytometry to provide quantitative effects of laser irradiation on chondrocyte viability [69]. Porcine septal cartilages were irradiated with Nd:YAG laser with wavelength of 1.32 μm at 25 W/cm^2, with exposure times of 6.7, 7.2, or 10 s. Samples were then examined immediately and at 5 days following laser exposure. Wong et al. determined that nearly 60% of chondrocytes were viable after one irradiation and that chondrocyte viability decreased to 31% and 16% after two and three exposures, respectively. A similar pattern was seen in samples 5 days following exposure, with the least amount of deterioration in untreated and singly irradiated samples.

Additional studies by Wong et al. demonstrated that thermal tissue damage is concurrent with shape change and that significant cell death occurs at laser dosimetry necessary to produce clinically relevant shape changes both in rabbit septal cartilage [69] and in human septal cartilage [16].

13.3.1.2 Long-Term Viability

To determine long-term changes, Wong et al. examined the in vivo effect of laser dosimetry on rabbit septal cartilage integrity, viability, and mechanical behavior over 7 months [70]. In the first study, cartilage samples were treated with Nd:YAG laser across a broad dosimetry range (4–8 W and 6–16 s) and then examined 7 months later. In all laser-irradiated samples, variable tissue resorption and calcification were observed to correlate with increases in dosimetry. Elastic moduli of specimens were observed to be significantly different from controls, and viability assays demonstrated a total loss of viable chondrocytes within laser-irradiated zones. These results provided evidence against the presence of a laser dosimetry parameter space where the competing objectives of shape change and cell viability are both achievable and thereby underscore the importance of spatially selective heating.

13.3.2 LCR of the Airway

Deformities in the cartilages of the upper airway are a common problem encountered by the head and neck surgeon. Whether acquired or congenital, the standard treatment calls for serial endoscopic dilation, cartilage grafting, laser ablation, endotracheal stenting, tracheostomy, or segmental resection. Such invasive procedures bring significant potential for morbidity and mortality. Endoscopic laser reshaping of the trachea has been demonstrated in multiple studies and is a promising minimally invasive solution.

Early reports by Shapshay and Wang et al. on the in vivo use of Nd:YAG on dog tracheal cartilage demonstrated the remarkable effect on laser cartilage reshaping [71]. Six weeks postoperatively, all subjects had an adequate airway lined by healthy mucosa. Later studies by Wong et al. on ex vivo rabbit tracheal cartilage, selected to simulate the human neonate trachea, by Er:glass laser determined that optimal parameters for shape change were at a wavelength of 1.54 μm and power of 1 W for a duration of 6–7 s [72]. At this setting, shape change was effected with minimal thermal injury. Subsequent studies by Wong et al. further investigated parameters for shape change, effect of temperature on the mechanical behavior of cartilage, and tissue viability, again in the rabbit model [73]. Shape change transition zones were observed between 62 °C and 66 °C in saline bath and above power densities of 350 J/cm^2. In line with previous results, a significant loss of viable chondrocytes within laser irradiation zones was observed.

Additional reports by Helidonis et al. show the potential of laser reshaping for the epiglottis, with applications for correcting laryngomalacia, obstructive sleep apnea resulting from epiglottal prolapse, and other congenital or acquired deformities of the epiglottis [74]. In a cadaveric model, they demonstrated the use of aCO_2 laser at 1560-nm wavelength and power density of 48 J/cm^2. Twenty to 30 pulses of 0.5 s or between 60 and 90 J were required to remodel the epiglottis.

13.3.3 LCR of Septal Cartilage

A patent nasal airway is critical for maintaining proper functioning of vocalization, humidification, filtration, heating of air, and adequate ventilation. Nasal airway obstruction can lead to subjective complaints while awake, as well as impairment while asleep, which potentially may lead to further complications such as reduced mentation, arrhythmia, and cor pulmonale.

Airflow through the upper airway can be approximated by Poiseuille's law, which states that flow is proportional to the fourth power of the radius of the tube. Therefore, even with small changes in airway radius, there may be a relatively large decrease in flow. Clinically, this reduction in flow may be observed at many levels of the upper aerodigestive tract. Nasal septum deviations are a common cause of airway obstruction, and until now, the standard of care for significant septal deviations has been through surgical correction.

The classical Indian textbook *Sushruta Samhita*, dating to around 600 B.C., was the first recorded description of nasal reconstruction [75]. Around this time, nasal fractures and gross septal deformities were corrected by manual manipulation. In the seventeenth century, Taglioacozzi and Brancas made advances in changing the external shape of the nose. Further advances were made in the eighteenth and nineteenth century including Freer and Killian's development of submucous resection of the nasal septum [76]. Contemporary septal surgery has evolved from Cottle, Loring, and Fisher's intranasal maxillary-premaxillary approach [77]. However, despite such advances, surgical correction of nasal septal deformities still requires most frequently general anesthesia and the potential for significant morbidity.

The development of laser cartilage reshaping brings the potential for a nearly bloodless procedure to achieve functional improvements in nasal airflow. The underlying principles of laser reshaping (discussed in greater detail at the beginning of this chapter) can be summarized in the steps of (1) mechanical deformation of tissue into desired shape and (2) laser irradiation of areas of highest internal stress, which results in (3) stress relaxation and stable shape change.

Historically, the use of laser-assisted cartilage reshaping was first utilized for septoplasty. Laser-assisted cartilage reshaping may be applied to native septal cartilage or, in cases where this is not possible, to autologous costal cartilage samples. Although costal cartilage is among the most suitable natural materials for transplantation, its natural semicircular curvature presents a challenge for obtaining a proper and stable shape. Optimal laser parameters have been extensively investigated and, in general, depend on multiple factors including thickness of tissue, its chemical composition, and structure.

13.3.3.1 Clinical Results of Laser Reshaping of Nasal Septal Cartilage

Advances in the clinical use of laser reshaping have been made by multiple groups within the past couple of decades. Starting in 2000, Sobol's group treated 40 patients with a holmium laser and followed the effects of reshaping throughout the course of 12 months [78]. Even from this initial study, the results have been very promising. Twenty-three patients showed excellent long-term reshaping effects, 12 patients acceptably good results, and five patients with only marginal reshaping effects achieved. Thirty-five of the 40 patients reported a marked improvement in breathing, and no patient enrolled in the study displayed any visible undesirable side effects. In 2002, Ovchinnikov et al. followed 110 patients treated with Ho:YAG laser for an average of 18 months. Eighty-four patients were observed to display stable improvement in septal shape change and noted disappearance of any attendant symptoms [79]. Later in 2008, Bourolias et al. treated 64 patients using an Er:glass laser and followed for 6 months while recording average NOSE scores and flow and resistance measurements. In all of these metrics, they noted significant improvement without any intraoperative pain or postoperative complications [80].

In 2010, Leclere et al. followed 12 patients undergoing laser reshaping with an Er:glass laser with integrated cooling (Fig. 13.5) for the duration of 3 months. They were careful to do preoperative examinations including nasomanometry and nasal endoscopy to exclude inferior turbinate or adenoid hypertrophy. NOSE score was calculated at 1 week, 1 month, and 3 months post-procedure, and rhinomanometry was performed at 3 months. They noted improvements in mean NOSE scores and improvements to air inflow resistance. Adequate septal reshaping was observed in seven adults, and in five adults incomplete septal reshaping was observed. Of the cases where the results were inadequate, anatomical variations such as a thick or a longer septum were hypothesized to be the causal factors. They also noted that inadequate local anesthesia prevented the completion of the procedure in two patients. However, following retreatment, all patients were able to achieve suitable reshaping [81].

These studies show that laser septal cartilage reshaping has the potential to be a safer alternative to surgical septoplasty that offers the potential for nearly painless and much less morbidity than conventional techniques.

13.3.4 LCR of Auricular Cartilage

Deformities in the external ear are estimated to occur in roughly one in every 5000 births. Common malformations include lack of antihelical folds or increased conchal-mastoid angles and have traditionally necessitated surgical correction by means of otoplasty. The technical difficulty of otoplasty is quite high, and as it requires precise placement of stitches or creation of cartilage-splitting incisions that precisely balance forces to resist deformation, otoplasty is

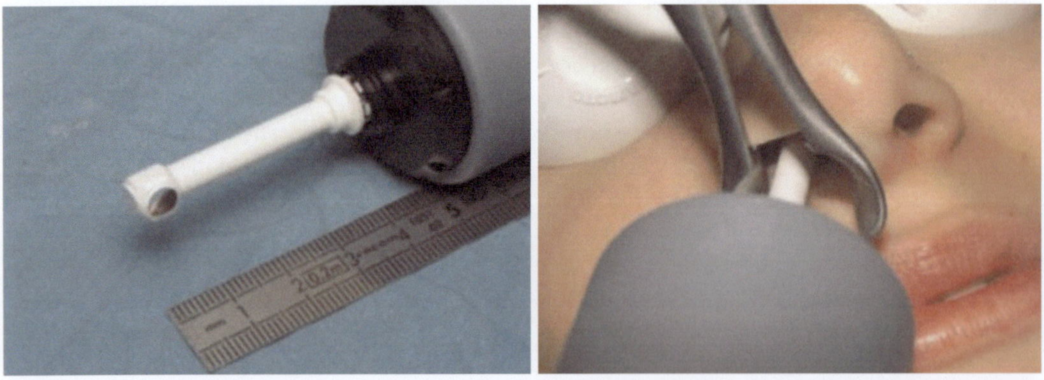

Fig. 13.5 Left image depicts handpiece allowing laser beam delivery at 90° and contact cooling (+5 °C) of the mucosa. Right image demonstrates treatment setup. Five stacked pulses (3 ms, 2 Hz, 50 J/cm^2 cumulative fluence) applied using 4-mm chilled handpiece at 5 °C temperature on both sides of the septum (After Leclere et al. Laser-assisted septal cartilage reshaping (LASCR): A prospective study in 12 patients. Lasers in Surgery and Medicine, 42(8), 693–698. 2010 [81])

regarded as among the most difficult surgical procedures to master. With the advent of laser-assisted cartilage reshaping, the correction of auricular deformities may now be performed with much greater ease and simplicity.

In 2004, Mordon et al. at the French National Institute of Health and Medical Research (INSERM) proposed a method for reshaping protruding ears through 1.54-μm Er:glass laser irradiation in the rabbit model [66]. Rabbit ears were treated at fifteen spots applied on ten contiguous parallel rows (with parameters of 3 ms, 7 pulses, 12 J/cm², 2 Hz, 84/cm² cumulative fluence) while using a perforated cylindrical guide to determine ear curvature. Thermal damage was assessed via biopsies taken from irradiated areas at 1, 3, and 6 weeks. This initial study showed that with the parameters above, the skin was not visibly affected by laser irradiation, and every ear in the study was successfully reshaped. Furthermore, the authors noted chondroblastic proliferation around the area of contracted cartilage at 3 weeks and observed significant thickening of the cartilage layer along with the presence of new chondrocytes at 6 weeks. Perhaps most remarkable is that these results were achieved despite the substantial musculature within the rabbit ear.

In 2006, Mordon et al. conducted trials of LACR on human patients using the same 1.54-μm Er:glass laser [82]. In later reviews, it would be determined that the 1.54-μm wavelength is ideal for cartilage reshaping of the ear, as the wavelength's penetration depth matches the thickness of the auricular cartilage, allowing for homogenous heat generation [83]. In this study, eight patients were treated with four undergoing LACR of both ears and four of only one ear. The entire concha and helix were irradiated on both sides with settings of 12 J/cm², seven pulses, 3 ms, 2 Hz, and 84/cm² cumulative fluence, applied with a 4-mm spot handpiece integrated in a cooling device. The integrated cooling, which resulted in about a 5 °C temperature drop, allowed for the procedure to be performed without the need for anesthesia. To produce shape change, a silicone elastomer mold was applied inside the helix and concha, and patients were asked to wear the resulting solid mold for 15 days using a bandage wrap. To assess for chondrocyte viability and epithelial damage, biopsies were taken immediately after LACR and subsequently at 1, 2, 3, and 4 weeks. The entire procedure could be performed in under 20 min per ear, was well tolerated, and was not associated with the development of hematomas or skin necrosis. Shape change was achieved in all patients, and all patients responded that the shape change met their expectations (Fig. 13.6). One patient had a mild recurrence of the upper antihelical fold; however, in all other cases, the reshaping was

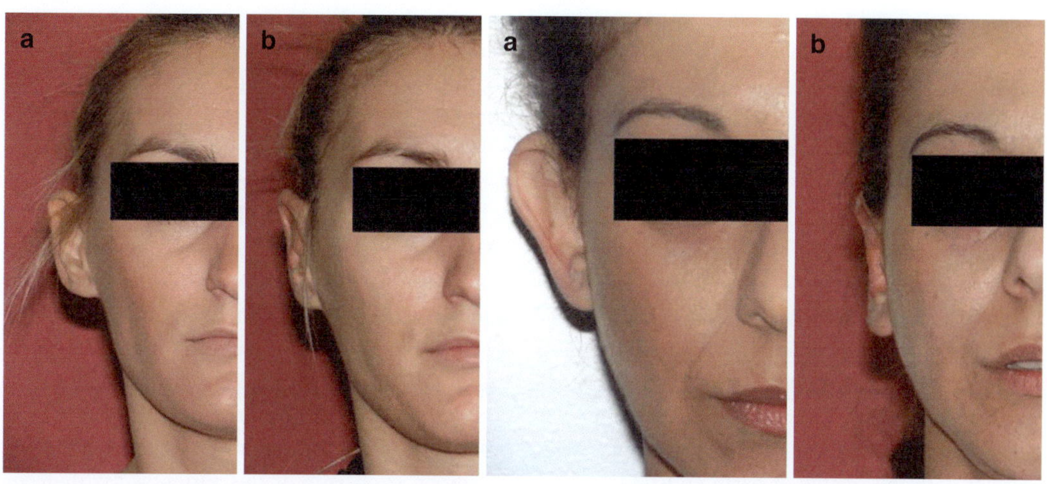

Fig. 13.6 Left and right series (**a**, **b**) show adult patient before (**a**) and 3 months after (**b**) LACR (After Leclere et al. Laser-assisted cartilage reshaping (LACR) for treating ear protrusions: A clinical study in 24 patients. Aesthetic Plastic Surgery 2010 [84])

found to be stable 6 months after LACR. Biopsy results showed discrete inflammatory reaction within the dermis at 1 week and a thickening of perichondrium and cartilage layers at 2 weeks, which was also observed at 3 and 4 weeks, along with viable chondrocytes.

A few years later, Leclere et al. presented their LACR results for treating protruding ears in 24 patients [84]. In order to determine optimal treatment parameters, the parameters used in this study were varied from those of previous studies by Mordon et al., with cumulative fluences ranging from 70 to 84 J/cm^2. In 21 of the patients, the 1.54-μm Er:YAG laser was set to 12 J/cm^2 per pulse with seven stacked pulses (3 ms, 2 Hz, 84 J/cm^2 cumulative fluence) applied using a 4-mm spot handpiece with integrated cooling. For the remaining three adult patients, the laser was set at fluence of 10 J/cm^2 per pulse for a total cumulative fluence of 70 J/cm^2. All patients were given NSAIDs for 3 days after LACR and instructed to wear an elastomer mold at all times for 3 weeks and only at night for an additional 3 weeks. The authors noted six cases of contact dermatitis which they presume may be due to inappropriate mold design. In these cases, the patients stopped wearing the mold and thus did not achieve shape change. Otherwise, the authors note no cases of infections, hematomas, or skin necrosis. The remaining 18 patients achieved the expected outcome. At the lower fluence of 70 J/cm^2, the authors noted that incomplete reshaping was observed. The three patients treated at the lower fluence were re-treated at 3 months with 84 J/cm^2 fluence, and all achieved stable reshaping.

In 2010, Ragab described an open approach to the use of carbon dioxide laser, whereby the LACR is performed via evaporation of the perichondrium and laser incisions [85]. Sixteen patients were treated with application of the CO2 laser directly onto the medial surface and posterior perichondrium of the auricular cartilages. A pair of parallel laser incisions was also created using a focused laser beam, reaching to a deeper thickness. Thirteen and 14 patients were pleased with the results at early and late assessment, respectively. McDowell's basic goals score was used as an objective measure of otoplasty success, and the score was 4–6, with a mean of 5, with 6 as the total score. Hyperpigmentation, thermal injury, and other complications were not observed, and no revision surgery was needed even after 2.4 years of follow-up. The advantages of this open approach are the reduced reliance on external molds, which must be worn over an extended period, and a reduced recurrence rate.

Additional LACR treatment protocols have been studied using 1064-nm Nd:YAG lasers [86]. At this wavelength, there is a broader spectrum of absorption relative to the 1540-nm wavelength, which would allow for greater penetration depth. However, a few significant adverse effects were observed at 1064 nm, including skin burn and damage to auricular cartilage. The 2015 study by Leclere et al. was conducted on 14 patients who underwent 1065-nm LACR for protruding ears (repetition pulse emission of 1 Hz, 25-ms pulse length, 70 J/cm^2 fluence per pulse), with a beam diameter of 6 mm, using a handpiece with integrated cooling spray. It was noted with the above parameters that local anesthesia was necessary despite dynamic cryogen cooling. Despite the need for anesthesia and adverse effects, ten patients were pleased with the results, two patients satisfied, and one patient not satisfied. Overall, there were eight cases of localized skin burn and one case of dermatitis. Therefore, the authors conclude that the 1540-nm wavelength is superior due to the following: (1) the wavelength matches the cartilage thickness, (2) treatment is tolerated without anesthesia as long as contact cooling is available, and (3) it can achieve adequate reshaping.

The longest follow-up period investigated to date was conducted by Leclere et al. in 2011 [87]. In this study, Leclere et al. performed 32 LACR procedures in 17 patients and followed outcomes over a period of 30 months. A 1540-nm Er:glass laser set at 12 J/cm^2 with seven stacked pulses (3 ms, 2 Hz, 84 J/cm^2 cumulative fluence) applied using a 4-mm spot handpiece with integrative cooling was used to perform LACR. The authors note that treatment requires at least 50 (×7) pulses on each side of the auricular cartilage to be effective. The outcomes in this set of patients were similar to those seen in previous studies, with no immediate complications seen. In the early postoperative period, two cases of contact dermatitis were noted due to inappropriate mold design. In five patients, a slight asymmetry was noticeable only by the surgeon after measuring cephalo-auricular distances. No other complications were noted, and overall satisfaction was 8.6/10 in the series.

13.3.4.1 Cryogen Spray Cooling in LCR

The development of a reliable cooling method was essential to bridge the gap between the bench and the bedside for LACR. As seen in the previous section, the success in applying LACR in the clinic depends on the ability to perform laser irradiation of the auricular cartilage without the need for anesthesia. This section will provide a concise overview of the development of cryogen spray cooling and explore its applications.

Early studies on the biomechanical properties of cartilage and material property changes due to laser irradiation determined that the critical temperature range of 60–70 °C marks the beginning of stress relaxation [27, 29, 34, 88]. Since protein denaturation occurs near 70 °C, this critical temperature range for cartilage reshaping must be precisely controlled, as extensive loss of cell viability may result in complete graft resorption, infection, and/or necrosis. Cryogen spray cooling (CSC) may be used to minimize excessive temperature elevations on the irradiated cartilage surfaces while allowing for homogenous axial temperature distributions within deeper portions of the irradiated cartilage. CSC involves the atomized delivery of a cryogen onto the skin surface 40–120 ms prior to laser irradiation. The evaporative cooling effect of the cryogen draws heat from the epidermis and allows for spatially selective thermal treatment of underlying cartilage.

In 2001, Karamzadeh et al. investigated the biophysical properties of cartilage and chondrocyte viability after LACR using CSC [89]. Chondrocyte viability was determined after 50 W/cm^2 Nd:YAG-mediated cartilage reshaping with and without CSC and correlated with dynamic measurements of tissue optical and thermal properties. This initial study found that after 2 s of laser exposure, specimens in both groups maintained shape change for up to 14 days. Chondrocyte viability was shown to correlate with the number of laser exposures. However, the relative viability in the cryogen controls was 99.58 ± 0.80%, suggesting that CSC along with the parameters used in this study do not contribute significantly to cell death.

In a later study by Cheng et al., optimization of laser and CSC parameters were determined on composite cartilage grafts (Fig. 13.7) from rabbit ears [90]. In this study, cryogen R134a (1,1,1,2-tetrafluoroethane) was applied to samples using a solenoid valve with a distance of 30 mm between the valve orifice to the sample. Cryogen was released at 50–70 mL/s spurts when surface temperatures on the outer portion of the bend exceeded 40 °C and ceased when thermocouple readings fell below 40 °C. Best results were obtained in specimens receiving 50 W with controlled CSC, with successful reshaping and minimal thermal damage.

The parameters for using CSC with LACR underwent further optimization with studies to determine therapy thresholds. Chlebicki et al. investigated optimal treatment parameters for laser output energy, CSC duration, and treatment cycles required to achieve shape change while limiting skin and cartilage injury [91]. Since this study attempted to identify therapy thresholds, aggressive parameters were used. Laser parameters resulting in acceptable skin injury to thick regions included the following parameters: 14 J/cm^2, a cryogen cooling spurt duration of 30–35 ms, and five to eight cycles. Unacceptable skin injury resulted from using 14 J/cm^2, a cryogen cooling spurt duration of 35 ms, and delivered in 10 cycles. When the CSC duration was reduced to 25 ms at 14 J/cm^2, unacceptable skin injury was also observed after six cycles. In thinner regions, parameters that resulted in unacceptable skin injury were the following: 13 J/cm^2 with CSC duration of 35 ms, delivered in six to seven cycles.

Since thicker tissues such as auricular cartilage may require higher laser power, and therefore increased cooling requirements, alternatives to conventional cryogens may provide a more

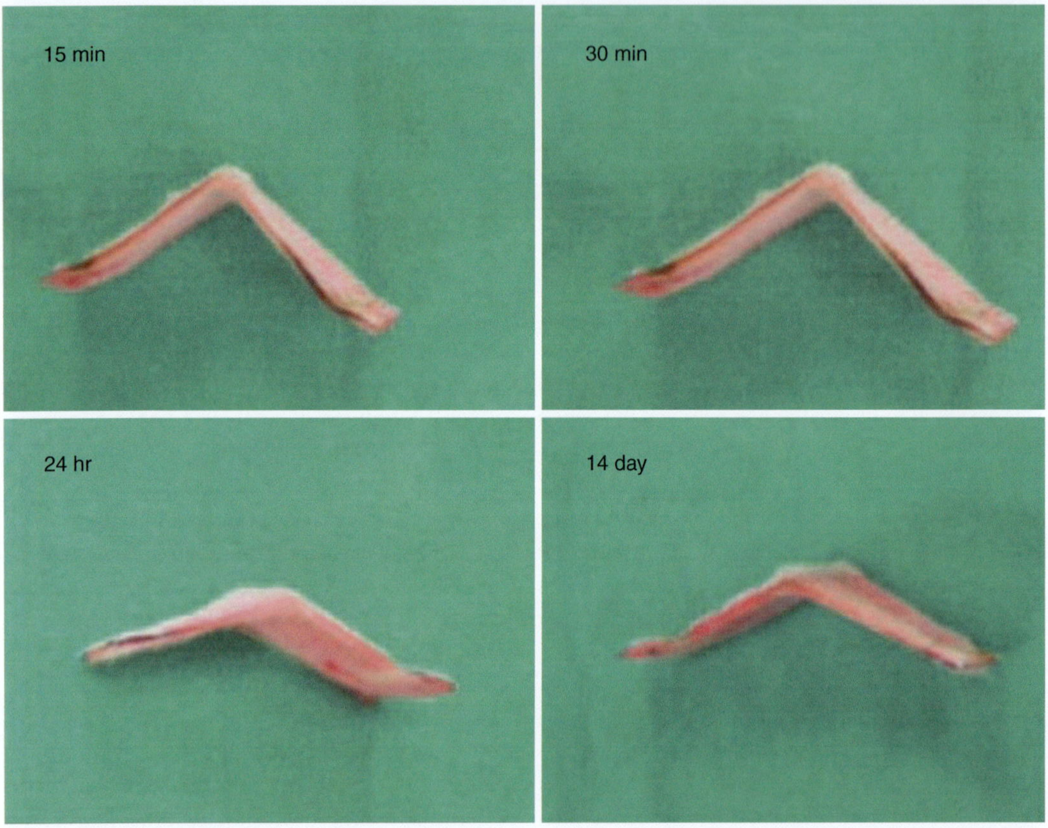

Fig. 13.7 A 50-W specimen shows most favorable deformation angle measuring 90° after initial elapsed time slot of 15 min. At the same wattage after 30 min post-illumination, the deformation angle remained at 90°. After 24 h, a small deformation angle of approximately 100° was measured. Deformation angle was maintained at about 100° and nonetheless produced a favorable angle, as with other specimens of this group, that closely measured to that calculation throughout the remaining 14 days. (After Cheng et al. Minimizing Superficial Thermal Injury Using Bilateral Cryogen Spray Cooling During Laser Reshaping of Composite Cartilage Grafts. Lasers in Surgery and Medicine, 2008 [90])

optimal cooling effect. Wu et al. investigated the use of CO_2 spray cooling in ex vivo rabbit auricular cartilage [92]. CO_2 has the advantage of leaving no residue on skin, which reduces the risk of frostbite, has a lower environmental impact, and is economically cheaper than conventionally used cryogens. Significant reshaping was achieved with all dosimetry tested, and with a 50–70 °C difference noted between controls and irradiated ears. The authors noted that increasing cooling pulse duration leads to progressively improved gross skin protection during irradiation.

The use of CSC in vivo 1has been investigated by Holden [93] and Kuan et al. [94] In 2009, Holden et al. showed that cartilage reshaping using 1450-nm diode laser combined with CSC may be used to safely perform LACR in the rabbit model. Parameters of 14 J/pulse with cryogen spray duration of 33 ms per cycle were used on experimental ears, with contralateral ears serving as internal controls. Adequate shape change was observed in all treated ears, and skin injury or post-procedural pain was not observed. In 2014, Kuan et al. used 1.45-µm wavelength diode laser along with CO_2 cooling in the in vivo rabbit model to show that shape change can be performed with minimal thermal cutaneous and cartilaginous injury (Fig. 13.8).

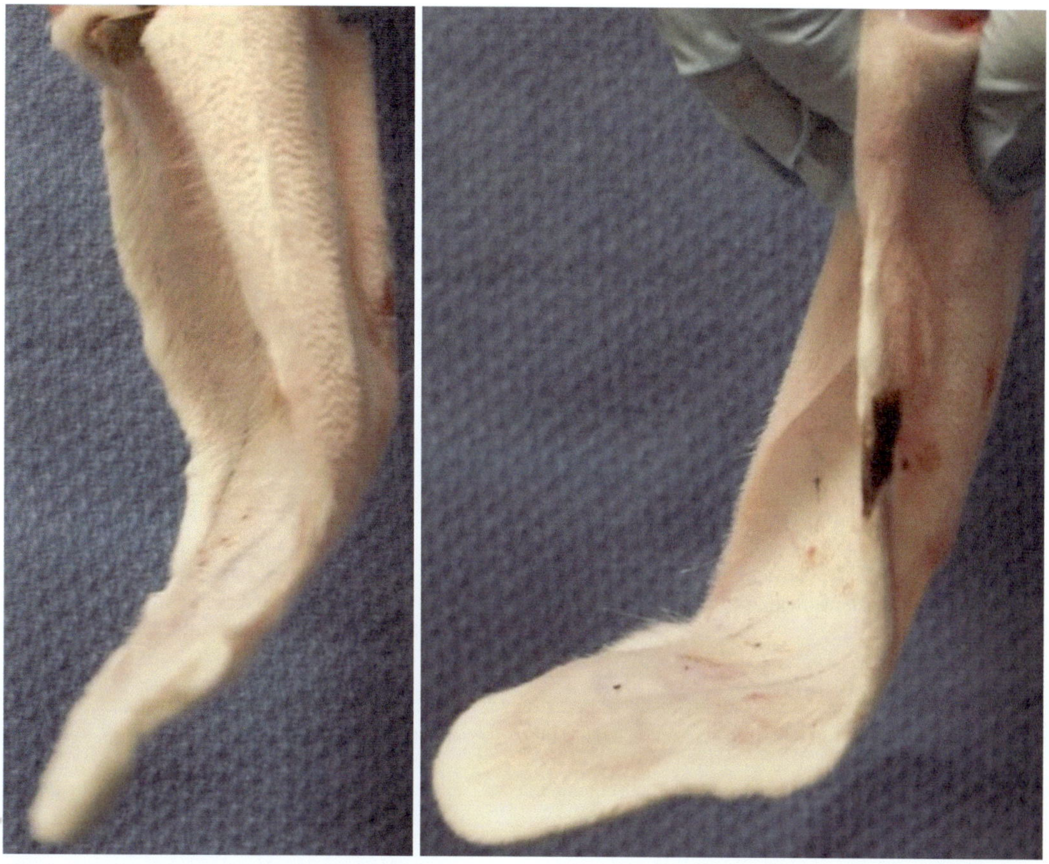

Fig. 13.8 Inversion of ears from same rabbit for bend angle measurement. This ear has been treated with laser and CO_2 (After Kuan et al. In Vivo Laser Cartilage Reshaping with Carbon Dioxide Spray Cooling in a Rabbit Ear Model: A Pilot Study. Lasers in Surgery and Medicine, 2015 [94])

13.4 Conclusions

There has been a tremendous amount of work over the past few decades in optimizing the use of laser cartilage reshaping for clinical use. As we have examined laser cartilage reshaping from its development, through its many improvements and finally its clinical applications, we remain incredibly optimistic for what future developments may bring.

References

1. Wan LQ, Jiang J, Arnold DE, Guo XE, Lu HH, Mow VC. Calcium concentration effects on the mechanical and biochemical properties of chondrocyte-alginate constructs. Cell Mol Bioeng. 2009;1(1):93–102. https://doi.org/10.1007/s12195-008-0014-x.
2. Gu WY, Lai WM, Mow VC. A triphasic analysis of negative osmotic flows through charged hydrated soft tissues. J Biomech. 1997;30(1):71–8.
3. Lu XL, Wan LQ, Edward Guo X, Mow VC. A linearized formulation of triphasic mixture theory for articular cartilage, and its application to indentation analysis. J Biomech. 2010;43(4):673–9.
4. Lux Lu X, Miller C, Chen FH, Edward Guo X, Mow VC. The generalized triphasic correspondence principle for simultaneous determination of the mechanical properties and proteoglycan content of articular cartilage by indentation. J Biomech. 2007;40(11):2434–41.
5. McCluskey RT, Thomas L. The removal of cartilage matrix, in vivo, by papain; identification of crystalline papain protease as the cause of the phenomenon. J Exp Med. 1958;108(3):371–84.
6. Thomas L. The effects of papain, vitamin a, and cortisone on cartilage matrix in vivo. Biophys J. 1964;4(2):207–13.

7. Thomas L. Papain, vitamin A, lysosomes, and endotoxin. Arch Intern Med. 1962;110:782–6.
8. Thomas L, Mccluskey RT, Potter JL, Weissmann G. Comparison of the effects of papain and vitamin A on cartilage I. The effects in Rabbits. J Exp Med. 1960;111(5):705–18.
9. Fell HB, Thomas L. Comparison of the effects of papain and vitamin A on cartilage. J Exp Med. 1960;111:719–44.
10. Sobol E, Bagratashvili V, Sviridov A, Omel'chenko A, Kitai M. Study of cartilage reshaping with holmium laser. SPIE. 1996;2623(95):544–7.
11. Helidonis E, Sobol E, Kavvalos G, Bizakis J, Christodoulou P, Velegrakis G, et al. Laser shaping of composite cartilage grafts. Am J Otolaryngol. 1993;14(6):410–2.
12. Frenzl M, Zuger BJ, Monin D, Weber HP, Schafffier T. Laser-induced cartilage damage: an ex-vivo model using confocal microscopy. SPIE. 1999;3601:115–20.
13. Sobol EN, Omelchenko AI, Mertig M, Pompe W. Scanning force microscopy of the fine structure of cartilage irradiated with a CO_2 laser. Lasers Med Sci. 2000;15:15–23.
14. Velegrakis GA, Papadakis CE, Volitakis ME, Nikolidakis AA, Naoumidi I, Prokopakis EP, Helidonis ES. In vitro ear cartilage shaping with carbon dioxide laser: an experimental study. Ann Otol Rhinol Laryngol. 2000;109(12):1162–6.
15. Johansen E, Burden M, Wong BJF. Determination of optimum laser parameters for cartilage reshaping in porcine septum using Nd:YAG Laser (λ = 1.32 μm). Proc SPIE. 2001;4257 https://doi.org/10.1117/12.434706.
16. Li C, Protsenko DE, Zemek A, Chae YS, Wong B. Analysis of Nd:YAG laser-mediated thermal damage in rabbit nasal septal cartilage. Lasers Surg Med. 2007;39(5):451–7. https://doi.org/10.1002/lsm.20514.
17. El Kharbotly A, El-Tayeb T, Mostafa Y, Hesham I. Diode laser (980 nm) cartilage reshaping. SPIE. 2011.
18. Lu XL, Mow VC. Biomechanics of articular cartilage and determination of material properties. Med Sci Sports Exerc. 2008;40(2):193–9. https://doi.org/10.1249/mss.0b013e31815cb1fc.
19. Gu WY, Lai WM, Mow VC. A mixture theory for charged-hydrated soft tissues containing multi-electrolytes: passive transport and swelling behaviors. J Biomech Eng. 1998;120:169–80.
20. Sobol EN. Phase transformations and ablation in laser-treated solids. New York: Wiley; 1995. p. 316–22.
21. Bagratashvi NV, Sviridov AP, Sobol EN, Kitai MS. Optical properties of nasal septum cartilage. SPIE. 1998;3254:398–406.
22. Wong BJF, Milner TE, Kim HK, Telenkov S, Chew C, Kuo T, Smithies DJ, Sobol EN, Nelson JS. Critical temperature transitions in laser mediated cartilage reshaping. Proc SPIE. 1998;3425:161–72.
23. Wong BJF, Milner TE, Anvari B, Sviridov A, Omel'chenko A, Bagratashvili V, Sobol EN, Nelson JS. Thermo-optical response of cartilage during feedback controlled laser-assisted reshaping. Proc SPIE. 1997;2970:380–91.
24. Wong BJF, Milner TE, Anvari B, Sviridov A, Omel'chenko A, Bagratashvili V, Sobol EN, Nelson JS. Measurement of radiometric surface temperature and integrated backscattered light intensity during feedback controlled laser-assisted cartilage reshaping. Lasers Med Sci. 1998;13:66–72.
25. Youn JI, Telenkov SA, Kim E, Bhavaraju NC, Wong BJ, Valvano JW, Milner TE. Optical and thermal properties of nasal septal cartilage. Lasers Surg Med. 2000;27(2):119–28. Retrieved from http://www.ncbi.nlm.nih.gov/pubmed/10960818
26. Wong BJF, Chao KKH, Kim HK, Chu BSEA, Gaon M, Sun C, et al. Laser mediated cartilage reshaping the porcine and lagomorph septal cartilages: models for tissue engineering and morphologic cartilage research. Am J Rhinol. 2001;15(2):109–16.
27. Sobol E, Sviridov A, Bagratashvili V, Omeltchenko A. Stress relaxation and cartilage shaping under laser radiation. SPIE. 1996;2681:358–63.
28. Bagratashvili VN, et al. Thermal and diffusion processes in laser-induced stress relaxation and reshaping of cartilage. J Biomech. 1997;30:813–7.
29. Sobol EN, et al. Mechanism of laser-induced stress relaxation in cartilage. SPIE. 1997; https://doi.org/10.1117/12.275495.
30. Sobol EN, et al. Theoretical modeling of heating and structure alterations in cartilage under laser radiation with regard of water evaporation an difusion dominance. SPIE. 1998; https://doi.org/10.1117/12.308207.
31. Wong BJF, Milner TE, Kim HH, Nelson JS, Sobol E. Stress relaxation of porcine septal cartilage during Nd:YAG (1.32 m) laser irradiation: mechanical, optical, and thermal responses. J Biomed Opt. 1998;3:409–14.
32. Bagratashvili V, et al. Kinetics of water transfer and stress relaxation in cartilage heated with 1.56um fiber laser. SPIE. 2000;3914:102–7.
33. Wong BJF, et al. Critical temperature transitions in laser mediated cartilage reshaping. SPIE. 1998;3245:161–72.
34. Wong BJF, et al. Characterization of temperature-dependent biophysical properties during laser mediated cartilage reshaping. IEEE J Sel Top Quantum Electron. 1999;5:1095–102.
35. Sobol EN, et al. Effect of wavelength on threshold and kinetics of tissue denaturation under laser radiation. SPIE. 1999;3601:122–9.
36. Gaon MD, Ho KHK, Wong BJF. Measurement of the elastic modulus of porcine septal cartilage specimens following Nd: YAG laser treatment. Lasers Med Sci. 2003;18:148–53.
37. Chao KKH, Ho K-HK, Wong BJF. Measurement of the elastic modulus of rabbit nasal septal cartilage

during Nd:YAG (l 1/4 1.32 lm) laser irradiation. Lasers Surg Med. 2003;32:377–83.
38. Chae Y, Aguilar G, Lavernia EJ, Wong BJF. Characterization of temperature dependent mechanical behavior of cartilage. Lasers Surg Med. 2003;32:271–8.
39. Wright R, et al. Effect of bath water temperature and immersion time on bend angle during cartilage thermoforming. SPIE. 2003;4949:293–9.
40. Wright R, Protsenko DE, Diaz S, Ho K, Wong B. Shape retention in porcine and rabbit nasal septal cartilage using saline bath immersion and Nd:YAG laser irradiation. Lasers Surg Med. 2005;37:201–9.
41. Chae Y, Protsenko DE, Lavernia EJ, Wong BJF. Effect of water content on enthalpic relaxations in porcine septal cartilage. J Therm Anal Calorim. 2009;95:937–43.
42. Diaz SH, Aguilar G, Lavernia EJ, Wong BJF. Modeling the thermal response of porcine cartilage to laser irradiation. IEEE J Sel Top Quantum Electron. 2001;7:944–51.
43. Diaz SH, et al. Rate process analysis of thermal damage. Phys Med Biol. 2003;48:19–29.
44. Protsenko DE, Wong BJF. Laser-assisted straightening of deformed cartilage: numerical model. Lasers Surg Med. 2007;39:245–55.
45. Sobol E, Sviridov A, Kitai MS. Time-resolved, light scattering measurements of cartilage and cornea denaturation due to free electron laser radiation. J Biomed Opt. 2003;8(2):216–22.
46. Sobol EN, Sviridov AP, Kitai MS, Edwards GS. Temperature alterations of infrared light absorption by cartilage and cornea under free-electron laser radiation. Appl Opt. 2003;42(13):2443–9. Retrieved from http://www.ncbi.nlm.nih.gov/pubmed/12737481
47. Ignat'eva NY, Sobol EN, Averkiev SV, Lunin VV, Grokhovskaya TE, Bagratashvili VN, Yantsen ES. Thermal stability of collagen II in cartilage. Dokl Biochem Biophys. 2004;395(1–6):96–8. https://doi.org/10.1023/B:DOBI.0000025555.66340.27.
48. Youn J-I, Vargas G, Wong BJF, Milner TE. Depth-resolved phase retardation measurements for laser-assisted non-ablative cartilage reshaping. Phys Med Biol. 2005;50(9):1937–50. https://doi.org/10.1088/0031-9155/50/9/001.
49. Hajioannou JK, Nikolidakis A, Naumidi I, Helidonis E, Tzanakakis G, Velegrakis GA. In vitro enzymatic treatment and carbon dioxide laser beam irradiation of morphologic cartilage specimens. Arch Otolaryngol Head Neck Surg. 2006;132:1363–70.
50. Ignat'eva NY, Averkiev SV, Lunin VV, Grokhovskaya TE, Obrezkova MV. Effect of supramolecular organization of a cartilaginous tissue on thermal stability of collagen II. Russ J Phys Chem. 2006;80(8):1336–41. https://doi.org/10.1134/S0036024406080292.
51. Sviridov AP, Kondyurin AV. Optical characteristics of cartilage at a wavelength of 1560 nm and their dynamic behavior under laser heating conditions. J Biomed Opt. 2010;15(5):055003.
52. Soshnikova YM, Keselman MM, Baum OI, Shults EV, Obrezkova MV, Lunin VV, Sobol EN. Effect of anisotropy and drying of costal cartilage on its optical transmittance in laser reshaping of implants with 1, 2, and 3 mm in thickness. Lasers Surg Med. 2016;48(9):887–92. https://doi.org/10.1002/lsm.22575.
53. Wong BJF, Mimer TE, Anvari B, Sviridov A. Thermo-optical response of cartilage during feedback controlled laser-assisted reshaping intrinsic tissue turgor termed the donnan osmotic pressure. SPIE. 1997;2970:13–5.
54. Wong BJ, Milner TE, Harrington A, Ro J, Dao X, Sobol EN, Nelson JS. Feedback-controlled laser-mediated cartilage reshaping. Arch Facial Plast Surg. 1999;1(4):282–7. Retrieved from http://www.ncbi.nlm.nih.gov/pubmed/11430436
55. Bagratashvili NV, Dmitriev AK, Omel AI, Sobol N. Acoustic control of laser shaping of cartilage. SPIE. 1999;3732:312–8.
56. Burden M, Johansen E, Wong BJF. Design and construction of a precision cartilage reshaping device. SPIE. 2001.
57. Sobol EN, Sviridov AP, Svistushkin VM, Vorobieva NN. Feedback controlled laser system for safe and efficient reshaping of nasal cartilage. SPIE. 2010.
58. Gibson T, Davis WB. Distortion of autogenous grafts: Its cause and prevention. Br J Plast Surg. 1958;10:257–74.
59. Thomas L. Reversible collapse of rabbits ears after intravenous papain and prevention of recovery by cortisone. J Exp Med. 1956;104:245–51.
60. De Palma RG, De Palma MT, De Forest M. Experimental alteration of the shape of rabbit ear cartilage. J Surg Res. 1964;4:2–6.
61. Rubin FF. Permanent change in shape of cartilage. Arch Otolaryngol. 1969;89:64–70.
62. Wang Z, Pankratov MM, Perrault DF, Shapshay SM. Laser-assisted cartilage reshaping: in vitro and in vivo animal studies. SPIE. 1995.
63. Sviridov A, Sobol E, Bagratashvili V, Omelchenko A. In vivo study and histological examination of laser reshaping of cartilage. SPIE. 1999.
64. Jones N, Sviridov A, Sobol E, Omelchenko A, Lowe J. A prospective randomised study of laser reshaping of cartilage in vivo. Lasers Med Sci. 2001;16(4):284–90. Retrieved from http://www.ncbi.nlm.nih.gov/pubmed/11702634
65. Chang JC, Diaz SH, Wong BJF. Preliminary investigations of laser mediated cartilage reshaping in the in vivo rabbit model. SPIE. 2002.
66. Mordon S, Wang T, Fleurisse L, Creusy C. Laser cartilage reshaping in an in vivo rabbit model using a 1.54 μm Er:Glass laser. Lasers Surg Med. 2004;34(4):315–22. https://doi.org/10.1002/lsm.20029.
67. Pullin JG, Collier MA, Das P, Smith RL, DeBault LE, Johnson LL, Walls RC. Effects of holmium: YAG laser energy on cartilage metabolism, healing, and biochemical properties of lesional and perile-

sional tissue in a weight-bearing model. Arthroscopy. 1996;12(1):15–25. Retrieved from http://www.ncbi.nlm.nih.gov/pubmed/8838724
68. Wong BJ, Milner TE, Kim HK, Chao K, Sun CH, Sobol EN, Nelson JS. Proteoglycan synthesis in porcine nasal cartilage grafts following Nd:YAG (lambda = 1.32 microns) laser-mediated reshaping. Photochem Photobiol. 2000;71(2):218–24. https://doi.org/10.1562/0031-8655(2000)071.
69. Rasouli A, Sun CH, Basu R, Wong BJF. Quantitative assessment of chondrocyte viability after laser mediated reshaping: a novel application of flow cytometry. Lasers Surg Med. 2003;32(1):3–9. https://doi.org/10.1002/lsm.10142.
70. Karam AM, Protsenko DE, Li C, Wright R, Liaw L-HL, Milner TE, Wong BJF. Long-term viability and mechanical behavior following laser cartilage reshaping. Arch Facial Plast Surg. 2006;8(2):105–16. https://doi.org/10.1001/archfaci.8.2.105.
71. Wang Z, Perrault DF, Pankratov MM, Shapshay SM. Endoscopic laser-assisted reshaping of collapsed tracheal cartilage: a laboratory study. Ann Otol Rhinol Laryngol. 1996;105(3):176–81.
72. Tsang W, Lam A, Protsenko DE, Wong BJF. Endoscopic laser reshaping of rabbit tracheal cartilage: preliminary investigations. SPIE. 2005;2150:345–54.
73. Chae Y, Protsenko DE, Holden PK, Chlebicki C, Wong BJF. Thermoforming of tracheal cartilage: viability, shape change, and mechanical behavior. Lasers Surg Med. 2008;40(8):550–61. https://doi.org/10.1177/0145721709355835.
74. Bourolias C, Hajiioannou J, Sobol E, Velegrakis G, Helidonis E. Epiglottis reshaping using CO2 laser: a minimally invasive technique and its potent applications. Head Face Med. 2008;4:15. https://doi.org/10.1186/1746-160X-4-15.
75. Donald PJ. Homographic cartilage in facial implantation. Facial Plast Surg. 1992;8(3):157–75. https://doi.org/10.1055/s-2008-1064646.
76. Rhinology. The collected writings of Maurice H. Cottle, MD. American Rhinologic Society. Editorial Board. Pat A. Barelli, Walter E.E. Loch, Eugene B. Kern, Albert Steiner; 1987. p 35–37.
77. Cottle NH, Loring RM. Fisher GC< Gaynon IE. The maxilla-premaxilla approach to extensive nasal septum surgery. Arch Otolaryngol. 1958;68:303–13.
78. Sobol EN, Sviridov AP, Bagratashvili VN, Omelchenko AI, Ovchinnikov Y, Shekhter A, et al. Laser reshaping of nasal septum cartilage: clinical results for 40 patients. SPIE. 2000.
79. Ovchinnikov Y, Sobol E, Svstushkin V, Shekhter A, Bagratashvili VN, Sviridov AP. Laser septochondrocorrection. Arch Facial Plast Surg. 2002;4:180–5.
80. Bourolias C, Prokopakis E, Sobol E, Moschandreas J, Velegrakis GA, Helidonis E. Septal cartilage reshaping with the use of an Erbium doped glass fiber laser. Preliminary results. Rhinology. 2008;46(1):62–5.
81. Leclère FM, Petropoulos I, Buys B, Mordon S. Laser assisted septal cartilage reshaping (LASCR): a prospective study in 12 patients. Lasers Surg Med. 2010;42(8):693–8. https://doi.org/10.1002/lsm.20958.
82. Trelles MA, Mordon SR. Correction of ear malformations by laser-assisted cartilage reshaping (LACR). Lasers Surg Med. 2006;38:659–62.
83. Leclère FM, Vogt PM, Casoli V, Vlachos S, Mordon S. Laser-assisted cartilage reshaping for protruding ears: a review of the clinical applications. Laryngoscope. 2015;125:2067–71.
84. Leclère FMP, Petropoulos I, Mordon S. Laser-assisted cartilage reshaping (LACR) for treating ear protrusions: a clinical study in 24 patients. Aesthet Plast Surg. 2010;34:141–6.
85. Ragab A. Carbon dioxide laser-assisted cartilage reshaping otoplasty for prominent ears. Adv Cosmet Otoplasty Art Sci New Clin Tech. 2010:249–65. https://doi.org/10.1007/978-3-642-35431-1_24.
86. Leclère FM, et al. 1064-nm Nd: YAG laser-assisted cartilage reshaping for treating ear protrusions. Laryngoscope. 2015;125:2461–7.
87. Leclère FM, Mordon SR, Trelles MA. Cartilage reshaping for protruding ears: a prospective long term follow-up of 32 procedures. Lasers Surg Med. 2011;43:875–80.
88. Helidonis A, Sobol E, Velegrakis G, Bizakis J. Shaping of nasal septal cartilage with the carbon dioxide laser—a preliminary report of an experimental study. Lasers Med Sci. 1994:51–4.
89. Karamzadeh AM, Rasouli A, Tanenbaum BS, Milner TE, Wong BJF. Laser-mediated cartilage reshaping with feedback-controlled cryogen spray cooling: biophysical properties and viability. Lasers Surg Med. 2001;28:1–10.
90. Cheng CJ, et al. Minimizing superficial thermal injury using bilateral cryogen spray cooling during laser reshaping of composite cartilage grafts. Lasers Surg Med. 2008;40:477–82.
91. Chlebicki C, Protsenko DE, Wong BJF. Preliminary investigations on therapy thresholds for laser dosimetry, cryogen spray cooling duration, and treatment cycles for laser cartilage reshaping in the New Zealand White Rabbit Auricle Cara. Lasers Med Sci. 2014;10:54–6.
92. Wu EC, et al. Ex vivo investigations of laser auricular cartilage reshaping with carbon dioxide spray cooling in a rabbit model. Lasers Med Sci. 2013;28:1475–82.
93. Holden PK, Chlebicki C, Wong BJF. Minimally invasive ear reshaping with a 1450-nm diode laser using cryogen spray cooling in New Zealand White Rabbits. Arch Facial Plast Surg. 2009;48:1–6.
94. Kuan E, et al. In vivo laser cartilage reshaping with carbon dioxide spray cooling in a rabbit ear model: a pilot study. Lasers Surg Med. 2015;19:161–9.

Laser Treatment of MEDICATION-Related Osteonecrosis of the Jaws

14

Paolo Vescovi

Contents

Abstract

MRONJ is a multifactorial disease, and it is therefore difficult to realize an aetiological therapy.

MRONJ management is controversial: there are no evidence-based guidelines in the literature, in particular with regard to surgical procedures possibly associated with good results during a long-term follow-up.

The literature recommends a conservative treatment as initial therapy for pain control and elimination of acute inflammatory signs before any surgical option, for all stages of disease.

Laser applications at low intensity (low-level laser therapy—LLLT) have been reported in the literature for the treatment of MRONJ. Biostimulant effects of laser improve reparative process, increase inorganic matrix of bone and **osteoblast mitotic index** and stimulate lymphatic and blood capillary growth. It has been reported that LLLT has anti-inflammatory actions and it can help to control pain as well. LLLT also holds biostimulatory properties with favourable actions on bacterial control and wound healing. The review of the literature confirmed the superiority of the LLLT association with antibiotic therapy in comparison to other noninvasive approach to MRONJ management.

In our experience, more than 60% of MRONJ patients treated with laser biostimulation and

P. Vescovi (✉)
Unit of Oral Medicine and Laser Surgery, Department of Medicine and Surgery, University Center of Dentistry, University of Parma, Parma, Italy
e-mail: paolo.vescovi@unipr.it

S. Stübinger et al. (eds.), *Lasers in Oral and Maxillofacial Surgery*,
https://doi.org/10.1007/978-3-030-29604-9_14

antibiotic therapy (2 g of amoxicillin and 1 g of metronidazole a day for 2 weeks) have had improvement of their symptomatology, and 35% have had complete mucosal healing during 6 months of follow-up.

This therapy is easy to administer and useful also for aged and compromised patients, and it is not associated with any known side effect.

A soft surgical approach performed with laser, in patients unresponsive to antibiotic therapy or LLLT, represents a good solution: it is rapid and poorly invasive and can be performed under local anaesthesia in day-surgery regimen. The erbium-doped yttrium aluminium garnet (Er:YAG) laser has emerged as a possible alternative to conventional methods of bone ablation as the main components of bone have a high absorption of laser light at the wavelength of 2.94 μm. The histological findings of bone treated with erbium laser highlighted vital lamellar bone at the lased margins without microscopic evidence of inflammation or osteoclastic activity. Some recent researches reported that Er:YAG laser irradiation stimulates the secretion of platelet-derived growth factor in osteotomy sites and has bactericidal effect against *Actinomyces* and anaerobes. Results confirm that the laser surgery represents the best therapeutic option for minimally invasive treatment of the early stages of the disease also in immunocompromised patients.

The association of the Er:YAG laser and autofluorescence examination seems to be highly useful in removing additional minimal necrotic bone after osteoplasty. It is possible to use laser evaporation in areas in which absence of fluorescence or hypofluorescence has been revealed. Moreover, the previously cited biological advantages of Er:YAG surgery combined with the biomodulation of the soft and hard tissues induced by LLLT seem to integrate a valid approach for MRONJ treatment.

Keywords

MEDICATION-related osteonecrosis of the jaw (MRONJ) · Low-level laser therapy (LLLT) · Laser jaw bone surgery · Erbium laser · Diode laser · Nd:YAG laser

14.1 Introduction

Robert Marx described in 2003 an unusual condition related to bisphosphonate therapy in cancer patients: diffuse or localized area of necrotic jaw bone [1].

In 2014, the American Association of Oral and Maxillofacial Surgeon (AAOMS) published an update of the 2009 Position Paper on Bisphosphonate-Related Osteonecrosis of the Jaws [2].

The term "MEDICATION-related osteonecrosis of the jaw (MRONJ)" has recently replaced the previous "bisphosphonate-related osteonecrosis of the jaw (BRONJ)". Such as a decision was taken to include in the definition the growing number of osteonecrosis cases involving the maxilla and mandible associated with drugs different than bisphosphonates (BP), such as antiresorptive (denosumab) and antiangiogenic (bevacizumab, sunitinib) medications [3–5]. Patients may be diagnosed with MRONJ if all of the following characteristics are present: (1) current or previous treatment with antiresorptive or antiangiogenic agents; (2) exposed bone or bone that can be probed through an intraoral or extraoral fistula (e) in the maxillofacial region that has persisted for more than 8 weeks; and (3) no history of radiation therapy or obvious metastatic disease to the jaws.

The prevalence of MRONJ in patients under BP therapy (BPT) for osteopenia, osteoporosis and Paget's disease is significantly lower (from 0.1% to 0.21%) than prevalence in those treated intravenously for multiple myeloma and bone metastases (from 0.7% to 6.7%) [6].

Many hypotheses concerning the pathophysiology of MRONJ have been put forward, but none could explain all of the peculiar features of this disease.

Many factors such as anatomic site and high concentration and release of bisphosphonates (BPs) in the jaw bone, bone remodelling suppression, inhibition of the vascularization, soft tissue toxicity, bacterial infection, local trauma and genetic predisposition are involved.

Denosumab, a monoclonal antibody that is used in the treatment of osteoporosis and bone metastasis, has been shown to have an equal or higher capacity to suppress bone turnover than bisphosphonates. It acts by inhibiting osteoclast activity, reducing bone resorption and increasing bone density. Its highly specific mechanism of action is the inhibition of receptor activator of nuclear factor-kappa B ligand (RANKL).

Local factors associated with ONJ appearance in patients receiving BPs or denosumab are dental extractions (or other surgical procedure in the jawbone), periodontal diseases and poor oral hygiene and trauma induced by dental removable prostheses [7–9].

Prevention of ONJ related to BPs or denosumab is still debated, although a combined approach seems to be beneficial: preventive measures for the elimination or reduction of the risk factors, including periodic clinical screening.

MRONJ is a multifactorial disease, and it is therefore difficult to realize an aetiological therapy.

MRONJ management is controversial: there are no evidence-based guidelines in the literature, in particular with regard to surgical procedures possibly associated with good results during a long-term follow-up. The first purposes of treatment should be the reduction of pain and infection and the interruption of the progression of disease. Within such a context, the literature supports a noninvasive approach especially for asymptomatic stages of MRONJ. Temporary suspension of BPs offers no short-term benefit, whilst long-term discontinuation (if feasible with patient systemic conditions) may be beneficial in stabilizing sites of ONJ and reducing clinical symptoms [10].

Patients with exposed bone are usually treated with systemic antibiotics (penicillin or clindamycin along with metronidazole), oral rinses (chlorhexidine gluconate or hydrogen peroxide) or antimycotic agents (nystatin, ketoconazole or fluconazole).

The main problem of local or systemic antibacterial therapy is the nonpersistent clinical result (abscess disappearance, pain, swelling improvement) which is usually followed by a recurrence after an mean time of 3 weeks. Such an approach has as main problem the usual advanced age of patients and their usual administration with chemotherapy, leading to poor health conditions, which make them not able to bear the side effects of a prolonged (and sometimes permanent) antibiotic schedule. The second issue is the possible evolution of the disease and the unpredictable shifting from stage I to advanced stages of MRONJ [11].

14.2 Conservative Management of MRONJ

The literature recommends a conservative treatment as initial therapy for pain control and elimination of acute inflammatory signs before any surgical option, for all stages of disease [12, 13].

Ozone therapy (OT) and hyperbaric oxygen therapy (HBO) may stimulate cell proliferation and soft tissue healing, thus reducing pain.

Laser applications at low intensity (low-level laser therapy—LLLT) have been reported in the literature for the treatment of MRONJ. Biostimulant effects of laser improve reparative process, increase inorganic matrix of bone and **osteoblast mitotic index** and stimulate lymphatic and blood capillaries growth. HBO, OT and LLLT are usually recommended in addition to medical or surgical therapy: frequently, the positive clinical result is associated with an improvement of results obtained with conventional treatments, supplemented by alternative therapies [14–16].

14.2.1 Low-Level Laser Therapy (LLLT) and MRONJ Treatment

The mechanism of action underlying the biological effect of laser therapy has been widely investigated by researchers, but it remains controversial.

Laser applications at low intensity (low-level laser therapy—LLLT) produce some changes in cellular metabolism: the light is absorbed by primary photoacceptors, and this event triggers a pathway on the existing cell regulation mechanism. The wide range of applications of low-power laser effects and the possibility of using different wavelengths for irradiation depend on the fact that the primary photoacceptors of monochromatic visible light are the respiratory chain components [17, 18]. A secondary reaction consists in the transduction of the signal outside the mitochondria leading to enhancement of cell differentiation and/or proliferation, which represent the ultimate effects of light irradiation. The modulation of macromolecular synthesis has been suggested as part of the secondary reaction at the tissue level, related to the laser irradiation [19].

The effects of LLLT with different wavelengths on the trophism of skin and mucosa and stimulation of blood capillaries have been reported by several authors, and these observations could, to some extent, give support for a possible usefulness of laser biostimulation in the prevention and treatment of MRONJ.

LLLT represents an effective option largely reported in the literature for the management of chemotherapy- and/or radiotherapy-induced oral mucositis and, during the last 12 years, for MRONJ management.

It has been reported that LLLT has anti-inflammatory actions and it can help to control pain as well. LLLT also holds biostimulatory properties with favourable actions on bacterial control and wound healing [20].

In in vitro studies, a stimulatory effect of many wavelengths (diode or Nd:YAG laser) on the cell viability and proliferation of human osteoblast-like cell culture exposed to BPs was reported [21–23].

Osteocalcin seems to have several functions in bone metabolism: it has an important role in the process of bone remodelling affecting both osteoblast and osteoclast activities, and it is also a regulator of bone mineralization. In vivo studies in animal models show that laser irradiation after tooth extraction can promote osteoblast differentiation. In the same studies, it has been also demonstrated a higher expression of bone markers osteopontin (OPN) and osteocalcin (OCN), 8 days after surgical interventions [24].

Clinical studies performed in cancer and noncancer patients under BPT reported an important reduction of pain, oedema, size of bone exposure, pus, fistulas and halitosis with significant improvement of quality of life [25].

In our experience, more than 60% of MRONJ patients treated with laser biostimulation and antibiotic therapy (2 g of amoxicillin and 1 g of metronidazole a day for 2 weeks) have had improvement of their symptomatology, and 35% have had complete mucosal healing during 6 months of follow-up [26, 27]. On the contrary, percentage of improvement after systemic antibiotic therapy and local antibacterial rinses (without the laser applications) can be estimated between 20% and 30%.

The association of laser biomodulation and antibiotic therapy leads, in many cases after few weeks, to elimination of bone sequestrum (Figs. 14.1, 14.2, 14.3, 14.4 and 14.5).

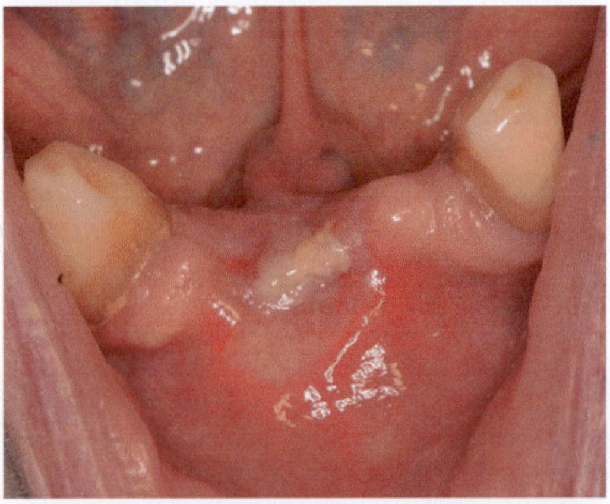

Fig. 14.1 An 87-year-old woman with osteoporosis treated with alendronate for 15 years without other known risk factors. Spontaneous form of MRONJ stage 1 (according to AAOMFS 2014) in edentulous ridge (possible prosthetic trauma)

LLLT was delivered through an Nd:YAG laser (1064 nm) with power of 1.25 W, frequency of 15 Hz and a fibre diameter 320 μm. The laser source was used at a distance of 1–2 mm from tissues for 1 min (PD 1555 W/cm^2, total fluence 167.94 J/cm^2) for five consecutive applications. Laser energy was widely applied by scanning the affected area. Each patient underwent five laser irradiation sessions (one during the first week of medical treatment and the other every 7 days after the first).

The review of the literature confirmed the superiority of the LLLT association with antibiotic therapy in comparison to other noninvasive approach [28, 29]. This therapy is easy to administer and useful also for aged and compromised patients, and it is not associated with any known side effect.

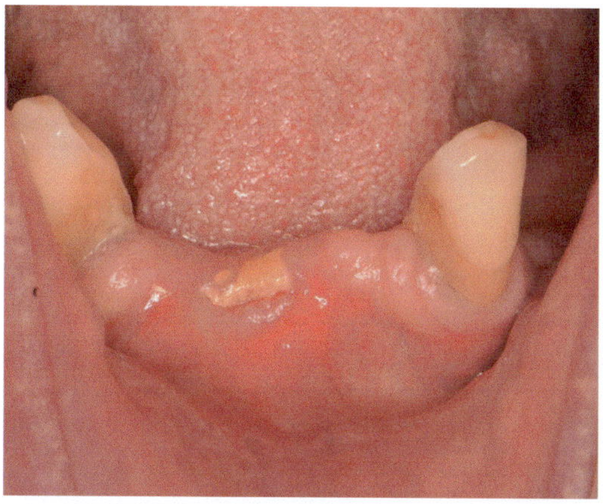

Fig. 14.2 Reduction of inflammation after 3 weeks of Nd:YAG laser (1064 nm) biomodulation at 1.25 W, 15 Hz (fibre diameter 320 μm) at a distance of 1–2 mm from the tissue for 1 min (fluence 167.94 J/cm^2) and antibiotic treatment (2 g of amoxicillin and 1 g of metronidazole a day)

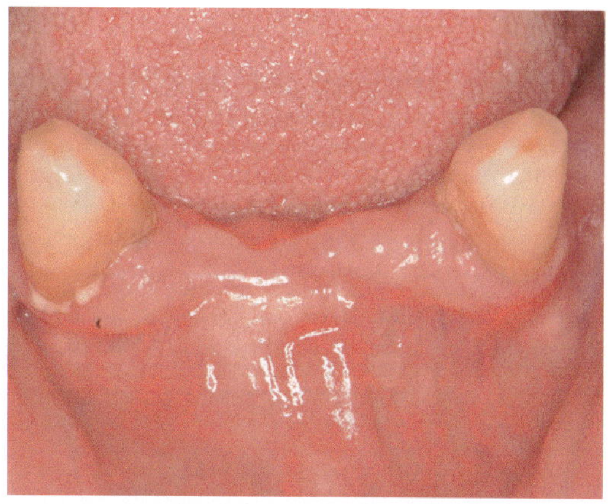

Fig. 14.5 Complete recovery after 4 weeks

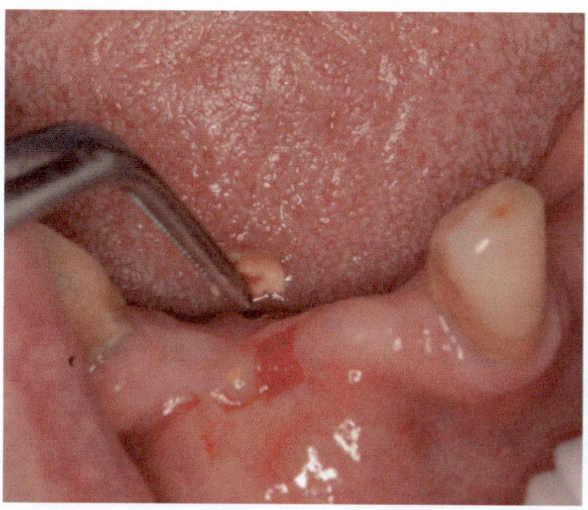

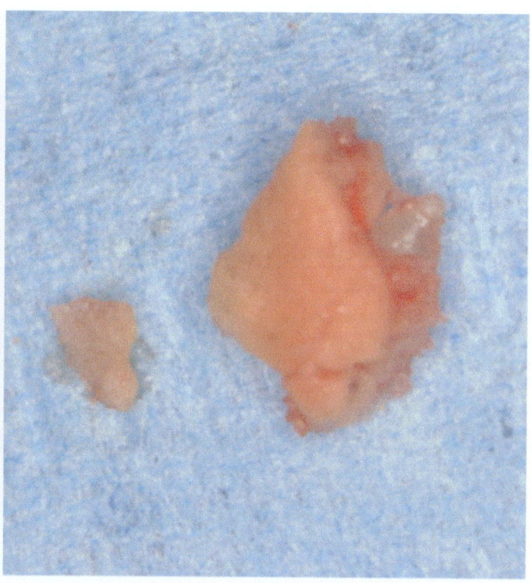

Figs. 14.3 and 14.4 Bone sequestrum elimination

14.3 Surgical Management of MRONJ

Surgery may be avoided if permanent mucosal repair appears after the conservative management; however, such an occurrence seems to be limited to very few cases. Surgical approach seems unavoidable in most of the cases of MRONJ, where complete healing or permanence of symptoms has not been obtained irrespectively by the stage of the disease.

The rate of remission reported in the literature is higher for MRONJ in non-cancer patients (osteoporosis) and those with multiple myeloma than for MRONJ in those with solid tumours and slightly higher for early stages than for late stages of disease [30–32]. Discontinuation of BPs or denosumab therapy can favour the surgical outcome, most probably for the reduction of the action of the drugs in the soft tissues.

Surgical debridement or resection in combination with antibiotic therapy may offer long-term palliation with resolution of acute infection and pain. Mobile segments of bony sequestrum and necrotic tissue should be removed extending surgery until unaffected bone [33]. In diffuse MRONJ, the resection of mandible and vascularized reconstruction with free fibula flaps have been proposed in the literature. In case of large and complex surgical interventions, a careful evaluation of the general conditions of each patient, including situation and evolution of disease, age, performance status and life expectancy, is advisable [34].

14.3.1 Laser Surgery of MRONJ

A soft surgical approach performed with laser, in patients unresponsive to antibiotic therapy or LLLT, represents a good solution: it is rapid and poorly invasive and can be performed under local anaesthesia in day-surgery regimen. Over the last decades, in several experimental and clinical studies, it has been reported the benefit of laser osteotomy in oral-maxillofacial surgery with efficient ablation rates and rare or absent carbonization phenomenon.

The erbium-doped yttrium aluminium garnet (Er:YAG) laser has emerged as a possible alternative to conventional methods of bone ablation as the main components of bone have a high absorption of laser light at the wavelength of 2.94 μm. The wavelength-dependent absorption coefficient for water is at its maximum peak at 2.94 μm. The Er:YAG laser theoretically has an absorption coefficient of water that is 10 being 15,000–20,000 times higher than the CO_2 and the Nd:YAG lasers, respectively. Air and water spray reduces overheating of both hard and soft tissues, but also it cleans the site of irradiation, increases ablation rate and efficiency and facilitates the ablation process. Water and air spray advantages include the prevention of tissue dessication and the excess of heat accumulation in tissues due to desiccation of bone surfaces, the improvement of bone ablation for photoacoustic effect and the improvement of surgical activity for increase of visibility due to smear layer elimination in aerosol [35].

Bone temperature during Er:YAG laser osteotomy has a mean increase of 3.3 °C. The mean biological advantage of erbium laser in comparison to other surgical devices is the bone and mucosal healing improvement. After Er:YAG laser ablation, red blood cell aggregate was noted over the treated bone surface. At 6 and 24 h and 3, 7 and 14 days, initial events of bone and soft tissue healing appear to progress earlier in comparison to CO_2 laser or traditional tungsten burr. Osteotomy sites after Er:YAG laser ablation exhibited more prominent inflammatory cell infiltration, revascularization and proliferation of fibroblasts and osteoblasts, indicating active osteoid tissue formation. The irregular surface structure after Er:YAG laser ablation, with no smear or char layers, provided a favourable surface for cell attachment and thus accelerated bone healing and formation [36]. The application of Er:YAG laser in the bone surface promotes the production of PGE2 and COX2 from fibroblasts of human gingiva promoting the early phases of wound healing [37].

Studies on bone damages induced through different cutting systems reported that all sections obtained with Er:YAG laser were better than those obtained with piezosurgery, high-speed drills and low-speed drills. Er:YAG laser showed poor peripheral carbonization with a regular incision without residual bone smear layer [38]. The histological findings of bone graft harvested from the mandibular ramus using an erbium laser highlighted vital lamellar bone at the lased margins without microscopic evidence of inflammation or osteoclastic activity [39–41]. Some recent researches reported that Er:YAG laser irradiation stimulates the secretion of platelet-derived growth factor in osteotomy sites [42].

The bactericidal effect of Er:YAG laser against periodontopathogens forms such as *Actinomyces* and anaerobes is well reported in the literature. The efficacy of erbium laser, in comparison to other wavelength, is described also for periodontopathogen bacteria, *Candida* spp., in biofilm models [43, 44].

Er:YAG laser could be used also for oral mucosa incision without thermal damage to the surrounding and underlying tissues inducing less pain and better healing than traditional scalpel.

Taking into account the possible MRONJ pathogenesis, the aim of intervention should be the elimination of the maximum of necrotic bone and the covering of the surgical field with a vascularized soft tissue.

In our experience, all surgical interventions were performed under local anaesthesia. Prophylactic antibiotics (amoxicillin and clavulanic acid 2 g a day—metronidazole 1 g a day) were administered starting 4 days before surgery and were continued postoperatively for 2 weeks. The surgical procedure begun with a detachment of an envelope flap through a linear mucoperiosteal cut around bone exposure, without lateral incisions to contain risk of reduction of vascularization. The inflamed margins of the mucosa were eliminated for at least 2 mm to obtain a better quality tissue to cover bone surgical area.

Laser can be used for conservative surgery through a vaporization of necrotic bone, until healthy bone is reached. The erbium laser penetrates only very slightly (0.1 mm), being therefore very safe and allowing a precise, minimally invasive treatment. The minimally invasive technique of evaporation allows us to obtain a regularity of the sectioned bone surfaces, and it can be used to create micro-perforations at the base for stimulating vascularization. The additional advantages of laser surgery are the bactericidal and biostimulatory action of the laser beam with a better postoperative recovery [45–49].

Bone spicule and defects can be eliminated to obtain a smooth surface to avoid local traumatisms and to facilitate soft tissue healing over the surgical site. The surgical sites were abundantly rinsed with iodopovidone solution.

Intraoral closure was achieved by a tension-free mucosal flap sitting passively over the bone with a 4–0 silk suture. The sutures were removed from 10 to 14 days after surgical intervention (Figs. 14.6, 14.7, 14.8, 14.9, 14.10, 14.11, 14.12, 14.13, 14.14, 14.15, 14.16 and 14.17).

In the postoperative period, non-steroid anti-inflammatory drugs (NSAID), in case of necessity, and chlorhexidine 0.12% gel, four times a day, were recommended.

Orthopantomography and TC scan, in all cases of complete mucosal healing, were requested after 6 months and 1 year from the surgical intervention, respectively [50].

Conservative nonsurgical treatment has demonstrated to be partially successful with a resolution rate reported in the literature of only 50% of cases particularly in stages 2 and 3. In contrast, surgical approach has proven to give good results for more than 80% of the patients [51–53]. The success of surgical management of MRONJ

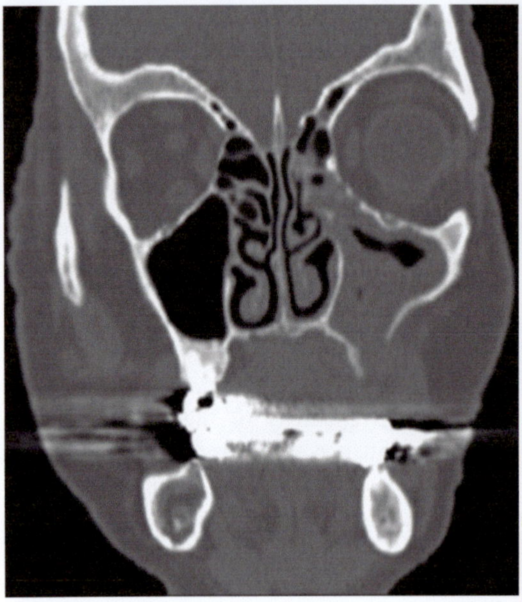

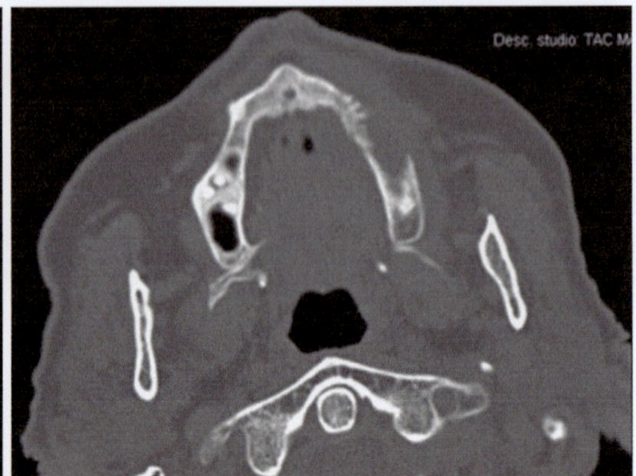

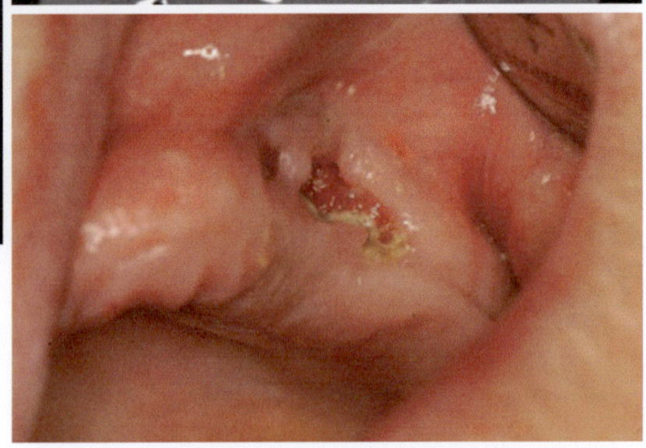

Figs. 14.6–14.8 A 74-year-old woman with osteoporosis treated for 8 years with alendronate. Other risk factors include diabetes, smoke and poor oral hygiene. Spontaneous MRONJ stage 3 (according to AAOMFS 2014) with large area of bone necrosis of edentulous ridge with involvement of paranasal sinuses

depends mainly on the stage of the disease and on the systemic conditions of patients; however, the individual patient status represents the only consideration guiding the choice of the surgical approach.

The literature confirms that patients having less severe disease were most likely to have improvement or complete healing of MRONJ lesions after surgical approach [54, 55].

Percentages of clinical success in MRONJ treatment with laser surgery are very high in comparison to conventional surgery reported in the literature [56]. Results confirm that the laser surgery represents the best therapeutic option for minimally invasive treatment of the early stages of the disease also in immunocompromised patients.

14.3.2 Autofluorescence-Guided Surgical Approach Performed with Er:YAG Laser

The clinical success of the surgical management of MRONJ lays on the precise individuation of the limits of the disease and on efficacy of necrotic bone elimination. The complete removal of osteonecrosis seems to be essential for avoid-

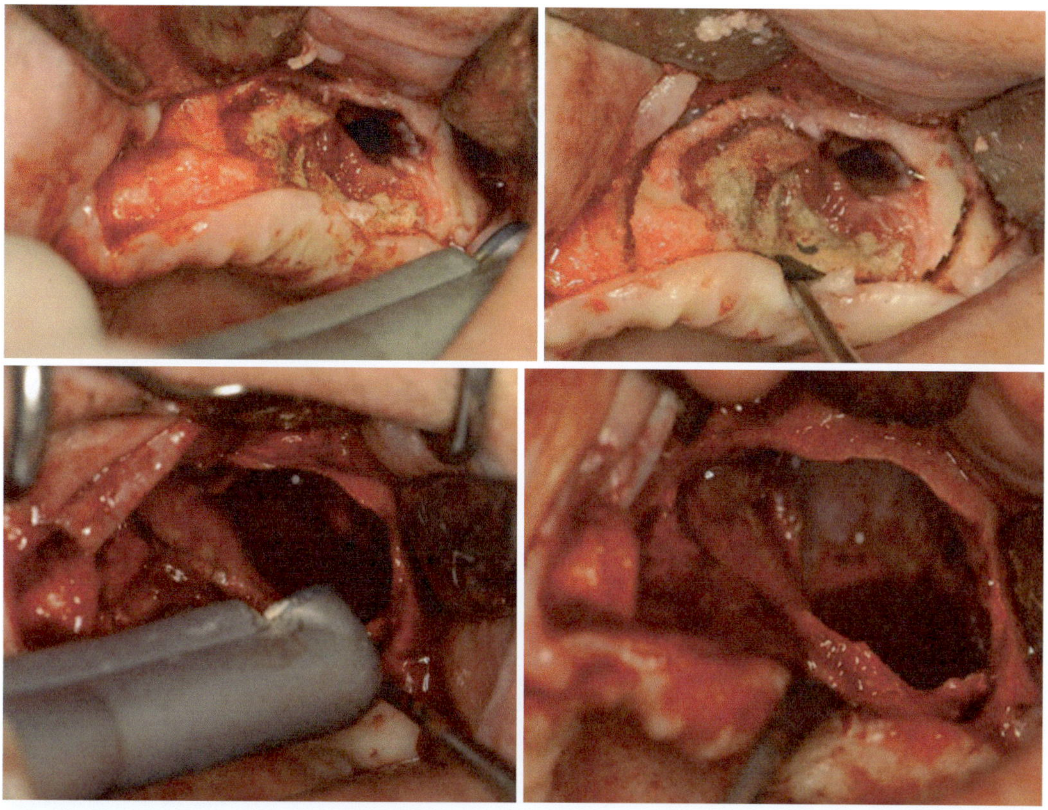

Figs. 14.9–14.12 Osteotomy performed with Er:YAG laser (2940 nm): extension at a distance of 1 cm around necrotic bone. Large communication with the maxillary sinus

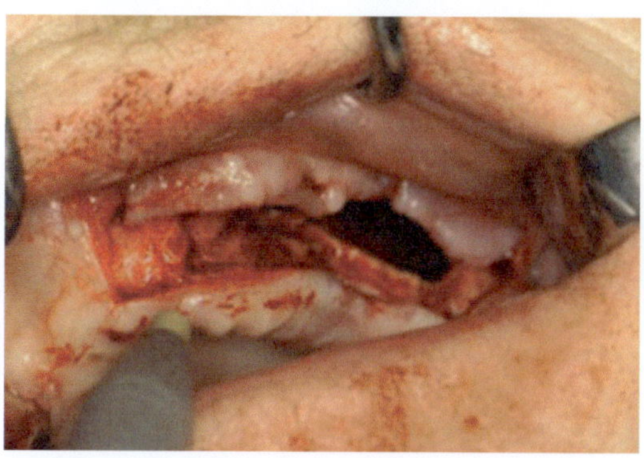

Fig. 14.13 Intraoperative Nd:YAG laser biostimulation

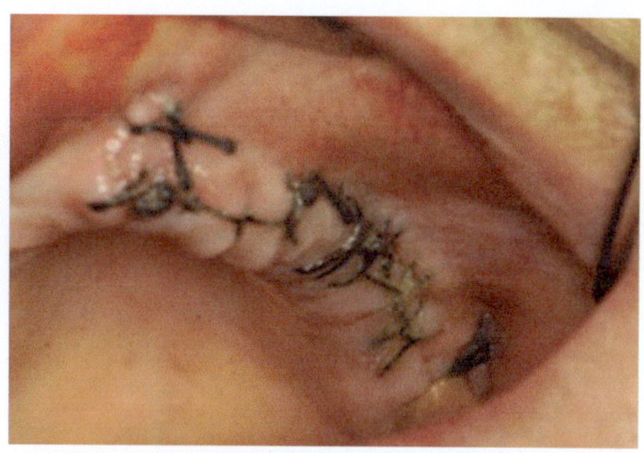

Fig. 14.14 Continuous suture

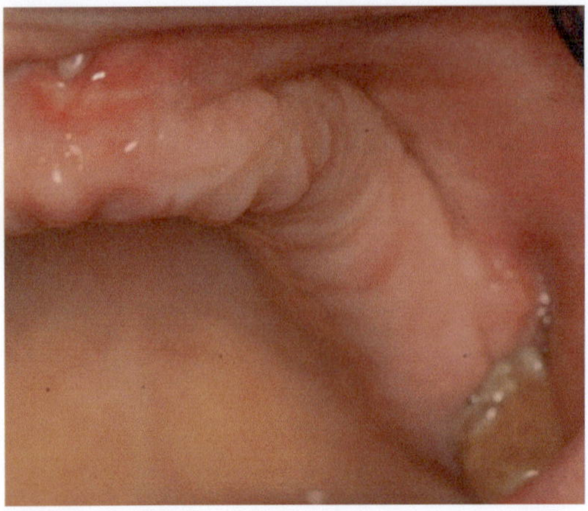

Fig. 14.15 Complete recovery after 2 months (maintained during 8 years)

ing recurrence or progression of the disease. The traditional systems to establish the extension of osteotomy are represented by radiological (computed tomography [CT], magnetic resonance imaging [MRI], fluoride positron emission tomography [PET] and orthopantomography [OPT]) or clinical (colour, consistence, bleeding or not bleeding bone) findings.

Recently, it has been reported in the literature a technique to discriminate necrotic from viable bone on the basis of fluorescence induced by tetracycline and stimulated by an appropriate excitation light. In order to standardize the surgical treatment and reduce its invasiveness, some authors proposed tetracycline fluorescence-

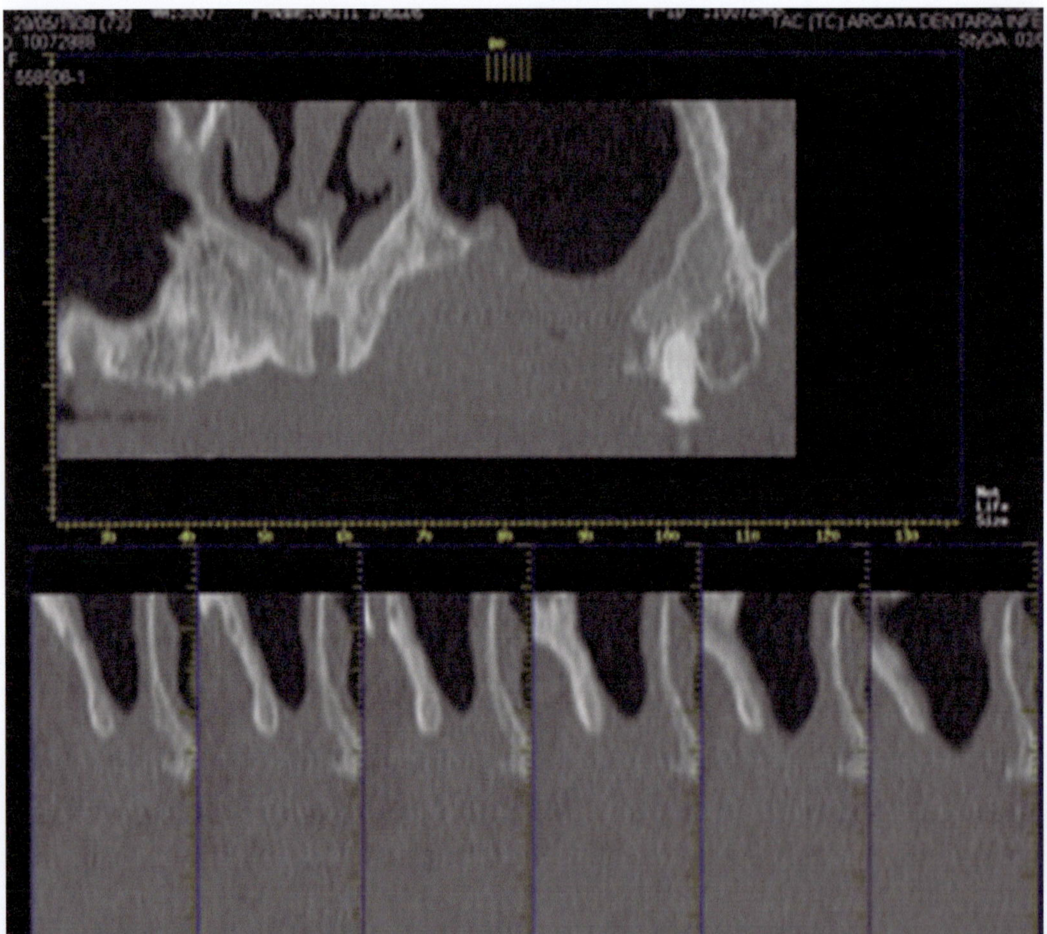

Figs. 14.16 and 14.17 TC scan. Complete resolution of MRONJ and regression of maxillary sinus involvement after 10 months from the surgical procedure

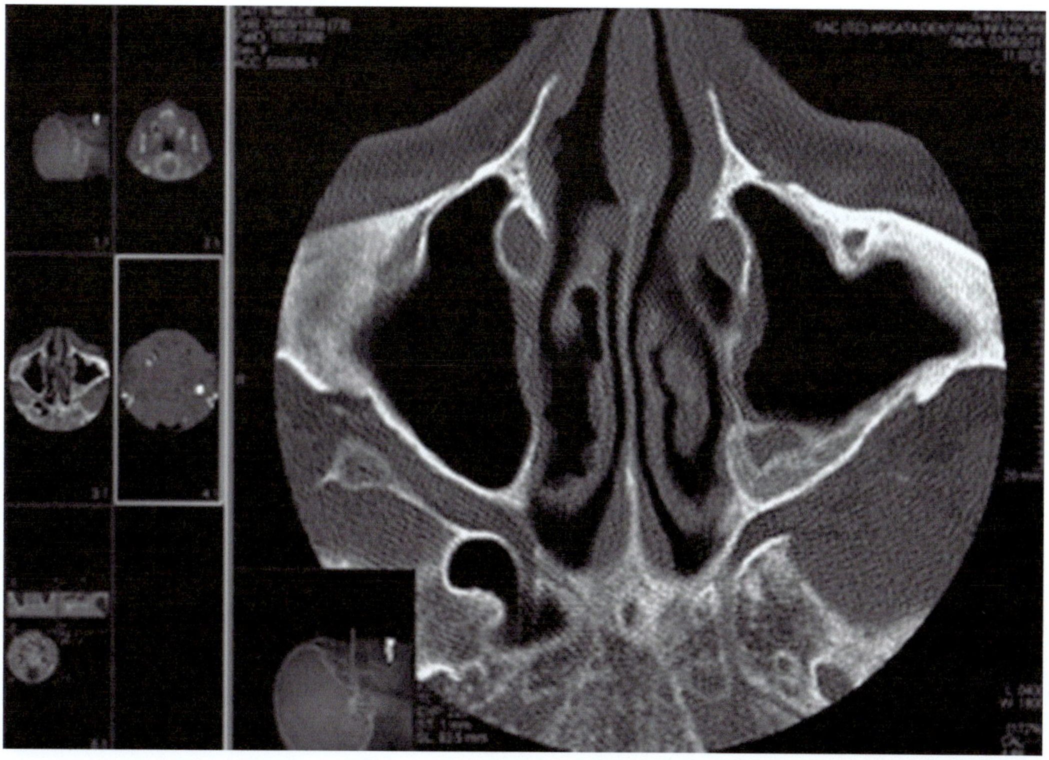

Figs. 14.16 and 14.17 (continued)

guided bone resection, with very high success rates [57, 58].

The autofluorescence (AF) examination is currently used to detect soft tissue dysplasia and malignancies, but the same protocol can be used for bone diseases. The fluorophores in the normal bone produce an emission of green AF. Alterations in stromal architecture are associated with a loss of autofluorescence (LAF). This phenomenon is obtained through a blue spectrum excitation light (400–460 nm). However, there are no explanations as to why necrotic bone seems to lose AF. It has been speculated that this could be caused by alterations in the extracellular calcified osteoid matrix or in the bone cells. Some authors reported the hypothesis that collagen matrix production of vital chondrocytes would correlate with AF intensity [59].

The intraoperative examination seems to be a suitable guide during surgical debridement/resection of MRONJ. The technique is not invasive, easy to apply and independent of the subjectivity of the surgeon [60, 61] (Figs. 14.18, 14.19, 14.20, 14.21, 14.22, 14.23, 14.24, 14.25, 14.26, 14.27, 14.28, 14.29, 14.30, 14.31, 14.32, 14.33, 14.34 and 14.35).

The association of the Er:YAG laser and AF seems to be highly useful in removing additional minimal necrotic bone after osteoplasty. It is possible to use laser evaporation in areas in which absence of fluorescence or hypofluorescence has been revealed. Moreover, the previously cited biological advantages of Er:YAG surgery combined with the biomodulation of the soft and hard tissues induced by LLLT seem to integrate a valid approach for MRONJ treatment [62–64].

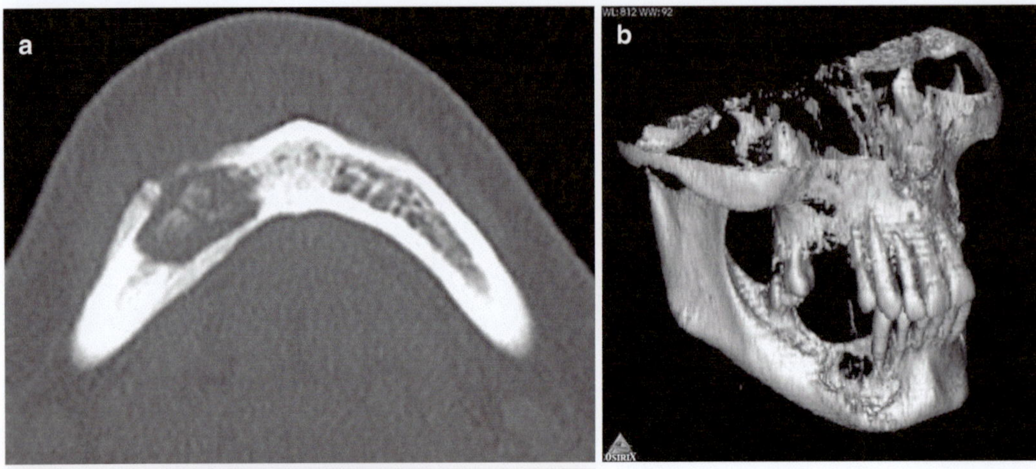

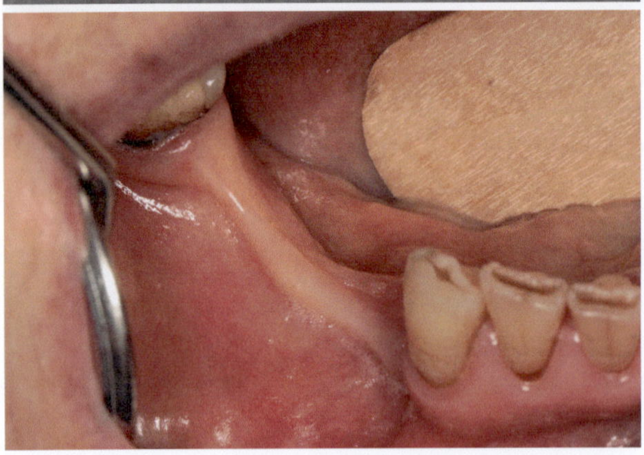

Figs. 14.18 and 14.19 A 69-year-old woman with osteoporosis treated for 6 years with alendronate without other known risk factors. MRONJ stage 2 (according to AAOMFS 2014): (**a**, **b**) computed tomography scan showing large osteonecrosis involving the vestibular and lingual plates. Non-exposed form of MRONJ appeared after teeth extraction (the premolars and the first molar)

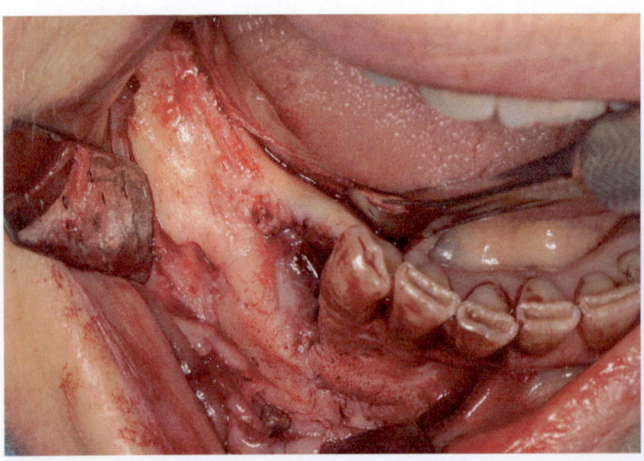

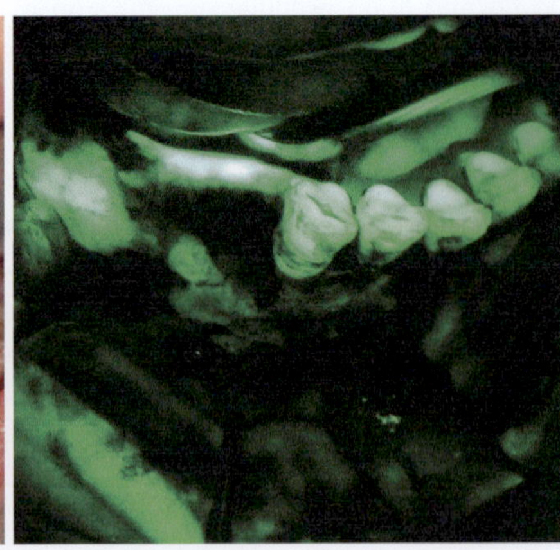

Figs. 14.20 and 14.21 Surgical field after mucoperiosteal flap elevation: necrotic bone and autofluorescence image showing hypofluorescent (dark) areas

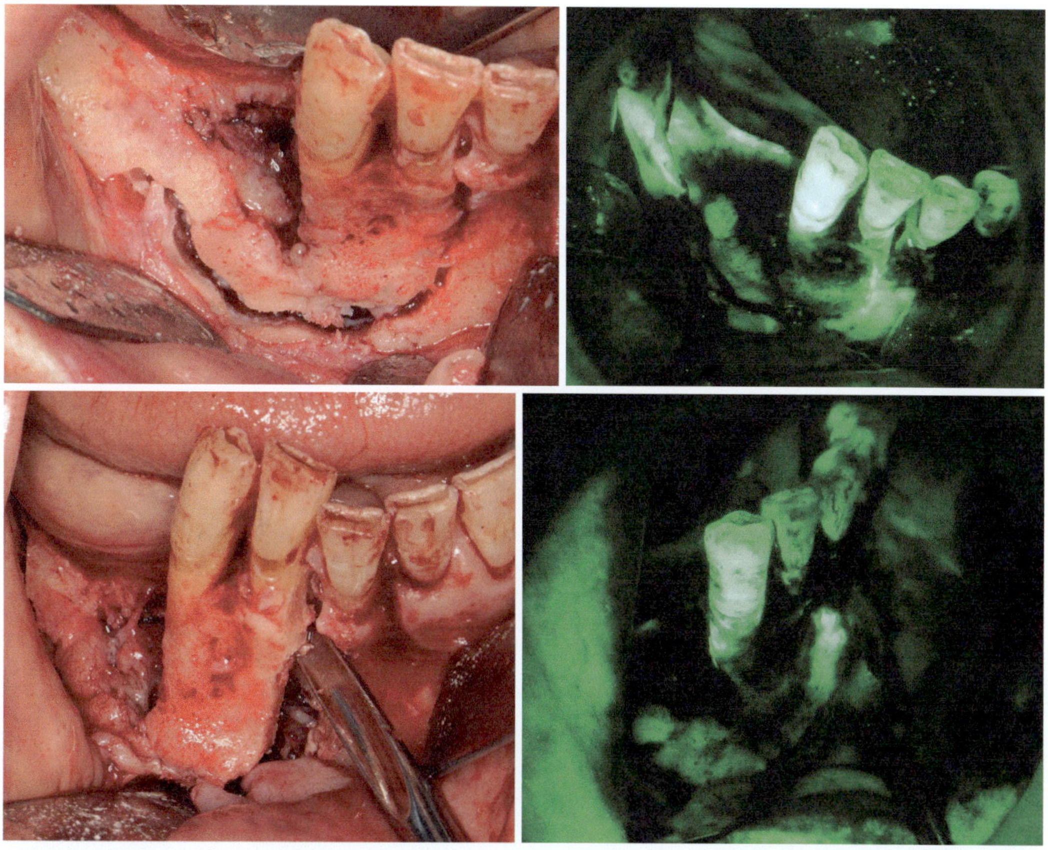

Figs. 14.22–14.25 Surgical field after osteotomy: clinical view and autofluorescent image showing hypofluorescent bone in the necrotic area and hyperfluorescent surfaces over the osteotomy line

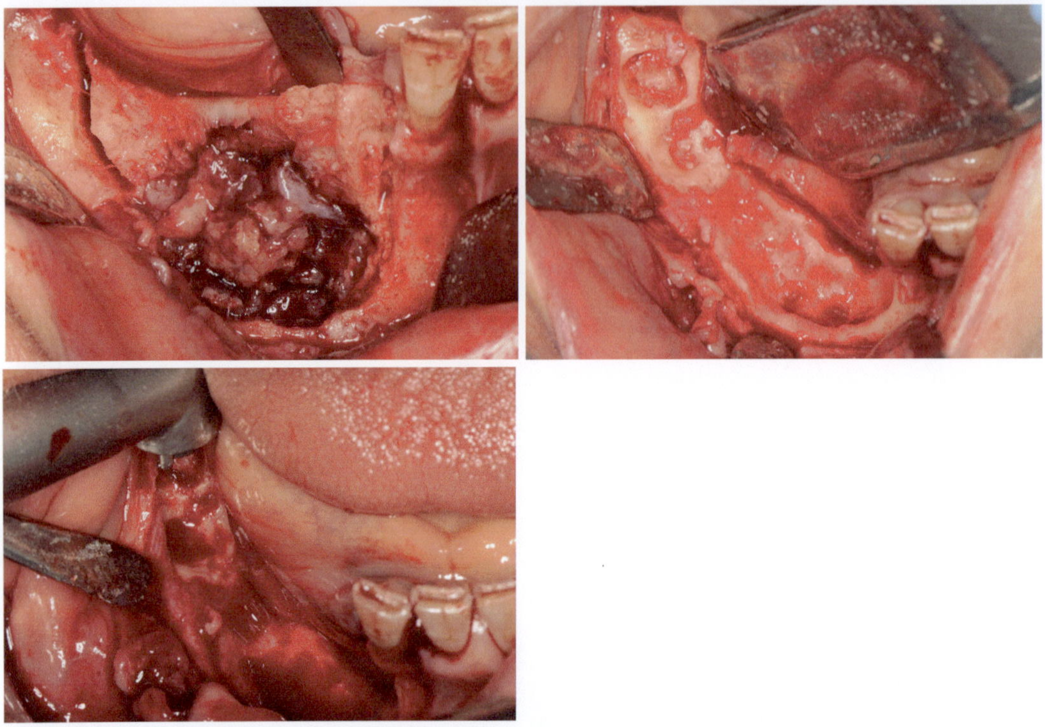

Figs. 14.26–14.28 Large area of necrotic bone removal and Er:YAG laser evaporation

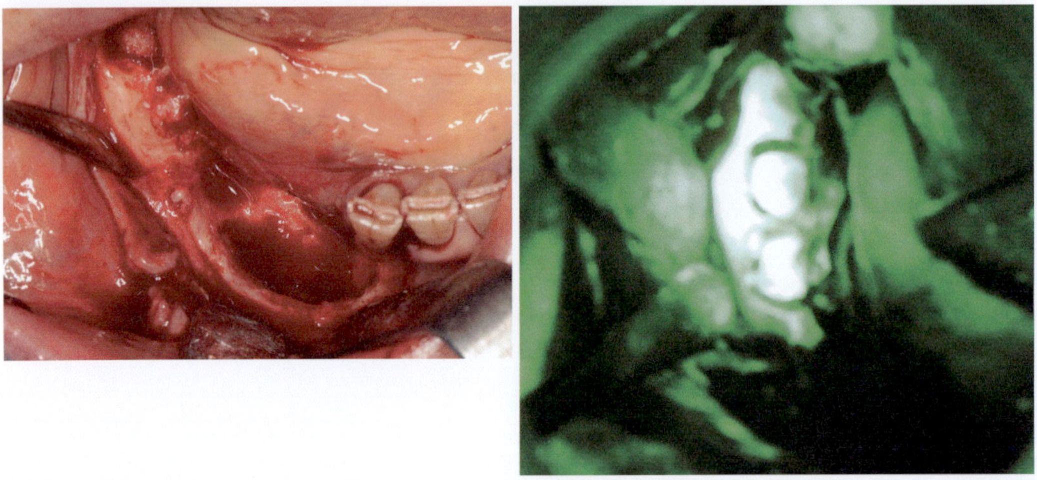

Figs. 14.29 and 14.30 Samples of hyperfluorescent bone collection (with Lindeman burr) in the area adjacent to necrosis. Clinical and autofluorescent view

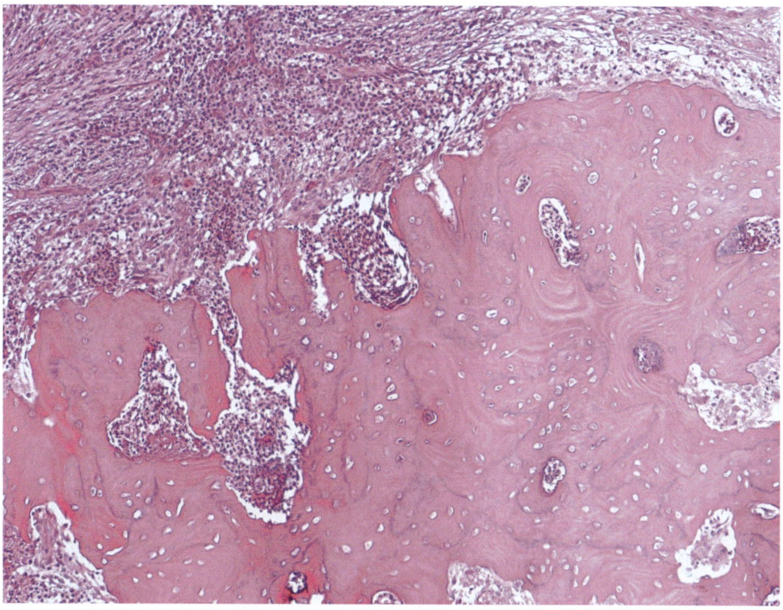

Fig. 14.31 Histopathological analysis of the hypofluorescent bone: large lacuna characterized by fibrous tissue with the coexistence of chronic and acute inflammation. Sparse residual bony trabeculae were present. This fibroinflammatory area was surrounded by necrotic bone

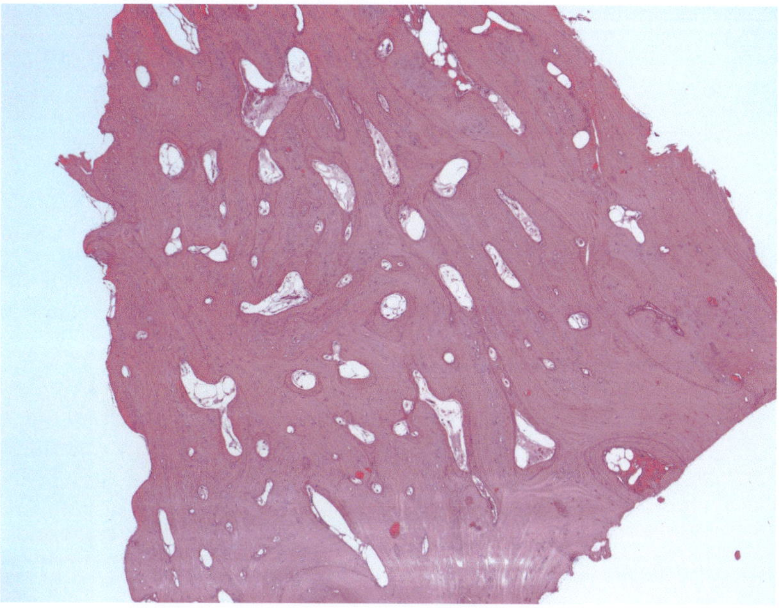

Fig. 14.32 Histopathological analysis of the hyperfluorescent bone: absence of necrosis signs, medullary bone with marked reactive changes in terms of hypertrophic trabeculae, in keeping with sclerotic bone

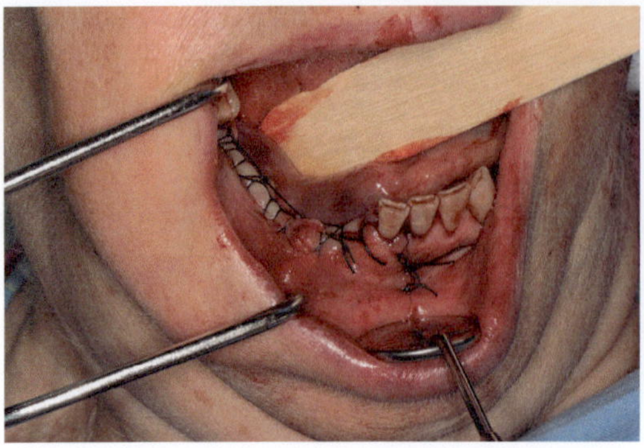

Fig. 14.33 Continuous suture

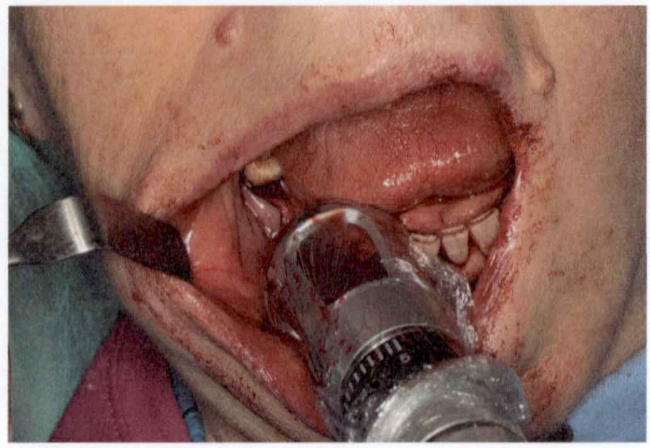

Fig. 14.34 Postoperative biomodulation session with diode laser

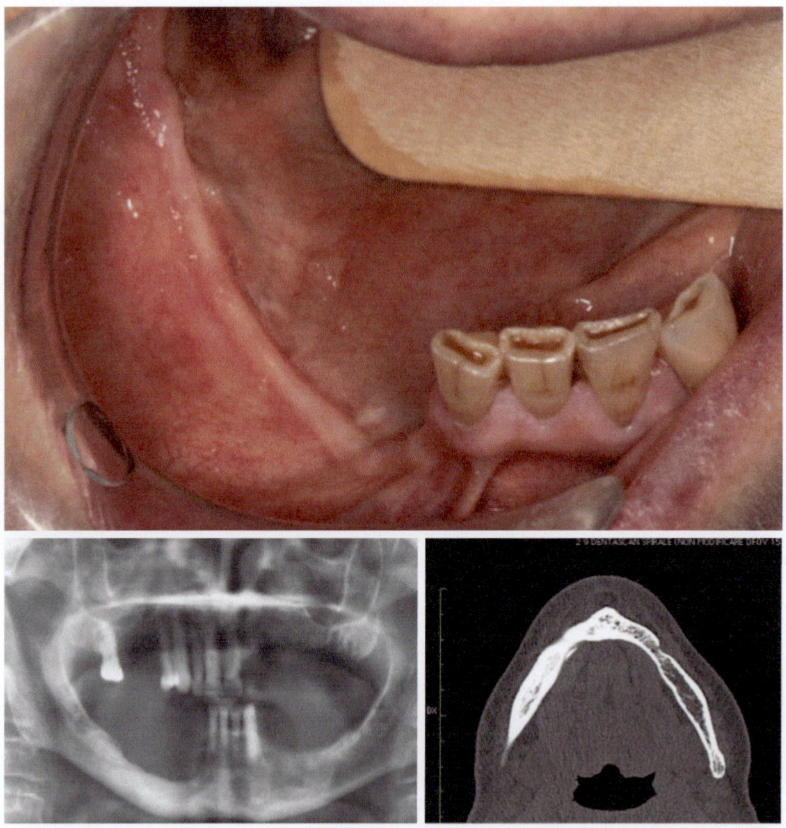

Fig. 14.35 Complete recovery after 2-year follow-up (last molar was extracted 1 year after the surgical intervention), without clinical and radiological signs of osteonecrosis

14.4 Conclusions

When making the decision to perform surgical procedures for the treatment of MRONJ, the deal between benefit and potential risks according to clinical features of each patient should be taken into account. Surgical operations for advanced stages of MRONJ are invasive and extensive and must be performed under general anaesthesia, usually for many hours. Only few patients may undergo this type of surgery. On the contrary, a minimal and faster intervention under local anaesthesia is useful also for aged and immunocompromised patients. Less invasive surgery may determine a complete mucosal healing reducing the microbial infection and the risk of disease progression.

The application of LLLT represents a noninvasive valid approach after invasive procedures such as tooth extractions, dental implant placement or oral surgical interventions, in patients under BPT, resulting in a possible way of MRONJ prevention.

Laser biostimulation (always associated with medical therapy) may offer an aid in the treatment of MRONJ, especially for those patients that cannot be treated with surgery (e.g. haemostasis impairment, immunodepression, age, comorbidities).

The treatment of patients affected by minimal bone exposition (as in the early MRONJ stages) with combined conservative surgical strategies can be useful to obtain a greater control of lesions for longer periods. Erbium laser allows a surgical debridement of jaw bone under local anaesthesia during a minimal invasive intervention with bactericidal and biostimulant action and better postoperative recovery.

On the basis of the previous considerations, antibiotic therapy combined with LLLT and the AF-guided surgical approach performed with Er:YAG laser and Nd:YAG biostimulation appears to be a promising modality of MRONJ prevention and treatment.

References

1. Marx RE. Pamidronate (Aredia) and zoledronate (Zometa) induced avascular necrosis of the jaws: a growing epidemic. J Oral Maxillofac Surg. 2003;61(9):1115–7.
2. Ruggiero SL, Dodson TB, Fantasia J, Goodday R, et al. American association of oral and maxillofacial surgeons position paper on medication-related osteonecrosis of the jaw-2014 update. J Oral Maxillofac Surg. 2014;72(10):1938–56.
3. Hoefert S, Yuan A, Munz A, Grimm M, et al. Clinical course and therapeutic outcomes of operatively and non-operatively managed patients with denosumab-related osteonecrosis of the jaw (DRONJ). J Craniomaxillofac Surg. 2017;45(4):570–8. https://doi.org/10.1016/j.jcms.2017.01.013.
4. Wynn RL. Bevacizumab (Avastin): an anti-angiogenic drug associated with osteonecrosis of the jaw. Gen Dent. 2011;59(6):410–3.
5. Fusco V, Porta C, Saia G, Paglino C, et al. Osteonecrosis of the jaw in patients with metastatic renal cell cancer treated with bisphosphonates and targeted agents: results of an italian multicenter study and review of the literature. Clin Genitourin Cancer. 2015;13(4):287–94.
6. Marx RE, Sawatari Y, Fortin M, Broumand V. Bisphosphonate-induced exposed bone (osteonecrosis/osteopetrosis) of the jaws: risk factors, recognition, prevention and treatment. J Oral Maxillofac Surg. 2005;63:1567–75.
7. Solomon DH, Mercer E, Woo SB, Avorn J, et al. Defining the epidemiology of bisphosphonate-associated osteonecrosis of the jaw: prior work and current challenges. Osteoporos Int. 2013;24:237–44.
8. Pichardo SE, van Merkesteyn JP. Bisphosphonate related osteonecrosis of the jaws: spontaneous or dental origin ? Oral Surg Oral Med Oral Pathol Oral Radiol. 2013;116(3):287–92.
9. Hinson AM, Smith CW, Siegel ER, Stack BC. Is bisphosphonate-related osteonecrosis of the jaw an infection? A histological and microbiological ten-year summary. Int J Dent. 2014;2014:452737. https://doi.org/10.1155/2014/452737.
10. Gallegro L, Junquera L. Consequence of therapy discontinuation in bisphosphonate-associated osteonecrosis of the jaws. Br J Oral Maxillofac Surg. 2009;47(1):67–8.
11. Vescovi P, Nammour S. Bisphosphonate-related osteonecrosis of the jaw (BRONJ) therapy. A critical review. Minerva Stomatol. 2010;59(4):181–213.
12. Bermúdez-Bejarano EB, Serrera-Figallo MA, Gutiérrez-Corrales A, Romero-Ruiz MM, et al. Prophylaxis and antibiotic therapy in management protocols of patients treated with oral and intravenous bisphosphonates. J Clin Exp Dent. 2017;9(1):e141–9.
13. Kühl S, Walter C, Acham S, Pfeffer R, Lambrecht JT. Bisphosphonate-related osteonecrosis of the jaws—a review. Oral Oncol. 2012;48(10):938–47.
14. Ripamonti CI, Cislaghi E, Mariani L, Maniezzo M. Efficacy and safety of medical ozone (O3) delivered in oil suspension applications for the treatment of osteonecrosis of the jaw in patients with bone metastases treated with bisphosphonates: preliminary results of a phase I-II study. Oral Oncol. 2011;47:185–90.
15. Freiberger JJ. Utility of Hyperbaric Oxygen in treatment of bisphosphonate-related osteonecrosis of the jaws. J Oral Maxillofac Surg. 2009;67(suppl 1):96–106.
16. Vescovi P, Meleti M, Merigo E, Manfredi M. Bisphosphonate-associated osteonecrosis (BON) of the jaws: a possible treatment? J Oral Maxillofac Surg. 2006;05:012.
17. Karu T. Mitochondrial mechanisms of photobiomodulation in context of new data about multiples roles of ATP. Photomed Laser Surg. 2010;28(2):159–60.

18. Belletti S, Uggeri J, Mergoni G, Vescovi P, Merigo E, Fornaini C, Nammour S, Manfredi M, Gatti R. Effects of 915 nm GaAs diode laser on mitochondria of human dermal fibroblasts: analysis with confocal microscopy. Lasers Med Sci. 2015;30:375–81.
19. McGee-Lawrence ME, Bradley EW, Dudakovic A, Carlson SW, Ryan ZC, Kumar R, Dadsetan M, Yaszemski MJ, Chen Q, An K-N, Westendorf JJ. Histone deacetylase 3 is required for maintenance of bone mass during aging. Bone. 2013;52:296–307.
20. Doeuk C, Hersant B, Bosc R, Lange F, SidAhmed-Mezi M, et al. Current indication for low level laser treatment in maxillo-facial surgery. Br J Oral Maxillofac Surg. 2015;53(4):309–15.
21. Basso FG, Turrioni AP, Soares DG, Bagnato VS, Hebling J, de Souza Costa CA. Low-level laser therapy for osteonecrotic lesions: effects on osteoblasts treated with zoledronic acid. Support Care Cancer. 2014;22(10):2741–8.
22. Pansani TN, Basso FG, Turirioni AP, Kurachi C, Hebling J, de Souza Costa CA. Effects of low-level laser therapy on the proliferation and apoptosis of gingival fibroblasts treated with zoledronic acid. Int J Oral Maxillofac Surg. 2014;43(8):1030–4.
23. Walter C, Pabst AM, Ziebart T. Effects of a low-level diode laser on oral keratinocytes, oral fibroblasts, endothelial cells and osteoblasts incubated with bisphosphonates: an in vitro study. Biomed Rep. 2015;3(1):14–8.
24. Mergoni G, Vescovi P, Sala R, Merigo E, Passerini P, Maestri R, Corradi D, Govoni P, Nammour S, Bianchi MG. The effect of laser therapy on the expression of osteocalcin and osteopontin after tooth extraction in rats treated with zoledronate and dexamethasone. Support Care Cancer. 2016;24(2):807–13.
25. Romeo U, Galanakis A, Marias G, Del Vecchio A, Tenore G, Palaia G, Vescovi P, Polimeni A. Observation of pain control in patients with bisphosphonate-induced osteonecrosis using low level laser therapy: preliminary results. Photomed Laser Surg. 2011;29(7):447–52.
26. Vescovi P, Merigo E, Meleti M, Fornaini C, Nammour S, Manfredi M. Nd:YAG laser biostimulation of bisphosphonate-associated necrosis of the jawbone with or without surgical treatment. Br J Oral Maxillofac Surg. 2007;45(8):628–32.
27. Vescovi P, Merigo E, Manfredi M, Meleti M, Fornaini C, Bonanini M, Rocca JP, Nammour S. Nd:YAG laser biostimulation in the treatment of Bisphosphonate-associated osteonecrosis of the jaws (BON): experience in 26 cases. Photomed Laser Surg. 2008;26(1):37–46.
28. Weber JB, Camilotti RS, Ponte ME. Efficacy of laser therapy in the management of bisphosphonate-related osteonecrosis of the jaw(BRONJ): a systematic review. Lasers Med Sci. 2016;31(6):1261–72.
29. Latifyan S, Genot MT, Klastersky J. Bisphosphonate-related osteonecrosis of the jaw: a review of the potential efficacy of low-level laser therapy. Support Care Cancer. 2016;24(9):3687–93.
30. Vescovi P, Merigo E, Meleti M, Manfredi M. Early surgical approach preferable to medical therapy for bisphosphonates related osteonecrosis of the jaw. J Oral Maxillofac Surg. 2008;66:931–3.
31. Urade M, Tanaka N, Furusawa K, Shimada J, et al. National survey for bisphosphonate-related osteonecrosis of the jaws in Japan. J Otal Maxillofac Surg. 2011;69:364–71.
32. Wutzl A, Pohl S, Sulzbacher I, Seemann R, Lauer G, Ewers R, Drach J, Klug C. Factors influencing surgical treatment of bisphosphonate-related osteonecrosis of the jaws. Head Neck. 2012;34(2):194–200.
33. Graziani F, Vescovi P, Campisi G, Favia G, et al. Resective surgical approach shows a high performance in the management of advanced cases of bisphosphonate-related osteonecrosis of the jaws: a retrospective survey of 347 cases. J Oral Maxillofac Surg. 2012;70(11):2501–7.
34. Caldroney S, Ghazali N, Dyalram D, Lubek JE. Surgical resection and vascularized bone reconstruction in advanced stage medication-related osteonecrosis of the jaw. Int J Oral Maxillofac Surg. 2017;46(7):871–6.
35. Stübinger S. Advances in bone surgery: the Er:YAG laser in oral surgery and implant dentistry. Clin Cosmet Investig Dent. 2010;2:47–62.
36. Pourzarandian A, Watanabe H, Aoki A, Ichinose S, Sasaki KM, Nitta H, et al. Histological and TEM examination of early stages of bone healing after Er:YAG laser irradiation. Photomed Laser Surg. 2004;22(4):342–50.
37. Poutzarandian A, Watanabe H, Ruwanpura M, Aoki A, Noguchi K, Ishikawa I. Er:YAG laser irradiation increase prostaglandin E2 production via the induction of cyclooxygenase-2 mRNA in human gingival fibroblasts. J Periodontol Res. 2005;40:182–6.
38. Romeo U, Del Vecchio A, Palaia G, Tenore G, Visca P, Maggiore C. Bone damage induced by different cutting instruments—an in vitro study. Braz Dent J. 2009;20(2):162–8.
39. Papadaki M, Doukas A, Farinelli WA, Kaban L, Troulis M. Vertical ramus osteotomy with Er:YAG laser: a feasibility study. Int J Oral Maxillofac Surg. 2007;36(12):1193–7.
40. Baek K-W, Deibel W, Marinov D, Griessen M, Dard M, Bruno A, et al. A comparative investigation of bone surface after cutting with mechanical tools and Er:YAG laser. Lasers Surg Med. 2015;47(5):426–32.
41. Gabrić D, Blašković M, Gjorgijevska E, Mladenov M, Tašič B, Jurič IB, et al. Evaluation of bone healing after osteotomies prepared with Er:YAG laser in contact and noncontact modes and piezosurgery—an animal study. J Oral Maxillofac Surg. 2016;74(1):18–28.
42. Kesler G, Shvero DK, Tov YS, Romanos G. Platelet derived growth factor secretion and bone healing after Er:YAG laser bone irradiation. J Oral Implantol. 2011;37:195–204.
43. Sennhenn-Kirchner S, Schwarz P, Schliephake H, Konietschke F, Brunner E, Borg-von

ZM. Decontamination efficacy of erbium:yttrium-aluminium-garnet and diode laser light on oral Candida albicans isolates of a 5-day in vitro biofilm model. Lasers Med Sci. 2009;24(3):313–20.
44. Aoki A, Mizutani K, Shwarz F, Sculean A, et al. Periodontal and peri-implant wound healing following laser therapy. Periodontol. 2000;2015(68):217–69.
45. Vescovi P, Merigo E, Manfredi M, Meleti M, Fornaini C, Bonanini M, Rocca JP, De Moor RJ, Nammour S. Surgical treatment of maxillary osteonecrosis due to bisphosphonates using an Er:YAG (2940 nm) laser. Discussion of 17 clinical cases. Rev Belg Med Dent. 2009;64(2):87–95.
46. Angiero F, Sannino C, Borloni R, Crippa R, Benedicenti S, Romanos GE. Osteonecrosis of the jaws caused by bisphosphonates: evaluation of a new therapeutic approach using the Er:YAG laser. Lasers Med Sci. 2009;24:849–56.
47. Stübinger S, Dissmann J-P, Pinho NC, Saldamli B, et al. A preliminary report about treatment of bisphosphonate related osteonecrosis of the jaw with Er:YAG ablation. Lasers Surg Med. 2009;41:26–30.
48. Rugani P, Acham S, Truschnegg A, et al. Bisphosphonate-associated osteonecrosis of the jaws: surgical treatment with ErCrYSGG-laser. Case report. Oral Surg Oral Med Oral Pathol Oral Radiol Endod. 2010;110(6):e1–6.
49. Vescovi P, Manfredi M, Merigo E, Meleti M, Fornaini C, Rocca JP, Nammour S. Surgical approach with Er:YAG laser on Osteonecrosis of the Jaws (ONJ) in patients under Bisphosphonate Therapy (BPT). Lasers Med Sci. 2010;25(1):101–13.
50. Vescovi P, Merigo E, Meleti M, Manfredi M, Guidotti R, Nammour S. Bisphosphonates-related osteonecrosis of the jaws: a concise review of the literature and a report of a single-centre experience with 151 patients. J Oral Pathol Med. 2012;41(3):214–21.
51. Holzinger D, Seeman R, Klug C, Ewers R, et al. Long-term success of surgery in bisphosphonate-related osteonecrosis of the jaw (BRONJs). Oral Oncol. 2013;49:66–70.
52. Gabriele M, La Ferla F, Cei S, Nisi M, Graziani F. Conservative surgical treatment in the management of BRONJ: a case series of 129 consecutive cases. Ann Stomatol. 2013;4(Suppl 2):18.
53. Vescovi P, Manfredi M, Merigo E, Guidotti R, Meleti M, Pedrazzi G, Fornaini C, Bonanini M, Ferri T, Nammour S. Early surgical laser-assisted management of bisphosphonate-related osteonecrosis of the jaws (BRONJ): a retrospective analysis of 101 treated sites with long-term follow-up. Photomed Laser Surg. 2012;30(1):5–13.
54. Ruggiero SL. Emerging concepts in the management and treatment of osteonecrosis of the jaw. Oral Maxillofac Surg Clin North Am. 2013;25(1):11–20.
55. Vescovi P, Merigo E, Meleti M, Manfredi M, Fornaini C, Nammour S, Mergoni G, Sarraj A, Bagan JV. Conservative surgical management of stage I bisphosphonate-related osteonecrosis of the jaw. Int J Dent. 2014;2014:107690. https://doi.org/10.1155/2014/107690.
56. Rupel K, Ottaviani G, Gobbo M, Contardo L, Tirelli G, Vescovi P, Di Lenarda R, Biasotto M. A systematic review of therapeutical approaches in bisphosphonates-related osteonecrosis of the jaw (BRONJ). Oral Oncol. 2014;50(11):1049–57.
57. Pautke C, Tischer T, Neff A, Horch HH, Kolk A. In vivo tetracycline labeling of bone: an intraoperative aid in the surgical therapy of osteoradionecrosis of the mandible. Oral Surg Oral Med Oral Pathol Oral Radiol Endod. 2006;102:e10–3.
58. Assaf AT, Zrnc TA, Riecke B, et al. Intraoperative efficiency of fluorescence imaging by Visually Enhanced Lesion Scope (VELscope) in patients with bisphosphonate related osteonecrosis of the jaw (BRONJ). J Craniomaxillofac Surg. 2014;42:e157–64.
59. Hoell T, Huschak G, Beier A, et al. Auto fluorescence of intervertebral disc tissue: a new diagnostic tool. Eur Spine J. 2006;15(Suppl 3):S345.
60. Ristow O, Pautke C. Auto-fluorescence of the bone and its use for delineation of bone necrosis. Int J Oral Maxillofac Surg. 2014;43(11):1391–3.
61. Ristow O, Otto S, Troeltzsch M, Hohlweg-Majert B, Pautke C. Treatment perspectives for medication-related osteonecrosis of the jaw (MRONJ). J Craniomaxillofac Surg. 2015;43(2):290–3.
62. Vescovi P, Giovannacci I, Otto S, Manfredi M, Merigo E, Fornaini C, Nammour S, Meleti M. Medication-Related Osteonecrosis of the Jaws: an auto-fluorescence guided surgical approach performed with Er:YAG laser. Photomed Laser Surg. 2015;33(8):437–42.
63. Giovannacci I, Meleti M, Manfredi M, Merigo E, Fornaini C, Bonanini M, Vescovi P. Autofluorescence as indicator for detecting the surgical margins of medication-related osteonecrosis of the jaws. Minerva Stomatol. 2016;65(4):248–52.
64. Giovannacci I, Meleti M, Corradi D, Vescovi P. Clinical differences in autofluorescence between viable and nonvital bone: a case report with histopathologic evaluation performed on medication-related osteonecrosis of the jaws. J Oral Maxillofac Surg. 2017;75(6):1216–22. https://doi.org/10.1016/j.joms.2016.12.011.

Laser Scanning in Maxillofacial Surgery

15

Britt-Isabelle Berg, Cornelia Kober, and Katja Schwenzer-Zimmerer

Contents

Abstract

Capturing three-dimensional (3D) imaging is essential in the broad field of cranio-maxillofacial surgery. Laser scanners and stereophotogrammetry are more and more relevant for capturing (facial) soft tissues. For this purpose, a 3D laser scanning imaging system, using a nonhazardous laser, with a precise texture reproduction and in some models with colour capturing, can replace 3D imaging with radiation in many cases. This chapter gives an overview on the different applications of laser scanning in maxillofacial surgery. The following topics will be pointed out: the method of laser scanning; the laser scanning of plaster models, impressions and skull models; the laser scanning for oral surgical planning and for the assessment of facial swelling after oral surgery; the laser scanning of malformations; the laser scanning in facial aes-

B.-I. Berg (✉)
Department of Cranio-Maxillofacial Surgery, University Hospital Basel, Basel, Switzerland
e-mail: britt-isabelle.berg@usb.ch

C. Kober
HAW Hamburg, Hamburg, Germany

K. Schwenzer-Zimmerer
Department of Oral and Maxillofacial Surgery, University Medical Center Hamburg-Eppendorf, Hamburg, Germany

S. Stübinger et al. (eds.), *Lasers in Oral and Maxillofacial Surgery*,
https://doi.org/10.1007/978-3-030-29604-9_15

thetics and epithetic procedures; and the laser scanning in orthodontic treatment and orthognathic surgery. 3D laser scanners are still commonly used, but recently other devices, often based on stereophotogrammetry or 3D camera systems, became often superior. Due to shorter acquisition times, these systems are less vulnerable to motion artefacts and, thereby, more suitable for capturing small children or less cooperative patients.

Keywords

Laser scanning · Stereophotogrammetry Photogrammetry · 3D imaging · Facial aesthetics · Epithetic procedures · Oral surgery · Malformations · Orthodontic treatment · Orthognathic surgery

15.1 Introduction

Once the machine is purchased for low cost, nowadays, short acquisition time and non-invasiveness are some of the advantages [1]. Following the ALARA (as low as reasonably achievable) principle, radiation for 3D acquisition should be avoided whenever possible. Radiation reduction is essential because the radiation dosage accumulates throughout a subject's lifetime. Publications, where dental X-rays and increased risk of intracranial meningioma [2] or computed topography (CT) imaging with possible influence to develop brain tumours or leukaemia [3, 4] were controversially discussed, lead to insecurity in patients. Magnetic resonance (MR) imaging would be another alternative to depict soft tissue, but the disadvantages prevail: long acquisition times and expensive and in the majority of magnetic resonance tomographs (MRT), the patient has to lie without moving. Therefore, due to gravidity, the soft tissue might be different to a sitting/standing position. Being able to offer a tool that allows 3D imaging without radiation is very helpful. A 3D laser scanning imaging system, using a nonhazardous laser, with a precise texture reproduction and in some models with colour capturing [5] can replace 3D imaging with radiation in large number of cases.

15.2 The Method of Laser Scanning

The laser scanning can be briefly described as follows: a laser beam is sent through a cylinder lens and a horizontal light beam is generated. This beam will be due to a Galvano mirror projected onto the object which should be scanned. The Galvano mirror enables to capture the object completely, and the reflected light beam will be captured with a CCD (charge-coupled device) sensor (Fig. 15.1).

Distances will be triangulated between the reflecting laser beam and the scanned surface, as shown in Fig. 15.2.

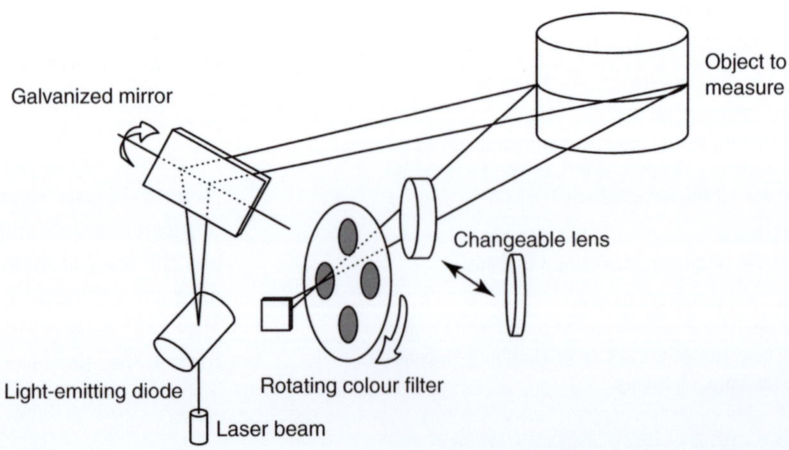

Fig. 15.1 Showing the operating principles of the laser. (Reproduced from, Fig. 1 in: Schwenzer-Zimmerer K, Chaitidis D, Borner BI, Kovacs L, Sader R, Zeilhofer HF, Holberg C. Lip, jaw, and palate clefts, Analysis of unilateral cleft lip using 3-D laser topometry. Mund Kiefer Gesichtschir. 2006;10:377–384)

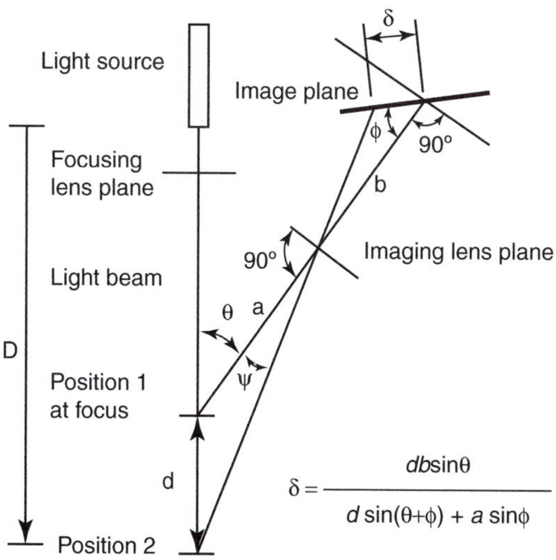

$$\delta = \frac{db\sin\theta}{d\sin(\theta+\phi) + a\sin\phi}$$

Fig. 15.2 Measurement principles of optical triangulation sensor. Reproduced from, Fig. 1 in: A robust signal processing algorithm for linear displacement measuring optical transmission sensors, Kim K.-C., Kim J.-A., Kim S., Kwak Y.K. August 2000, Review of Scientific Instruments 71(8):3220–3225. https://doi.org/10.1063/1.1304870

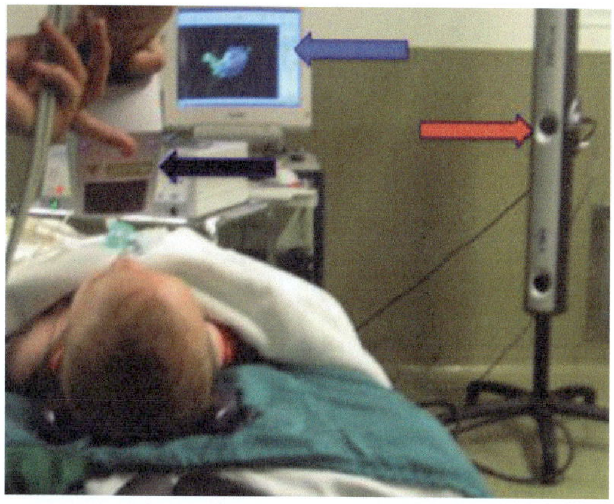

Fig. 15.3 Arrangement and handling of the scanning device T-scan® (Steinbichler, Carl Zeiss Optotechnik GmbH, Neubeuern, Germany) in operating theatre. In front, the baby's head with the handheld scanning device above (black arrow). The scan is acquired before start of the surgical procedure. The tracking camera (red arrow) is positioned on the right. The screen/PC with the image representation of the scan (blue arrow) is on the left. The child is under general anaesthesia. The scanning process takes 10–20 s with a minimal amount of practice

When two points with a known distance to the laser exist, it is possible to calculate the angle of a triangle due to angle measurements between the points and based on this the distance to the unknown point. The laser scanner can detect length, width and the depth of the scanned object [6]. Depending on whether the laser is a handheld, mobile or non-mobile device, a tracking camera is necessary, too. In Fig. 15.3, you see exemplarily the setup of the mobile (handheld) T-scan®, (Steinbichler, Carl Zeiss Optotechnik GmbH, Neubeuern, Germany). It uses a laser with 670 nm (class II). The handheld device has 29 infrared markers. Three of these markers are used for the precise spatial position when using an optical tracking system. The technical data as published by the manufacture [7] are as follows: resolution of distance measurement, 1 mm; accuracy of distance measurement *þ/e*, 30 mm; and sensor weight, <1500 g. The tracking system seen in Fig. 15.3 is an Optotrak Pro 1000 (Northern Digital Inc., Ontario, Canada) [8]. The advantage of the T-scan is that the scanner does not have to struggle with shadowing effects due to undercut as in other non-handheld devices. Sometimes multiple images from different angles must be acquired to compensate for missing surface parts. It is desirable to have complex areas as ear, nostril or cleft region complete without large data holes [9]. In Fig. 15.4, a screenshot is shown, as it is visible in real time on the PC monitor. The scan can be manually rotated to ensure that the desirable facial areas are captured completely.

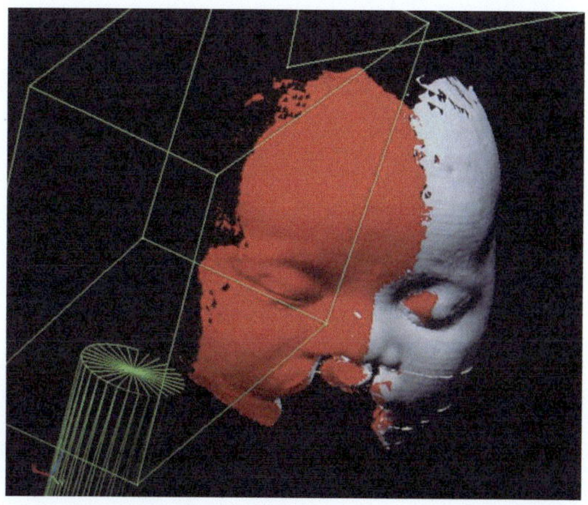

Fig. 15.4 A screenshot taken from the PC monitor. Scan of a facial plaster cast. In white, the first layer; in red, a second layer to complete the image process. This process is shown in real time. The green lines show the position of the scanning device. (Courtesy Boris Brun [10])

Below, the different usage of 3D laser scanning will be introduced: the scanning of plaster cast models and facial impressions, oral surgical interventions [11], orthognathic treatment and surgery [12], malformation, epithetic, aesthetics and facial movements [13–15]. Overlapping themes will be discussed depending on the aspect.

15.3 The Laser Scanning of Plaster Models, Impressions and Skull Models

The reliability of laser scanners in reproducing 3D objects has already been described [6], the accuracy and reproducibility having been tested on geometrical models and (facial/dental) plaster casts [6]. The comparison of laser scanner and stereophotogrammetry for nasal plaster casts showed no significant differences between these two different techniques [1], whereas measurements on stone casts were somewhat smaller than values obtained directly from subjects (differences between −0.05 and −1.58 mm) [16]. These findings were also detected by Holberg et al. [17]. In their study, the accuracy of facial plaster casts and suitability for 3D mapping was investigated. From 15 adult volunteers, a facial alginate impression was taken. These impressions were poured with plaster resulting in facial plaster casts. The plaster casts and the probands' faces were captured using a 3D laser scanner operating with structured light. They found – depending on the area of the face – deviations between 0.95 and 3.55 mm. Especially, soft tissue areas as lips, cheeks or tip of the nose as well as the lower face area showed marked differences. Areas with less soft tissue mass which could be shifted showed less deviations, e.g. forehead (1 mm) or nasal base (1.4 mm) [17].

An even better scanning quality can be achieved if a robot arm is used (Fig. 15.5).

In Fig. 15.6, both plaster cast scans (manual and robot arm) seem to be smooth, but looking more precisely, the ear of the manually scanned patient is not captured in its complexity and has to be recaptured.

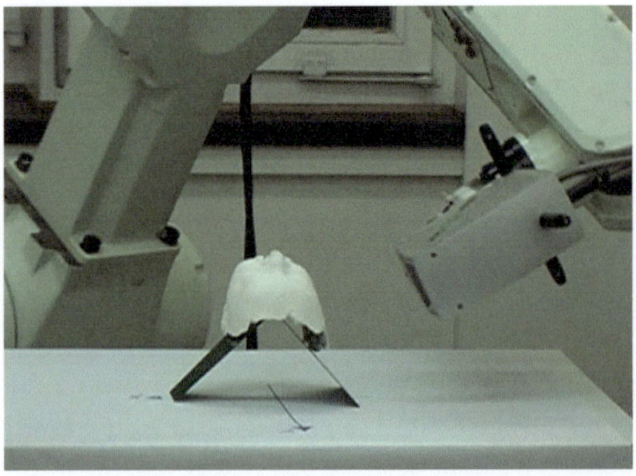

Fig. 15.5 Robot arm in the process of scanning a facial plaster cast by T-scan. (Courtesy Boris Brun [10])

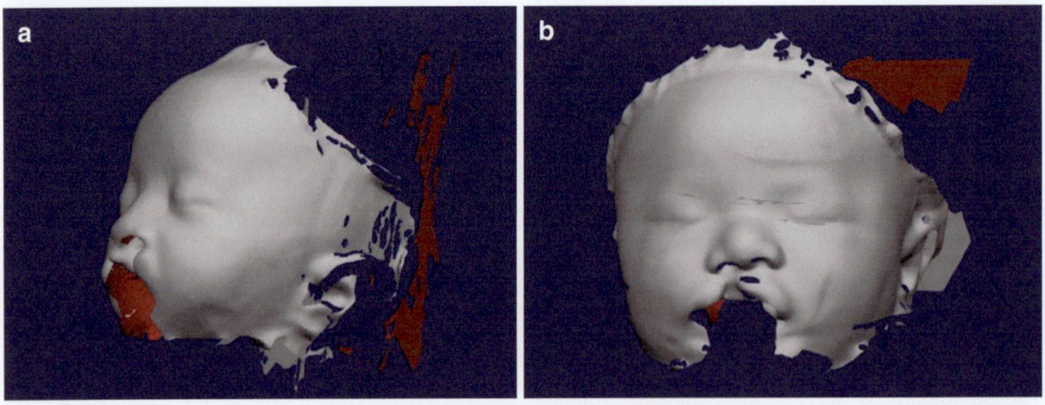

Fig. 15.6 T-scan images acquired manually (**a**) or with the use of a robot arm (**b**). (Courtesy Boris Brun [10])

15.4 The Laser Scanning for Oral Surgical Planning and for the Assessment of Facial Swelling After Oral Surgery

Jung et al. compared four intraoral scanners. One of them was a laser scanner (iTero; Cadent, Align Technology, San Jose, CA, USA). They compared the accuracy using models with buccal brackets and orthodontic wires where they found that the scanning results acquired by iTero were among the most reliable ones.

Buccal brackets and orthodontic wires were not clinically significant on the 3D image [18]. The same scanner was used in a study, comparing different intraoral scanners as well as a lab scanner regarding the accuracy of scanbodies on dental implants. If computer-aided design or a computer-assisted manufacture process for implant prosthetics is requested, the digitization of the scanbodies is necessary. The precision of the intraoral scanners decreased with increasing distance between the scanbodies in contrast to the dental lab scanner. Independent of the increasing distance, a continuous precision was observed [19]. All studies mentioned above were conducted with models. Lee et al. described the use of an intraoral laser scanner (iTero) for capturing the spatial position, surrounding tissue and a special scanning abutment of tooth implants in 36 patients. The acquired data were stored in STL format and used to produce a custom computer-aided design abutment and crown. Adjustments of contact and occlusion were required in six and seven patients, respectively, but the time for the adjustments was below 15 min [20]. Another study, evaluating data from 100 patients, was published by San José V et al. [21]. They were interested in comparing the reliability and accuracy of direct and indirect dental measurements using intraoral laser scanning (iTero), segmented cone beam computed tomography (CBCT) and a scanner for capturing plaster cast models. These results showed that both the iTero and the models segmented from CBCT are usable and accurate enough for dental measurements [21].

A different field is the evaluation of facial swelling after wisdom tooth removal. Before laser scanner and stereophotogrammetry became widely available, tape measurements were performed. Schultze-Mosgau et al. in their study about ibuprofen and methylprednisolone described how to measure the facial swelling by tape and ultrasound. They took distances from the lateral corner of the eye to the mandibular angle, from tragus to the outer corner of the mouth and from the tragus to the pogonion which they marked with a water-resistant pen [22]. The use of an optical 3D scanner (FaceScan3D; 3D-Shape GmbH, Erlangen, Germany) for volumetric measurements of facial swelling is described by Rana et al. [23]. They assessed the swelling after the use of different cooling mechanisms. For calculation of the volume, the patients were photographed while looking into a mirror with standard horizontal and vertical lines simulating a red cross marked on it. Harrison et al. [11] described the use of a laser scanner for the assessment of facial scanning. They evaluated a handheld laser surface scanner (FastSCANTM; Bruker Corporation, MA, USA) for the assessment of postoperative facial swelling. In their study, 20 patients were scanned before and 2 days after wisdom tooth removal. They detected the variability of the position as a source of inaccuracy. Otherwise, they found that the FastSCANTM is a simple, accurate and non-invasive method for the measurement of soft tissue volume changes.

15.5 The Laser Scanning of Malformations

Depending on the kind of malformation, a huge variety of 3D deviations to "normal" anatomy is seen. Just looking at cleft lip and palate patients, the cleft can vary widely. Lips with strong pouting and strong vermillion are seen, but it is also possible that the columella is short in combination with a severely contorted alar wing. Lip length differences also show a broad spectrum of variation, and so does the philtrum. For all of these variations, the non-cleft side (in unilateral clefts) is taken as the normal anatomy. The surgeon aims to establish anatomical symmetry as far as possible [24]. The method of choice to perform the closure of the cleft varies between surgeons; therefore, a 3D tool for assessment of the surgical outcome is of high relevance in this field of maxillofacial surgery. It is also necessary to use standardized, reliable facial landmarks so a comparison is easier achievable. Literature about 3D facial landmarks is available [25, 26]. The identifications of landmarks need a certain amount of practice, but taking the same landmarks will show a learning effect and therefore higher accuracy in less time. For measurements, the patient's presence is not necessary which is an advantage towards measurements taken directly/manually on the patient's face.

Since operations in the field of facial malformation are also performed at an early age, the compliance of children is not always given. Mori et al. published in their laser scanning study that, from the age of 5 years, most children showed enough compliance for the scanning procedure [27]. Usable data sets of noncompliant babies can therefore only be captured by using sedation. A sedation for this purpose on its own cannot be justified. Scanning the babies just before the surgical procedure (see Fig. 15.1) is possible with minimal extra amount of time. The setup of the scanner can be done in the absence of the baby so that there is no loss of time regarding this aspect. In Fig. 15.7, you see the preoperative and 7 days postoperative pictures of a patient with a unilateral cleft lip. Figure 15.8 shows the belonging 3D laser scans. For these scans, the Vivid 900 (Konika Minolta Co., Tokyo, Japan) was used. In this case, only one scanner was built up. If only one scanner is available, for a complete 3D view, two separate 3D data sets, one from each side, have to be captured and fused. The Vivid 900 parameters are as follows: resolution, x = 0.17 mm, y = 0.17 mm and z = 0.047 mm; input time, 0.3–2.5 s; and data size, 1.6–2.4 MB, mobile system (11 kg).

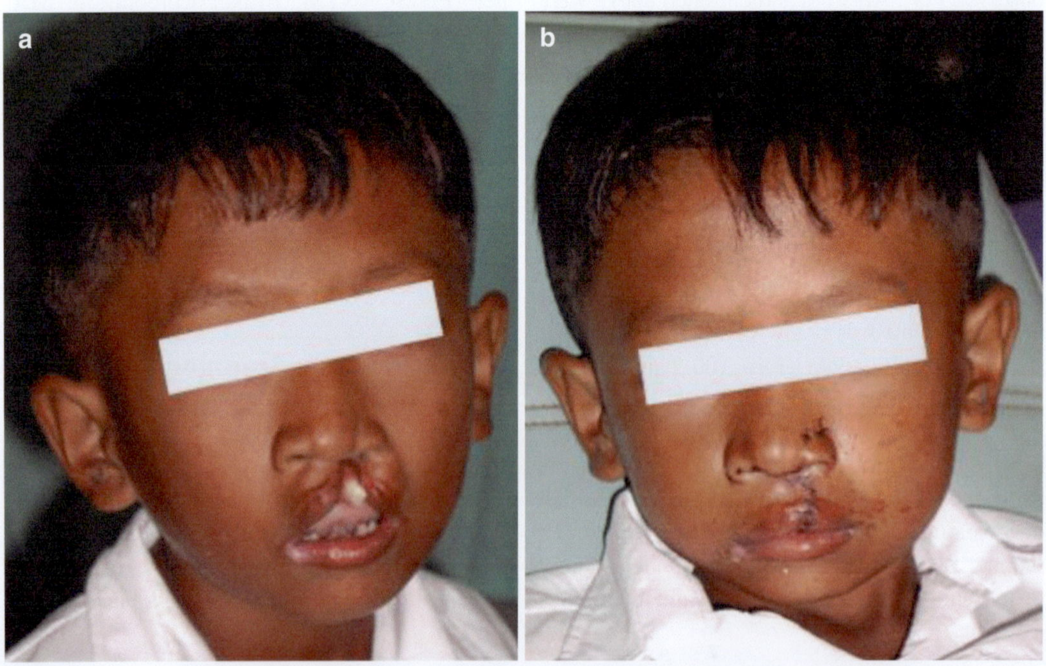

Fig. 15.7 Child with unilateral cleft preoperatively (**a**) and 7 days postoperatively (**b**)

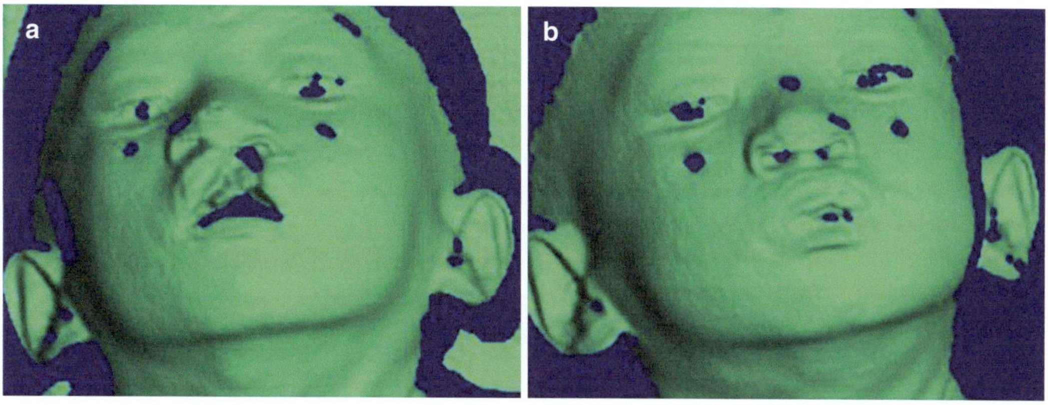

Fig. 15.8 Preoperative (**a**) and 7 days postoperative (**b**) laser scans of the patient from Fig. 15.7 captured with the Vivid 900 (Konika Minolta,Tokyo, Japan)

15.6 The Laser Scanning in Facial Aesthetics and Epithetic Procedures

The face is a complex region where alterations regarding form, volume and shape are of great importance when assessing the surgical outcome [28]. This aspect can have an even stronger input if the procedure is elective and involves strong expectations from the patient's side. For comparison of pre- and postoperative results, a high quality and a standardized face/head position are indispensable. Also the cooperation of the patient is required. Even short scanning times of, e.g. 5 s can be a long time to keep a "frozen" position. This can be expected from adults, but young children will have difficulties to stay in one position without moving at all for such a period of time. In the study by Kovacs et al., they assessed that the best precision was reached when the Frankfort was angled +10° relative to the horizontal. A stronger reclination of the head was more precise for areas as the mouth and the nose [28].

One of the regions which has been investigated by laser scanning is the philtrum. The philtrum, the central unit of the upper lip, can be separated into following parts: the dimple, both columns, the tubercle and the white roll between the two high points of Cupid's bow [29]. The shape of the philtrum is not only of great importance in cleft surgery but also for interventions after Botox injections or cheiloplasties. Kishi et al. published a study investigating the depth of the philtral dimple using the VIVID910 laser scanner (Konika Minolta, Tokyo, Japan) [29]. When assessing their laser scans using the Uemura classification [30], they found a sex difference concerning the shape: the parallel type was often visible. The triangular type seems to be the most common one in men and rarely seen in women. The unclear type was never found in men.

Another use of laser scanning in aesthetic surgery is imaging the nose for evaluation of the nasal shape following rhinosurgery or for preoperative planning and quality control in rhinosurgery [31]. It can also be used as a follow-up tool for control after reconstructive rhytidectomy. Objective measurements regarding wrinkles (i.e. the cheek and malar region) were possible [32].

Another possible application of laser scanners is the documentation of the effect of either one or two botulinum toxin injections regarding the volume of masseter muscles (Vivid 9i; Konika Minolta, Tokyo, Japan) before the injection and 6 months after. Bilateral masseteric hypertrophy, leading to a broad-looking face, is considered as aesthetically unpleasant, especially in Asia. The use of botulinum toxin leads to a significant reduction of the masseter muscle. By laser scanning, these findings could be objectively validated [33].

As another aspect, laser scanning can be used for aesthetic aspects of the face in patients who suffer from facial lipoatrophy. This can occur when highly active antiretroviral therapy has to be taken. It is seen in people infected by the human immunodeficiency virus (HIV). Although the medication has very much improved the quality of life, facial lipoatrophy is a severe complication [34]. When a polylactic acid (PLA) facial filler is inserted, a strong improvement of the normal facial appearance can be achieved. Performing scans with the University College London (UCL) optical face scanner, it was possible to detect that mean 12-month and 18-month cheek volumes are higher than the mean posttreatment (6-month) scans, but the laser scans also detected a significant drop in cheek volume from 18 to 24 months. The cheek volumes at 24 months were similar to the volumes immediately after treatment and significantly higher than baseline (pretreatment) volume measurements [34]. An explanation might be a relatively slow process of new collagenous tissue generation in response to the inserted filler rather than direct volume increase due to the filler volume on its own [34].

Another use of laser is in patients with missing parts of the face who are showing a major stigma. Especially, nose and ear are worth mentioning due to malformation, trauma or oncological resection; either a part or the complete nose/ear can be missing. In some cases, a complete surgical solution is possible; in others, rehabilitation can only be achieved by a manufactured prosthesis. Coward et al. [35] pointed out that positioning is an important aspect of successful rehabilitation. The positioning of the ear prostheses can be observational. Measuring these distances on the ear and if available the healthy ear can result in gross differences compared to 3D measurements since distance measurements alone give no information on the precise 3D location of a landmark of the ear. For data acquisition, Coward et al. applied a laser scanner developed at the University College London, London, UK [36]. They defined landmarks in probands with normal facial symmetry that can also be found in patients with facial asymmetry (e.g. hemifacial microsomia) [35]. If the loss of the external ear was due to trauma or tumour, the external auditory canal can be used as a guide, but, in malformation cases, the external auditory canal might be absent or displaced. In the healthy probands assessed by these authors, only small differences between the left and right sides of the face were found [35]. Ciocca et al. described how to use rapid prototyping to fabricate a mirrored volume of the healthy ear [37]. In their department, the authors have a virtual ear-nose library at their disposal, which enables them to design a facial part. For the ear, this can be useful in cases with malformations such as Treacher Collins syndrome [38] and, for the nose, if no impression was made before surgery [39] or a trauma case occurred which is unforeseeable. In the publication by Mueller et al., the margins of the epithesis were scanned using the VI-910 (Konika Minolta, Tokyo, Japan) before and after the adaptation of the margin. The scans were superimposed for an analysis of the extent of essential reduction of the margins [40]. If a nasal prosthesis needs stabilization through mechanical support (e.g. eyeglasses) rather than implants, it is important to follow up the connecting system [41]. Ciocca et al. [41] published about eyeglass-supported nasal prosthesis using a 3D laser scanner (3dMDface System; 3dMD Ltd., London, UK) and rapid prototyping techniques. By means of their technique, they achieved a reduction in prosthesis weight leading to a flexible prosthesis with a consistency similar to natural skin when touched. The prosthesis will be able to follow natural facial movements that occur during eating, smiling, speaking or chewing [41].

After loss of all teeth, patients suffer from a concave face which is disturbing from an aesthetic point of view. Jivănescu et al. [42] evaluated the lower face morphology changes in edentulous patients after prosthodontic rehabilitation with upper and lower complete dentures. They could objectify the soft tissue changes very precisely by using a conventional method (the digital caliper) and the 3D laser scanning system (NextEngine 3D Laser Scanner; NextEngine, Santa Monica, CA, USA). The system comprised a digital imaging system, a structured laser light source and a light projection system. Three scans from different angles were required in order to obtain the complete 3D surface scan. They highlighted that 3D laser scanning offers several advantages over direct anthropometry: reduced invasiveness, increased data collection speed and the possibility to create 3D databases [42]. Depending on the publication, facial measurements should have an accuracy of 0.1 up to 0.5 mm [43, 44].

15.7 The Laser Scanning in Orthodontic Treatment and Orthognathic Surgery

A key aspect of orthodontic diagnostics is the recording of facial soft parts, not only for documentation but also for the analysis of facial aesthetics [17]. Contact-free 3D digitalization of the face is nowadays the gold standard. As previously described in "the laser scanning of plaster models, impressions and skull models", inaccuracies occur when facial plaster casts are made, but if no scanner or stereophotogrammetry is available, it is still a low-cost procedure that can be easily achieved and has been applied successfully for quite some time [17]. In orthodontic treatment, not only the hard tissue but also the soft tissue is of great importance. Patients often judge the outcome of orthodontic treatment or orthognathic surgery by visible soft tissue changes [45]. Notably, improved facial aesthetics are highly desired [46]. 2D soft tissue analysis using lateral cephalographs is still a common tool but with decisive limitations. 3D soft tissue analysis has the advantage of showing the soft tissue changes in its complexity. Techniques for 3D soft tissue analysis in the field of orthodontic treatment and orthognathic surgery nowadays include photogrammetry alone [47–49], photogrammetry in combination with CBCT [50], CBCT on its own [51, 52], CT [53, 54] and 3D laser scanning.

In orthodontic treatment, tooth extraction is a common procedure. Whether a change of facial fullness or flattening of the profile can occur due to tooth extraction is widely discussed [55, 56]. According to Moss et al., laser scanning data sets were compared preoperatively, after 9 months and at the end of treatment [57]. In their prospective study, Caucasians with a skeletal class I pattern in the age from 11 to 19 years were included. None of the included participants had received orthodontic treatment or suffered from facial asymmetry [57]. In their results, no evidence of a decrease in the size of the lips was found. In contrast, the soft tissues had increased. No change of facial size when comparing the two groups of patients was visible. Therefore, they concluded that the treatment made no difference between both groups [57]. By comparison of the facial shape using laser scanning, they showed that neither adverse changes nor any evidence of flattening of facial soft tissues occurred due to tooth extraction as part of orthodontic treatment [57]. This research group further reported that they installed a database of healthy children without orthodontic treatment in the age between 5 and 18 years. These data can be used, e.g. for comparison with treated patients for evaluation of abnormal growth [57].

To plan orthognathic surgery, the application of two different laser scanning systems might be reasonable, namely, one for the facial soft tissue and one for the dental cast models. The scanning pitch varies. So, Noguchi et al. chose 1.00 mm for the scanning device used to capture the facial aspect and 0.25 mm for the dental cast scans. The scans were part of a study to estimate facial shape changes without CT [58].

In orthodontic surgery, a change of the facial soft tissues can be expected. When facial deformities are presented, orthognathic surgery is often the only therapeutic option to achieve an acceptable aesthetic outcome. In a study with 46 patients presenting a class III dentoskeletal relationship, markers were placed in the face before scanning. Five markers were used to register pre- and postoperative optical surface scans over facial parts not affected by surgery. All patients received bimaxillary orthognathic surgery to achieve a class I dentoskeletal relationship. Optical surface scans were obtained again 6 months postoperatively. Additionally, pre- and postoperative cephalographs were acquired and digitized. They were used to assess whether the preoperative planning was achieved during surgery. By this information, the soft tissue changes could be compared with actual skeletal movements. In this study, precise details of the change of the upper lip for the subalar, subcommissural and supracommissural regions were assessable.

The soft tissue movement of the upper lip is tightly related to the underlying skeletal tissue, although other factors play an important role as elasticity of the lip or proximity and contour of the alveolar bone. In Le Fort I osteotomies, changes of the nasal morphology are detectable by 3D laser scanning. Widening of the nasal alae was well detected, whereas flattening of the lips was not found in a study with 12 female patients who received either an advancement or a horizontally/vertically rotation [59]. Furthermore, laser scanning can assess facial movements. After application of facial landmarks, laser scans were acquired before surgery and after 3, 6 and 12 months in bimaxillary surgery for class III patients. The following facial movements were evaluated: frowning, eye closure, grimace, smiling and lip purse. It could be shown that after surgery there was a change, but after 1 year, the movements were statistically similar to the presurgical registration [14]. To conclude, soft tissue changes follow the shift of the underlying skeletal structures. Prediction of the final result is still a challenge. However, it is possible to illustrate and quantify the soft tissue changes [60].

As another aspect, laser scanning can be used in the field of obstructive sleep apnoea syndrome (OSAS). OSAS is a common problem, showing narrowing and/or collapsing of the upper airway. Due to daytime sleepiness, the concerned patients often show a notable reduction in quality of life. Additionally, cardiovascular derangements or neurocognitive impairment is observed [61]. If conservative treatment by CPAP (continuous positive airway pressure) is not sufficient, surgery can be considered. In these cases, maxilla-mandibular advancement can be indicated [62]. The advancement can have a serious impact on the facial aesthetics especially in the case of previous disproportion [61]. Gerbino et al. published a prospective study about 3D analysis of the soft tissue changes in typical OSAS patients before and after maxilla-mandibular advancement [61]. Their inclusion criteria include white males, middle age (range 30–60 years), overweight (BMI > 25), normal cephalometric measurements (SNA°: 82 ∓ 3.5; SNB°: 80.9 ∓ 3.4) and severe OSAS (AHI > 30). Patients with facial deformity were not included. Maxilla-mandibular advancements were performed by one surgeon [61]. For 10 patients, laser scans were acquired (3030RGB; Cyberware, Inc., Monterey, CA, USA). The pre- and postoperative cephalograms showed a maxillary change of +9.2 ∓ 1.2 mm and a mandibular change of +10.4 ∓ 2.2 mm. By matching pre- and postoperative scans, the following changes were detected: increase of inter-cheilion width and increased bulking of the upper lip. No alar flaring was found. An overall increase in the sagittal projection of soft tissue points was found postoperatively and, when assessing the axial sections, a forward displacement of the alar base position. Asked about their feeling towards their facial appearance, 60% of the patients gave a favourable response to the changes, whereas 40% responded in a neutral way [61]. Facial mobility after maxilla-mandibular advancement in patients with OASA was also assessed using data sets acquired before and 1 year after surgery.

15.8 Conclusion

For a certain period of time, 3D laser scanners were very effective tools, which could capture 3D images without radiation. However, recently, other devices, often based on stereophotogrammetry or 3D camera systems, became often superior. Inter alia thanks to much shorter acquisition times, they are less vulnerable to motion artefacts and, thereby, more suitable for capturing small children or less cooperative patients.

References

1. Codari M, Pucciarelli V, Pisoni L, Sforza C. Laser scanner compared with stereophotogrammetry for measurements of area on nasal plaster casts. Br J Oral Maxillofac Surg. 2015;53(8):769–70. https://doi.org/10.1016/j.bjoms.2015.05.007.
2. Claus EB, Calvocoressi L, Bondy ML, Schildkraut JM, Wiemels JL, Wrensch M. Dental x-rays and risk of meningioma. Cancer. 2012;118(18):4530–7. https://doi.org/10.1002/cncr.26625.
3. Pearce MS, Salotti JA, Little MP, McHugh K, Lee C, Kim KP, Howe NL, Ronckers CM, Rajaraman P, Sir Craft AW, Parker L, Berrington de González

A. Radiation exposure from CT scans in childhood and subsequent risk of leukaemia and brain tumours: a retrospective cohort study. Lancet. 2012;380(9840):499–505. https://doi.org/10.1016/S0140-6736(12)60815-0.
4. Mathews JD, Forsythe AV, Brady Z, Butler MW, Goergen SK, Byrnes GB, Giles GG, Wallace AB, Anderson PR, Guiver TA, McGale P, Cain TM, Dowty JG, Bickerstaffe AC, Darby SC. Cancer risk in 680,000 people exposed to computed tomography scans in childhood or adolescence: data linkage study of 11 million Australians. BMJ. 2013;346:f2360. https://doi.org/10.1136/bmj.f2360.
5. https://www.creaform3d.com/de. Accessed 4 Feb 2018.
6. Kusnoto B, Evans CA. Reliability of a 3D surface laser scanner for orthodontic applications. Am J Orthod Dentofac Orthop. 2002;122:342–8.
7. http://optotechnik.zeiss.com/unternehmen. Accessed 18 Jan 2018.
8. https://www.ndigital.com/msci/products/optotrak-certus/. Accessed 18 Jan 2018.
9. Schwenzer-Zimmerer K, Boerner BI, Schwenzer NF, Müller AA, Juergens P, Ringenbach A, Schkommodau E, Zeilhofer HF. Facial acquisition by dynamic optical tracked laser imaging: a new approach. J Plast Reconstr Aesthet Surg. 2009;62(9):1181–6. https://doi.org/10.1016/j.bjps.2007.11.080.
10. Brun B. Robotergestützte Digitalisierung in der Kiefer- und Gesichtschirurgie; Diplomarbeit, Autumn semester 2007. Switzerland: HSR Hochschule für Technik, Rapperswil; 2007.
11. Harrison JA, Nixon MA, Fright WR, Snape L. Use of hand-held laser scanning in the assessment of facial swelling: a preliminary study. Br J Oral Maxillofac Surg. 2004;42(1):8–17.
12. Miller L, Morris DO, Berry E. Visualizing three-dimensional facial soft tissue changes following orthognathic surgery. Eur J Orthod. 2007;29(1):14–20.
13. Sidequersky FV, Verzé L, Mapelli A, Ramieri GA, Sforza C. Quantification of facial movements by optical instruments: surface laser scanning and optoelectronic three-dimensional motion analyzer. J Craniofac Surg. 2014;25(1):e65–70. https://doi.org/10.1097/SCS.0000000000000379.
14. Verzé L, Bianchi FA, Dell'Acqua A, Prini V, Ramieri GA. Facial mobility after bimaxillary surgery in class III patients: a three-dimensional study. J Craniofac Surg. 2011;22(6):2304–7. https://doi.org/10.1097/SCS.0b013e318232a7f0.
15. Verzé L, Nasi A, Quaranta F, Vasino V, Prini V, Ramieri G. Quantification of facial movements by surface laser scanning. J Craniofac Surg. 2011;22(1):60–5. https://doi.org/10.1097/SCS.0b013e3181f6c46d.
16. Ferrario VF, Mian F, Peretta R, Rosati R, Sforza C. Three-dimensional computerized anthropometry of the nose: landmark representation compared to surface analysis. Cleft Palate Craniofac J. 2007;44(3):278–85.
17. Holberg C, Schwenzer K, Mahaini L, Rudzki-Janson I. Accuracy of facial plaster casts. Angle Orthod. 2006;76(4):605–11.
18. Jung YR, Park JM, Chun YS, Lee KN, Kim M. Accuracy of four different digital intraoral scanners: effects of the presence of orthodontic brackets and wire. Int J Comput Dent. 2016;19(3):203–15.
19. Flügge TV, Att W, Metzger MC, Nelson K. Precision of dental implant digitization using intraoral scanners. Int J Prosthodont. 2016;29(3):277–83. https://doi.org/10.11607/ijp.4417.
20. Lee CY, Wong N, Ganz SD, Mursic J, Suzuki JB. Use of an intraoral laser scanner during the prosthetic phase of implant dentistry: a pilot study. J Oral Implantol. 2015;41(4):e126–32. https://doi.org/10.1563/AAID-JOI-D-13-00132.
21. San José V, Bellot-Arcís C, Tarazona B, Zamora NO, Lagravère M, Paredes-Gallardo V. Dental measurements and Bolton index reliability and accuracy obtained from 2D digital, 3D segmented CBCT, and 3d intraoral laser scanner. J Clin Exp Dent. 2017;9(12):e1466–73. https://doi.org/10.4317/jced.54428. eCollection 2017 Dec.
22. Schultze-Mosgau S, Schmelzeisen R, Frölich JC, Schmele H. Use of ibuprofen and methylprednisolone for the prevention of pain and swelling after removal of impacted third molars. J Oral Maxillofac Surg. 1995;53(1):2–7; discussion 7-8
23. Rana M, Gellrich NC, Ghassemi A, Gerressen M, Riediger D, Modabber A. Three-dimensional evaluation of postoperative swelling after third molar surgery using 2 different cooling therapy methods: a randomized observer-blind prospective study. J Oral Maxillofac Surg. 2011;69(8):2092–8. https://doi.org/10.1016/j.joms.2010.12.038.
24. Schwenzer-Zimmerer K, Chaitidis D, Berg-Boerner I, Krol Z, Kovacs L, Schwenzer NF, Zimmerer S, Holberg C, Zeilhofer HF. Quantitative 3D soft tissue analysis of symmetry prior to and after unilateral cleft lip repair compared with non-cleft persons (performed in Cambodia). J Craniomaxillofac Surg. 2008;36(8):431–8. https://doi.org/10.1016/j.jcms.2008.05.003.
25. Farkas LG, Hajnis K, Posnick JC. Anthropometric and anthroposcopic findings of the nasal and facial region in cleft patients before and after primary lip and palate repair. Cleft Palate Craniofac J. 1993;30:1e12.
26. Schwenzer-Zimmerer K, Chaitidis D, Boerner BI, Kovacs L, Sader R, Zeilhofer HF, Holberg C. Lip, jaw, and palate clefts: Analysis of unilateral cleft lip using 3-D laser topometry. Mund Kiefer Gesichtschir. 2006;10(6):377–84.
27. Mori A, Nakajima T, Kaneko T, Sakuma H, Aoki Y. Analysis of 109 Japanese children's lip and nose shapes using 3-dimensional digitizer. Br J Plast Surg. 2005;58:318–29.
28. Kovacs L, Zimmermann A, Brockmann G, Gühring M, Baurecht H, Papadopulos NA, Schwenzer-Zimmerer K, Sader R, Biemer E, Zeilhofer HF. Three-dimensional recording of the human face

with a 3D laser scanner. J Plast Reconstr Aesthet Surg. 2006;59(11):1193–202.
29. Kishi N, Tanaka S, Iida S, Kogo M. Comprehensive evaluation of three-dimensional philtral morphology. J Craniofac Surg. 2011;22(5):1606–11. https://doi.org/10.1097/SCS.0b013e31822e5ebf.
30. Uemura T. A study of the figures of Japanese philtrum by measurement. J Jpn PRS. 1993;13:55Y67.
31. Largo RD, Wettstein R, Fulco I, Tremp M, Schaefer DJ, Gubisch W, Haug MD. Three-dimensional laser surface scanning in rhinosurgery. Facial Plast Surg. 2013;29(2):116–20. https://doi.org/10.1055/s-0033-1341587.
32. Wettstein R, Kalbermatten DF, Rieger UM, Schumacher R, Dagorov P, Pierer G. Laser surface scanning analysis in reconstructive rhytidectomy. Aesthet Plast Surg. 2006;30(6):637–40.
33. Lee HH, Kim ST, Lee KJ, Baik HS. Effect of a second injection of botulinum toxin on lower facial contouring, as evaluated using 3-dimensional laser scanning. Dermatol Surg. 2015;41(4):439–44. https://doi.org/10.1097/DSS.0000000000000291.
34. Ong J, Clarke A, White P, Johnson MA, Withey S, Butler PE. Objective evidence for the use of polylactic acid implants in HIV-associated facial lipoatrophy using three-dimensional surface laser scanning and psychological assessment. J Plast Reconstr Aesthet Surg. 2009;62(12):1627–35. https://doi.org/10.1016/j.bjps.2008.07.046.
35. Coward TJ, Scott BJ, Watson RM, Richards R. Identifying the position of an ear from a laser scan: the significance for planning rehabilitation. Int J Oral Maxillofac Surg. 2002;31(3):244–51.
36. Coward TJ, Watson RM, Scott BJ. Laser scanning for the identification of repeatable landmarks of the ears and face. Br J Plast Surg. 1997;50(5):308–14.
37. Ciocca L, Scotti R. CAD-CAM generated ear cast by means of a laser scanner and rapid prototyping machine. J Prosthet Dent. 2004;92:591–5.
38. Ciocca L, De Crescenzio F, Fantini M, Scotti R. CAD/CAM bilateral ear prostheses construction for Treacher Collins syndrome patients using laser scanning and rapid prototyping. Comput Methods Biomech Biomed Engin. 2010;13(3):379–86. https://doi.org/10.1080/10255840903251304.
39. Ciocca L, Mingucci R, Gassino G, Scotti R. CAD/CAM ear model and virtual construction of the mold. J Prosthet Dent. 2007;98(5):339–43.
40. Mueller AA, Paysan P, Schumacher R, Zeilhofer HF, Berg-Boerner BI, Maurer J, Vetter T, Schkommodau E, Juergens P, Schwenzer-Zimmerer K. Missing facial parts computed by a morphable model and transferred directly to a polyamide laser-sintered prosthesis: an innovation study. Br J Oral Maxillofac Surg. 2011;49(8):e67–71. https://doi.org/10.1016/j.bjoms.2011.02.007.
41. Ciocca L, Tarsitano A, Marchetti C, Scotti R. Updates on the construction of an eyeglass-supported nasal prosthesis using computer-aided design and rapid prototyping technology. J Prosthodont. 2016;25(1):61–5. https://doi.org/10.1111/jopr.12332.
42. Jivănescu A, Bratu DC, Tomescu L, Măroiu AC, Popa G, Bratu EA. The assessment of lower face morphology changes in edentulous patients after prosthodontic rehabilitation, using two methods of measurement. Romanian J Morphol Embryol. 2015;56(2 Suppl):753–7.
43. Gäbel H, Kakoshke D. Photogrammetric quantification of changes of soft tissue after skeletal treatment of the facial part of the skull. In: Kraus K, Waldhäusl P, editors. IAPRS. Technical Commission V: close range techniques and machine vision. Vol. 31, Part B5. Horn: Druckerei Berger; 1996. p. 188–93.
44. Ayoub AF, Siebert P, Moos KF, Wray D, Urquhart C, Niblett TB. A vision-based three- dimensional capture system for maxillofacial assessment and surgical planning. Br J Oral Maxillofac Surg. 1998;36(5):353–7.
45. Baik HS, Jeon JM, Lee HJ. Facial soft-tissue analysis of Korean adults with normal occlusion using a 3-dimensional laser scanner. Am J Orthod Dentofac Orthop. 2007;131(6):759–66.
46. Baik HS, Kim SY. Facial soft-tissue changes in skeletal Class III orthognathic surgery patients analyzed with 3-dimensional laser scanning. Am J Orthod Dentofac Orthop. 2010;138(2):167–78. https://doi.org/10.1016/j.ajodo.2010.02.022.
47. Kulczynski FZ, Andriola FO, Deon PH, Melo DADS, Pagnoncelli RM. Postural assessment in class III patients before orthognathic surgery. J Oral Maxillofac Surg. 2018;76(2):426–35. https://doi.org/10.1016/j.joms.2017.07.157.
48. Masoud MI, Bansal NC, Castillo J, Manosudprasit A, Allareddy V, Haghi A, Hawkins HC, Otárola-Castillo E. 3D dentofacial photogrammetry reference values: a novel approach to orthodontic diagnosis. Eur J Orthod. 2017;39(2):215–25. https://doi.org/10.1093/ejo/cjw055.
49. Manosudprasit A, Haghi A, Allareddy V, Masoud MI. Diagnosis and treatment planning of orthodontic patients with 3-dimensional dentofacial records. Am J Orthod Dentofac Orthop. 2017;151(6):1083–91. https://doi.org/10.1016/j.ajodo.2016.10.037.
50. Freudlsperger C, Rückschloß T, Ristow O, Bodem J, Kargus S, Seeberger R, Engel M, Hoffmann J, Mertens C. Effect of occlusal plane correction on lip cant in two-jaw orthognathic surgery—a three-dimensional analysis. J Craniomaxillofac Surg. 2017;45(6):1026–30. https://doi.org/10.1016/j.jcms.2017.03.014.
51. Seo SW, Jung YS, Baik HS. Three-dimensional analysis of midfacial soft tissue changes after maxillary posterior impaction and intraoral vertical ramus osteotomy for mandibular setback in class III patients. J Craniofac Surg. 2017;28(7):1789–96. https://doi.org/10.1097/SCS.0000000000003754.
52. Lin CW, Wang YC, Chen YH, Ko EW. Dentoskeletal parameters related to visual perception of facial asymmetry in patients with skeletal class III malocclusion after orthognathic surgery. Int J Oral Maxillofac

Surg. 2018;47(1):48–56. https://doi.org/10.1016/j.ijom.2017.06.031.
53. Kim JH, Park YC, Yu HS, Kim MK, Kang SH, Choi YJ. Accuracy of 3-dimensional virtual surgical simulation combined with digital teeth alignment: a pilot study. J Oral Maxillofac Surg. 2017;75(11):2441.e1–2441.e13. https://doi.org/10.1016/j.joms.2017.07.161.
54. Song HS, Choi SH, Cha JY, Lee KJ, Yu HS. Comparison of changes in the transverse dental axis between patients with skeletal Class III malocclusion and facial asymmetry treated by orthognathic surgery with and without presurgical orthodontic treatment. Korean J Orthod. 2017;47(4):256–67. https://doi.org/10.4041/kjod.2017.47.4.256.
55. James RD. A comparative study of facial profiles in extraction and non-extraction treatment. Am J Orthodont Dentofac Orthop. 1998;114:265–76.
56. Boley JC, Pontier JP, Smith S, Fulbright M. Facial changes in extraction and non-extraction patients. Angle Orthod. 1998;68:539–46.
57. Moss JP, Ismail SF, Hennessy RJ. Three-dimensional assessment of treatment outcomes on the face. Orthod Craniofacial Res. 2003;6(Suppl 1):126–31; discussion 179-82
58. Noguchi N, Tsuji M, Shigematsu M, Goto M. An orthognathic simulation system integrating teeth, jaw and face data using 3D cephalometry. Int J Oral Maxillofac Surg. 2007;36(7):640–5.
59. Yamada T, Mishima K, Moritani N, Janune D, Matsumura T, Ikeya Y, Yamamoto T. Nasolabial morphologic changes after a Le Fort I osteotomy: a three-dimensional anthropometric study. J Craniofac Surg. 2010;21(4):1089–95. https://doi.org/10.1097/SCS.0b013e3181e1e6ff.
60. Soncul M, Bamber MA. Evaluation of facial soft tissue changes with optical surface scan after surgical correction of Class III deformities. J Oral Maxillofac Surg. 2004;62(11):1331–40.
61. Gerbino G, Bianchi FA, Verzé L, Ramieri G. Soft tissue changes after maxillo-mandibular advancement in OSAS patients: a three-dimensional study. J Craniomaxillofac Surg. 2014;42(1):66–72. https://doi.org/10.1016/j.jcms.2013.02.004.
62. Aurora RN, Casey KR, Kristo D, Auerbach S, Bista SR, Chowdhuri S, Karippot A, Lamm C, Ramar K, Zak R, Morgenthaler TI, American Academy of Sleep Medicine. Practice parameters for the surgical modifications of the upper airway for obstructive sleep apnea in adults. Sleep. 2010;33(10):1408–13.

Holographic 3D Visualisation of Medical Scan Images

16

Javid Khan

Contents

Abstract

Following decades of research and development, three-dimensional (3D) holographic visualisation and display technologies are ready to emerge. A 3D image can be described in terms of capturing the light field of a scene, which can be recreated by a surface that emits rays of light as a function of both intensity and direction. This may be realised via integral imaging or holography or a combination of these. Holographic technology relies on lasers to create diffractive interference patterns that enable encoding of amplitude and phase information within an optical medium. This is in the form of transmission or reflection holograms that act as gratings to deflect light. Suitable illumination of these patterns can form a 3D representation of an object in free space. Printed digital reflection holograms with static 3D images are now sufficiently mature for the depiction of volumetric data

J. Khan (✉)
Holoxica Ltd, CodeBase, Argyle House,
Edinburgh, UK
e-mail: jk@holoxica.com

S. Stübinger et al. (eds.), *Lasers in Oral and Maxillofacial Surgery*,
https://doi.org/10.1007/978-3-030-29604-9_16

from computed tomography, magnetic resonance imaging or ultrasound scans. The physiology of 3D visual image perception is introduced along with tangible benefits of 3D visualisation. Image processing and computer graphics techniques for medical scans are summarised. Next-generation holographic video displays for dynamic visualisation are on the horizon, which are also being designed for medical imaging modalities. Case studies are also presented in facial forensics and surgical planning.

Keywords

3D · Holography · Interference · Diffraction
Display · Light field · Hologram
Visualisation · CT · MRI · Medical imaging
Holoxica

16.1 Introduction

The most advanced medical imaging technologies including CT, MRI and ultrasound have been pioneered over the past few decades by many scientists and engineers, winning Nobel Prizes in 1979 (Cormack and Hounsfield for CT) and 2003 (Lauterbur and Mansfield for MRI). These scanning machines are highly sophisticated and expensive devices, performing 3D scans by taking 2D slices through the body using ionising (X-rays for CT) and non-ionising radiation (magnetic fields/radio waves for MRI) or acoustic energy (USS). The pace of innovation has been tremendous in terms of size, safety, speed, accuracy and image resolution amongst other parameters. However, it is somewhat surprising to find that corresponding advances in three-dimensional displays for the visualisation of this data have not matched this rapid pace of scanner development.

The human visual perceptual system is inherently tuned to interpret the visual field in three spatial dimensions in addition to the temporal aspect. However, the conventional presentation of digital imaging information is largely constrained to just two spatial dimensions. For medical images, surgeons are often required to interpret individual 2D scan slices to build a 3D mental picture of the stack of such slices. This is counter-intuitive, even for a highly trained radiologist, and can lead to inaccurate or inconsistent interpretations. It becomes even more of a challenge to use this information for surgical planning, and explaining pathologies to patients can also be difficult. Most of these issues can be overcome with 3D visualisation techniques, which are seen as a grand challenge for display industry which has thus far fallen short of expectations.

16.2 Physiology of Human Visual Perception

The human visual system captures continuous images of the 3D world as a pair of two-dimensional images projected on to the back of the retina through the cornea, lenses and pupils of the eyes. The retina comprises photoreceptor cells including colour-sensitive rods and photosensitive cones that convert the incident photons into neural impulses that are relayed to the visual cortex of the brain via the optic nerve. The pair of 2D images is processed by the visual cortex, which utilises a combination of binocular and monocular information as so-called depth cues to recreate a 3D scene. The binocular depth cues are:

- Stereopsis.
- Vergence.

Stereopsis is responsible for binocular vision due to the lateral displacement of the eyes, in which the similarities and differences between a pair of offset 2D images are used to synthesise depth information about the scene. *Vergence* is the ability of both eyes to triangulate and focus on an object where the eyes converge on objects nearby or diverge on objects further away.

While binocular depth cues are the dominant means of 3D perception, there are a surprising number of monocular visual cues that enhance the experience [1]:

- Accommodation.
- Motion parallax.
- Linear perspective.
- Occlusion.
- Familiar size and relative size.
- Lighting and shadows.
- Texture and shading.

Accommodation is the ability of the eye to focus on objects at different distances by changing the focal length of the lens via the muscles. Widening (and thus flattening) the lens increases the focal length and flattening causes it to be decreased. Using this mechanism, the eye can typically accommodate objects from about 7 cm to infinity in about 350 ms. Vergence and accommodation go hand-in-hand and any conflicts between the two lead to problems with 3D perception [2–4], which can be the case with conventional stereoscopic display implementations involving 3D glasses and headwear. *Motion parallax* is another related depth cue associated with the motion of the viewer across a scene where objects in the foreground appear to move more quickly than those in the background.

Figure 16.1 depicts a 2D image with a large number of 3D depth cues. *Linear perspective* is a geometric effect where parallel lines appear to triangulate towards a distant vanishing point located on the horizon. *Occlusion* of some objects by others provides depth cues about the relative distance of those objects, where background objects tend to be hidden or obscured by foreground objects. *Known size* implies that if we are familiar with the physical size of an object such as a person or a bicycle, then its perceived size in the visual field tells us how far away it is; *linear size* perceived in the visual field is inversely proportional to distance. Furthermore, the perceived relative size of two or more objects of known physical size informs the viewer regarding their relative distance. Finally, lighting, shading and texturing all enhance the perception of depth within a scene. Indeed, all of these factors are used to great effect in conveying 3D information in 2D imagery and artwork.

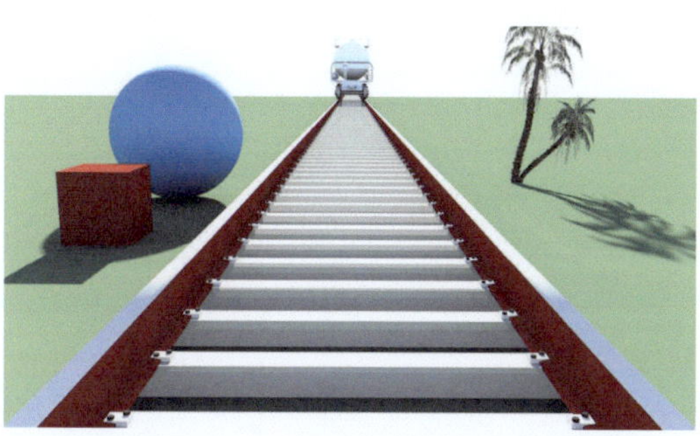

Fig. 16.1 Depth cues including perspective, occlusion and shadows

Apart from the monocular and binocular depth cues presented here, a number of other factors are important for the creation of high-quality 2D as well as 3D display imagery including persistence of vision, colour, etc. which are tackled in other texts [5, 6]. For colour perception, there are three types of rods within the eye whose lengths correspond to spectral peaks, leading to the red, green and blue (RGB) colour model. Hence it is important to have laser and other light sources (e.g. LED) around these peak wavelengths for colour display systems.

16.2.1 Benefits of 3D Visualisation

A US Air Force Research Laboratory study discusses the relative benefits of 3D visualisation vs. 2D [7]. This is a comprehensive review that summarises the results of over 160 publications describing over 180 experiments spanning 51 years. The research covers human factors psychology, engineering, human–computer interaction, vision science, visualisation and medicine. The study concluded that 3D is overall 75% better than 2D for specific applications including spatial manipulation, finding, identifying or classifying objects [7]. The US Army Research Laboratory looked at training with medical hologram vs. traditional 2S methods [8]. This showed significant improvement in retention and reduced cognitive load for recalling complex 3D anatomy.

These features are important for the interpretation of medical imaging data, where specific benefits of 3D visualisation include:

- Learning anatomy: increase retention and recall by over 20% [8].
- Diagnostics: 40% faster interpretation of CT/MRI scans [9].
- The speed of surgical procedures is increased by 15% [10].
- Improve accuracy of surgery by up to 20% (incisions, stitching, navigation) [10].

There are clear advantages to viewing 3D information using 3D techniques, as quantified by these studies.

16.3 Light Field Synthesis

The scientific literature suggests that the best means of 3D reconstruction is to recreate the light field of an object or a scene [11, 12]. This can be achieved by holographic and similar approaches such as integral imaging. The concept of a light field describes the all rays of light for a scene as an array of vectors comprising the colour intensity $I(\lambda)$, direction (θ, φ) and timing (t) of each ray of light, which can be described by the plenoptic function, L:

$$L = f\left(I(\lambda),\theta,\varphi,t\right) \tag{16.1}$$

16.3.1 Integral Imaging

Integral imaging was first proposed over a 100 years ago by Lippmann [13], who won the 1908 Nobel Prize. Integral imaging is a method of 3D image formation method based on ray optics by integrating a set of rays emerging from 2D elemental images recorded from slightly different perspectives across the scene. The arrangement consists of a matrix of lenslets or pinholes located just behind a similar arrangement of miniature 2D photos. Each tiny lens views the 3D object from a slightly different perspective than a neighbouring lens, resulting in simultaneous reconstruction from an array of discrete perspectives. This enables the viewer to perceive a 3D representation of the object, depicted in Fig. 16.2. Here, the tiny photos are replaced by a display panel, which can recreate the array of smaller images. The 3D image resolution is determined by the size of the lenslet matrix, whereas the angular resolution or parallax depends on the diameter and pitch as well as the pixel density of the display panel.

Although the idea has been around for a long time, integral imaging has proven to be difficult to implement in practice. Capturing the 3D image and transferring it to a display panel is not trivial, involving lenslet arrays and camera sensors. Additional optical or image processing is required to convert between pseudoscopic and orthoscopic and virtual and real images. Pseudoscopic images are essentially inside-out

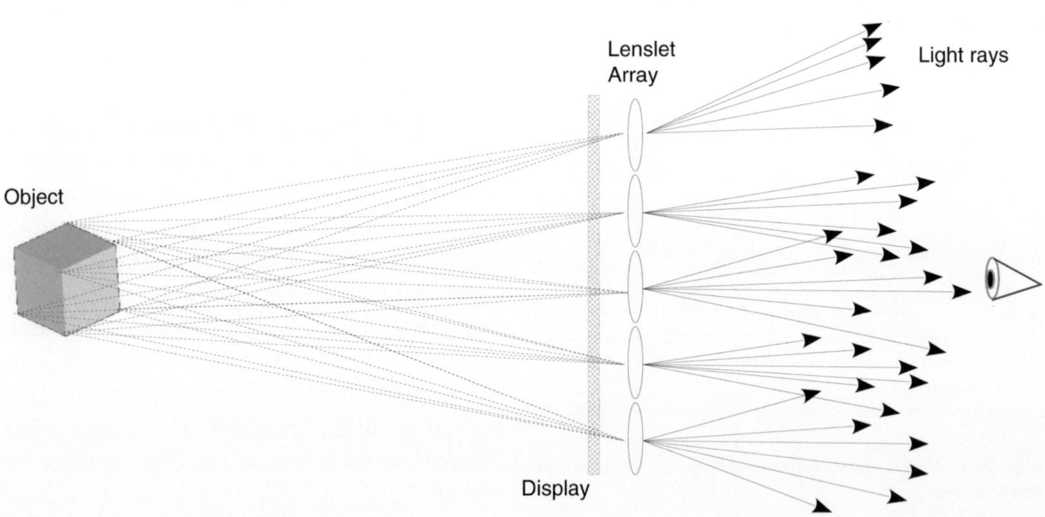

Fig. 16.2 Integra imaging with a lenslet array

(phase reversed) requiring conversion to orthoscopic viewpoint for presentation to the viewer. A virtual image is behind the screen, whereas a real image is in front of it, i.e. in mid-air. These issues have been researched extensively in an attempt to improve the performance of the technology using spatial and temporal multiplexing [14].

An increasingly popular approach is computational integral imaging that borrows techniques from 3D computer graphics. The advantage is that the object or scene can be generated completely synthetically from 3D model descriptions by the computer. The rendering of multiple 2D views of the 3D scene can be done using a 'virtual' camera that can pan around the object in any direction. These methods can leverage commodity graphics processing units (GPUs) to render the 3D views in hardware, described in Sect. 16.4.

16.3.2 Holography and Laser Interference

This section presents the basic principles and theoretical foundations of holograms and holography. The term hologram is derived from the Greek, meaning 'whole image'. Holograms are able to encode both amplitude and phase information about the 3D object or scene. This information is encoded such that the light field can be reconstructed to give a true 3D representation corresponding to the original subject. This is in contrast with a photograph, which only stores amplitude information, thus yielding a 2D representation.

The foundations of holography were laid by Dennis Gabor, a Hungarian scientist working in the UK, in a patent [15] and a series of papers written between 1948 and 1951 that were aimed at microscopy [16–18]. These introduced the notion of storing 3D information as a diffractive interference pattern that can subsequently be reconstructed through illumination. Holography remained somewhat obscure owing to its dependence on special coherent light sources. However, things changed dramatically after the invention of the laser in 1960 [19], which generates coherent light, leading to a revival of the field. Leith and Upatnieks reached a key milestone with the off-axis transmission hologram [20]. At about the same time, Denisyuk pioneered the reflection hologram [21] viewable using ordinary light rather than lasers. Dennis Gabor was awarded the Physics Nobel Prize in 1971.

The majority of holographic applications today can be found in security and authentication for credit cards, banknotes, passports or product packaging. These simple holograms are mass-produced using industrial-scale printing press-like machines. This is a billion-dollar industry, but which is currently not aimed at general 3D imaging as such.

16.3.2.1 Transmission and Reflection Holograms

Static holograms are formed by recording interference patterns in a photosensitive holographic material. Holograms use spatial variations in the absorption and/or the optical thickness to alter the amplitude and phase of an incident wave front. The modulation is due to interference patterns derived from the interaction of two laser beams: a reference beam and a beam reflected off an object.

There are two main types of holograms: transmission and reflection. Transmission holograms are formed by exposing the holographic material from the same side, whereas reflection holograms expose it from opposite sides. Transmission holograms are the simplest forms of holograms (Fig. 16.3) where a collimated laser beam is split in two, one path hitting the object which interferes with the other reference beam, thus exposing photographic plate. Details of practical recording considerations for transmission and reflection holograms (not shown) can be found in [22].

Holographic recording media are usually based on organic photosensitive materials such as dichromated gelatine (DCG) or silver halide, similar to traditional photographic film [23]; modern materials are based on photopolymers with organic dyes [24]. DCG and silver halide require further chemical processing (bleaching

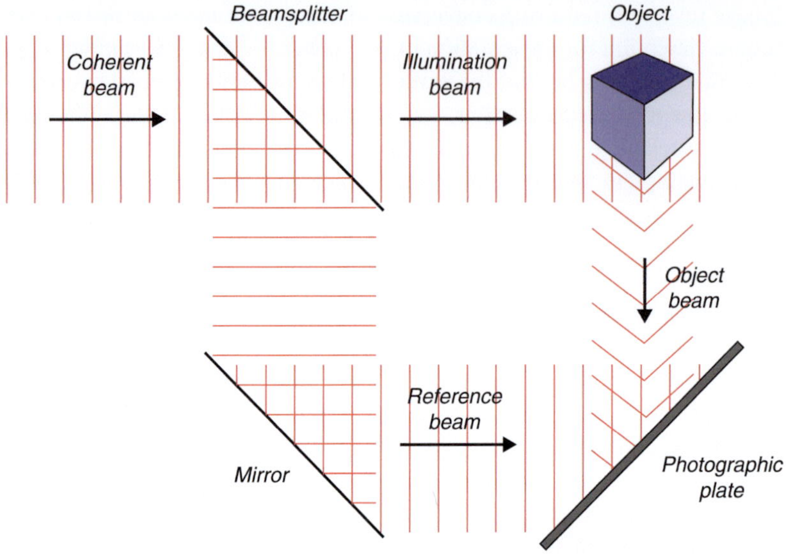

Fig. 16.3 Recording a transmission hologram

and developing) after exposure, whereas the latest photopolymers use the light itself to develop the photosensitive material. Additionally, in some cases, bleaching requires illumination with UV radiation.

A holographic image is reconstructed by transmission or reflection of light through this recording medium. The replay of a transmission hologram is shown in Fig. 16.4, where the reference beam is replaced with a laser illumination beam.

Transmission holograms behave rather like gratings, requiring coherent illumination through the hologram, based on the principles of Fresnel diffraction from Fourier optics theory [25], Fig. 16.5 (left). The average fringe spacing, or spatial frequency of the interference patterns, within a transmission hologram is given by the grating equation:

$$\Lambda = \frac{\sin\theta}{\lambda} \quad (16.2)$$

where θ is the angle between the object and the reference beam and λ is the wavelength of the recording laser. Reflection holograms can be regarded as tiny wavelength-selective micro-mirrors, requiring ordinary non-coherent illumination on the front surface, based on the principles of Bragg's diffraction theory [26], Fig. 16.5 (right). The average spatial frequency of the Bragg grating structures within a reflection hologram is given by:

$$\Lambda = \frac{2\sin\theta}{\lambda} \quad (16.3)$$

which is simply twice the spatial resolution of the transmission case. Reflection holograms require higher-resolution holographic media for

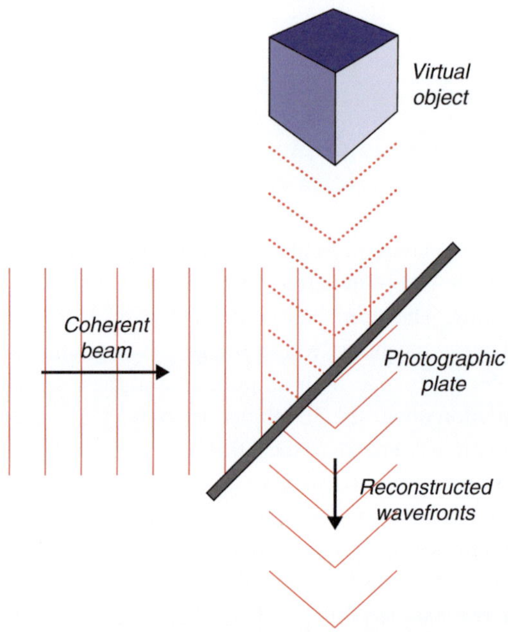

Fig. 16.4 Reconstructing a transmission hologram

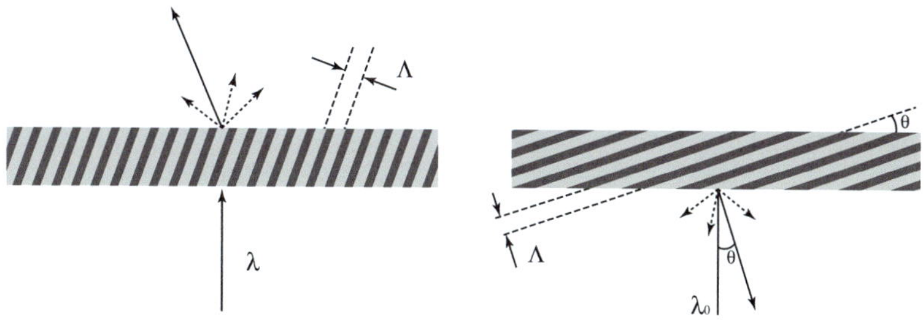

Fig. 16.5 Diffraction through transmission (left) and reflection (right) holograms

recording, and they are also highly angular and wavelength sensitive, while transmissions generally diffract many wavelengths. For replay and viewing the 3D image, transmission holograms require laser (coherent) illumination, whereas reflection holograms can use incoherent ordinary white light sources including LEDs.

The main characteristics of transmission and reflection holograms are shown in the table below:

Hologram type	Transmission	Reflection
Diffraction	Fresnel	Bragg
Recording lasers	Same side	Opposite sides
Resolution (lines/mm)	~2000	>5000
Transmission/reflection	Insensitive to λ and θ	Sensitive to λ and θ
Illumination	Laser (coherent)	Incoherent white light
Applications	Analogue mastering Holographic video display	Analogue/digital holograms

16.3.3 Static 3D Imaging and Digital Holography

Digital holograms are fabricated using holoprinter or holographic printing devices. These are industrial-scale machines that can manufacture full-colour, purely digital reflection holograms in a manner that is repeatable and reliable. They are available from a handful of manufacturers including Geola (LT), Ceres Holographics (UK), Zebra Imaging (USA) and HoloTech (HU).

The basic principles behind digital holography stem from integral imaging as described in Sect. 16.3.1, where a 3D scene or object can be decomposed into a series of tiny 2D images viewed through an array of micro-lenses. A digital hologram essentially combines the 2D image and lenslet into a single holographic pixel, also known as a holopixel or hogel. The digital hologram comprises a matrix of these holopixels created by the interference of red, green and blue (RGB) lasers in a holographic medium such as a photopolymer (manufactured by Bayer or DuPont) or silver halide film.

A holoprinter, Fig. 16.6, includes RGB lasers, a spatial light modulator (SLM) microdisplay, beam-steering optics, and a computer to depict the images on the SLM as well as a control system for the entire assembly. The laser-writing scheme uses an object and reference beam pair to create the interference pattern, which can be considered as a modified Fourier transform of the scene viewed through the holopixel aperture. The object beam is modulated via the SLM with 2D information synthesised from the scene. Optics are held stationary, whereas the holographic medium is mounted on an x-y translation stage and moved relative to the lasers, which are usually arranged vertically in-line and operate on different holopixels in parallel. The stage is moved continuously in a raster-scan fashion.

Holopixels are written with three (RGB) pulsed lasers with pulse widths around 40 ns and energies up to 10 mJ. The RGB holopixels

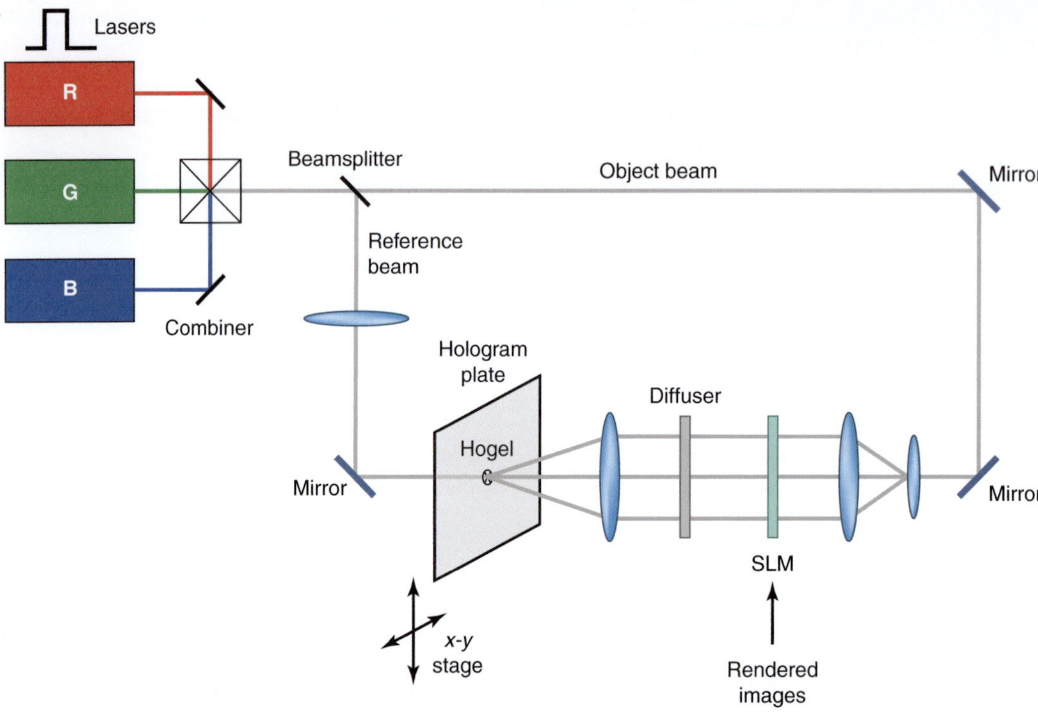

Fig. 16.6 Optical architecture of a holoprinter system

are spatially overlaid, with holopixel dimensions now shrinking to submillimetre diameters, currently around 0.7 mm, and trending even smaller to 0.5 mm or even 0.25 mm. At such small dimensions, the holopixels are no longer visible to the human eye, making it possible to create photorealistic digital holograms. The Zebra Imaging holopixel is 0.7 mm wide, imaging 512 × 512 pixels giving over half a million rays of light per square mm and a field of view of 90° full parallax. An A4 page-sized (200 × 300 mm) digital hologram has over 47 Gb of data and fabrication typically takes several hours.

The holograms produced in this manner are high-quality, full-colour reflection holograms. For replay (viewing) of the 3D image, digital holograms only require a simple, bright point light source for illumination. It is even possible to produce digital holograms that can lie flat, allowing the viewer to walk 360° around the image. Printing a small page-sized digital hologram costs a few hundred dollars to produce, with larger images, up to a square meter, scaling in price accordingly to thousands of dollars. For volume production, the price can be reduced by an order of magnitude via holographic replication technology that works like a 'holographic photocopier', using RGB lasers to make copies of digital holograms in just minutes. This is attractive given that the master hologram takes many hours to produce.

Current holoprinters are somewhat bulky devices with large and powerful lasers as well as mechanics, costing up to a million dollars. However, portable devices are not far off. Companies like Pioneer and Samsung are working to develop a desktop unit using RGB laser diodes that can produce smaller format digital holograms up to A4 page size. There is every reason to expect desktop-sized holoprinters no larger than a standard laser printer within the next few years. Some analogies can be drawn between holoprinter technology and physical 3D printing, where the latter was initially used in high-end industrial applications but is now available to anyone.

16.3.3.1 Digital Hologram Channelling and Animation

The digital hologram encoding mechanism means it is possible to control the light rays emanating from each holopixel. This means that it is feasible to include several distinct images within the digital hologram, each of which appears over a specific range of viewing angles. Holoxica developed a number of techniques that allow the 3D image to reveal layers, as the viewer moves past the hologram, thus revealing otherwise hidden aspects of the image. As most of the images are synthetic, it is also possible to include opacity and fading to highlight features that would otherwise be obscured.

16.3.4 Case Study: Facial Forensics for Archaeology

In 1857, Scottish archaeologist Alexander Rhind excavated a mummy from a tomb in Thebes and transported it to Edinburgh. The mummy was unusual because it was completely intact in its original wrappings when it was donated to the National Museum of Scotland, under the condition that it never be opened. The secrets of the Rhind Mummy were finally revealed over 150 years later when it was scanned by the Clinical Research Imaging Centre (CRIC) at The University of Edinburgh, Toshiba Aquilion One CT scanner.

The scan data was processed using a series of volume rendering software (Fovia, Toshiba Vitrea and Voxar 3D) to isolate the various layers through the wrapping to reveal underlying detail. Bone can easily be extracted using standard tools and techniques including the open source 3D Slicer application. The initial analysis also revealed further hidden artefacts, most significantly an embossed metal plate (possibly gold) with a flying scarab, placed on the forehead during mummification. Facial reconstruction detail was extracted from the CT data using similar methods via the Amira tool. Finally, the sarcophagus, or outer wrapping, was isolated. Forensic analysis determined that the mummy was in her late 20s and approximately 158 cm in height. The cause of death could not be inferred from the scan data.

Holoxica produced a 30 × 30 cm animated hologram of the face and head, all from the various volumetric and segmented models derived from the CT data. The digital hologram, Fig. 16.7, reveals different layers of information as the viewer moves from left to right. The first layer is the sarcophagus wrapping (Fig. 16.7, left), peeling away to reveal the face (centre) followed by the skull (right). The outer wrapping is encrusted with jewels and gold amulets, which are visible from all angles. The metal cap is revealed towards the right.

The Rhind Mummy will never be opened, so the best way to look inside and appreciate this

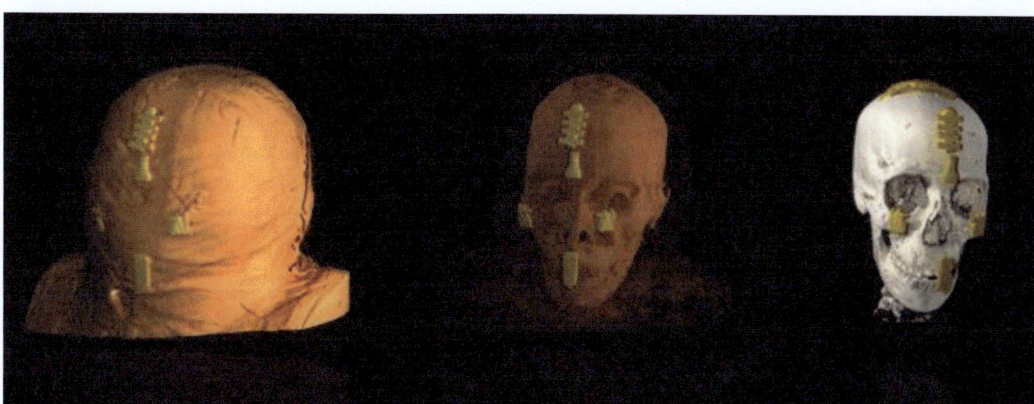

Fig. 16.7 The Rhind Mummy hologram with three channels (views)

artefact in 3D is to use advanced visualisation techniques. The colour-animated hologram is life-sized and shows a level of depth, detail and realism that is difficult to demonstrate to the public in other ways. The hologram has been shown in science museums including the MIT Museum, National Museum of Scotland and Saint Petersburg Museum of Optics.

16.4 Graphics Processing Medical Data for 3D Visualisation

In principle, it is possible to turn any type of 3D dataset into a digital hologram or a holographic/light field display. The data can be a scan, a mathematical description, molecular data, map/contour data, point cloud, volume data or a CAD model. Provided there is sufficient data to extract an acceptable 3D model, it is possible to generate a hologram. Visualisation of 3D data from medical scanners is based on two main techniques: surface rendering and volume rendering. The choice of an appropriate technique is often operator-selectable and depends on the clinical application.

Surface rendering is the most common and least computationally demanding 3D visualisation method. It is based on the identification and extraction of boundaries or edges that define organs, tissues, vessels, bones or other anatomical regions of interest within the scan volume. The boundaries can be identified either manually via simple thresholding voxels and their neighbours or automatically using algorithms such as marching cubes [27] or its derivatives [28] to identify isometric surfaces. Once the surface structures of the organ or region are classified and identified, they can be mapped to polygonal meshes to represent the geometry. This brings the scan data within the realm of computer graphics where standard techniques can be applied to the mesh model including lighting, shading, reflection, diffusivity, etc. Finally, specialised graphics hardware (GPUs) can be used to speed up rendering.

Volume rendering is an alternative technique enabling direct visualisation through the entire volume of the data, rather than the selected geometries from surface rendering. Volume rendering is a ray-tracing method in which virtual light rays are back-propagated through the 3D volume data and projected on to a viewing plane. Each ray intercepts a series of voxels along a linear path where they are weighted and summed to achieve a semi-transparent render through the volume. A simple rendering algorithm [29] is based on translucent/opacity propagation where the pixel value is given by the expression:

$$V_i = V_{i-1}\left(1-\alpha_i\right)+\gamma\alpha_i \quad (16.4)$$

where V_i is the value of the ray exiting from the ith voxel and V_{i-1} is the ray entering the voxel emitted from the preceding voxel. The parameter α describes the opacity and γ controls the luminance of the voxel, based on the local gradient. Volume rendering has the advantage that the final image is derived from the original data without information being discarded. However, this technique requires far more computation than surface rendering, scaling with the linear physical dimensions of (or number of voxels within) the dataset. In some ways, this casting of light rays through a volume and capturing the projections within a viewing zone is analogous to the tomographic techniques that acquired the volume in the first place.

16.4.1 Data and File Formats

Given the rising popularity of solid 3D printing, surface models are increasingly important not just for visualisation but also for physical implementation. Indeed, such models are used to make prosthetics and even fabricate certain organs [30, 31]. This has given rise to the STeroLithography (STL) file format, which is rapidly becoming a de facto means of disseminating 3D information. This file format is now supported by many 3D scanning, CAD and visualisation tools. Fortunately, in this context, the STL file format is also amenable to the production of digital holograms. However, there are some limitations with the format, namely, the lack of opacity and colour information, that can be overcome through use of the OBJ file format that combines surface mesh data with textures. This is also a de facto means of more complex 3D data representations. Unfortunately, OBJ is designed for single objects and does not contain scene information (camera position) or animation. Other formats such as Collada (DAE) and FilmBox (FBX) from Autodesk can be used for full-scale animations. Volume data from medical scanners is stored in the popular DICOM (Digital Imaging and Communications in Medicine) format. DICOM is the industry standard for the interchange of information between computers and medical devices, based on a non-proprietary protocol, image format and file structure.

16.5 Dynamic 3D Imaging: Video Displays

An ideal 3D display needs to be able to recreate the depth cues discussed in Sect. 16.2 in order for the human brain to perceive the scene correctly. The technologies employed within 3D displays can be broadly defined across the categories listed below.

- Stereoscopic displays.
- Auto-stereoscopic displays.
- Head-mounted displays.
- Volumetric displays.
- Light field displays.
- Holographic displays.

Currently, the most popular panel technologies for most of the above are based on variants of LCD or organic light-emitting diode (OLED) screens viewed through stereoscopic glasses per viewer or lenticular arrays. Prolonged viewing of such stereoscopic displays leads to discomfort and disorientation due to the vergence-accommodation conflict (Sect. 16.2). Wearing glasses is cumbersome and uncomfortable, whereas lenticulars limit the number of viewers. Head-mounted displays have been around for a long time, but they have never really caught on, largely because of inconvenience, technical, mechanical and cost issues. Holographic displays are still difficult to make and are still at the research stage.

The following sections outline a review of some emerging 3D light field and holographic display technologies with commercial potential. The coverage is by no means exhaustive and only reflects a subset of the technological spectrum. The key design parameters and specifications of the displays are considered, together with performance criteria.

16.5.1 Light Field Displays

A light field display (LFD) is a surface that emits rays of light at different intensities and directions according to Eq. (16.1). There are two main architectures for LFDs: lenslet arrays from Sect. 16.3.1 and arrays of spatially overlapping projectors. Important parameters to consider are spatial resolution (pixel density) and angular resolution (across a field of view), which can be expressed as a rays-per-unit area metric. A good place to start is to consider the angular and spatial resolution of the human eye, which depend on the viewing distance from the screen, typically 300–500 mm. A reasonable field of view is 90° in at least one parallax direction, and an angular resolution of around 1° is acceptable at this distance. For example, a 1 × 1 mm hogel that images 100 × 100 pixels within an FoV of 90° has an angular resolution 0.9° with 10,000 rays/mm^2 (in two dimensions). This implies that the underlying display needs to have a 2D resolution of 2,450 ppi or a pixel pitch of just 10 μm. Compare this with a current smartphone display of 500 pixels/in., which is rather challenging over a large surface area. In terms of storage, a 50 × 50 mm display requires 75 Mb of data for a single image and a bandwidth of 1.88 Gb/s for streaming video at 25 fps. These figures are challenging but possible with current computation (GPU) and network/interconnect technologies. The display resolution, computation, memory and bandwidth can be reduced considerably by constraining the parallax of the display to the horizontal dimension given that human eyes are mounted horizontally and visualisation is in this plane is acceptable for a vertically mounted display.

16.5.1.1 Zebra Imaging and FoVI3D

One of the most advanced 3D light field displays was initially developed by Zebra Imaging, a military contractor and manufacturer of holoprinter and 3D display technologies. The latest 3D display is being developed by its spin-out, FoVI3D. Zebra Imaging/FoVI3D have a long history of developing dynamic 3D LF displays funded by series of US military DARPA projects. The military requirements are for a tabletop or sandbox format for terrain and battlefield scenario visualisation with an FoV of 90° (360° walk around), full parallax, colour and video rate refresh capabilities.

A first demonstrator was presented in 2006, which was a 300 × 300 mm monochrome display with 10 mm resolution. The first colour display, known as the Gen1 display, was built in 2010, with a 0.5 m diagonal comprising 216 projectors and 27 computing nodes [32], with an FoV of 90° and ~5700 rays/mm², Fig. 16.8 (left). The Gen2 display is monochrome yellow with a 90 × 90 mm screen, 160 × 160 hogels with an FoV of 60° with almost 10 k rays/mm², Fig. 16.8 (right). Both of these rely on arrays of micro-displays with relay optics to the lenslet array.

16.5.1.2 Multi-projector Arrays

A commercially available 3D displays is the HoloVizio family made by Holografika [33, 34], which can show high-resolution horizontal parallax full-colour images. It is based on light field imaging where the light rays that form the 3D image are produced by a large array of 2D projectors through a holographic diffusion screen. Each point of the screen can emit rays of different colours in different directions, depending on the projector, all under computer control. The screen is a holographic diffuser with a randomised (non-periodic) surface structure that is independent of wavelength. For a horizontal parallax configuration, the screen ensures that each incident light beam is diverged by an angle of around 1° horizontally and 90° vertically. The light beams generated by the projectors hit the screen at various angles, and the screen blends these beams into a continuous 3D view. The 80WLT prototype, Fig. 16.9, has 80 projectors (each 1280 × 768 resolution) behind a 63 × 39 cm holographic screen with a remarkable 180° FoV (horizontally). The system has 78 M rays of light, with ~320 rays/mm² and an angular resolution of 0.9°.

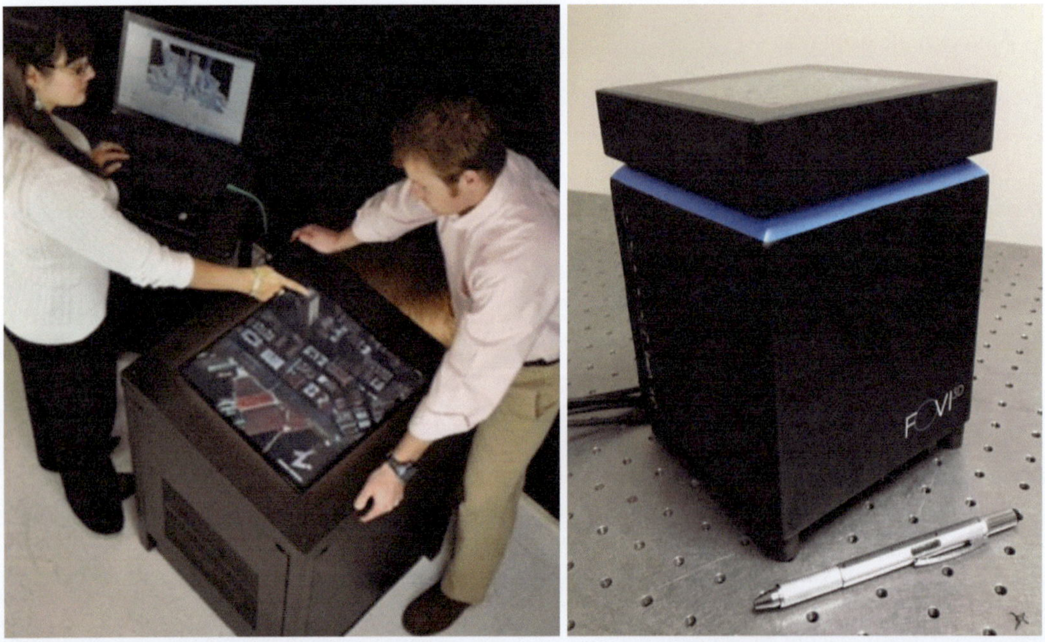

Fig. 16.8 Zebra Imaging Gen1 and FoVI3D Gen2 displays

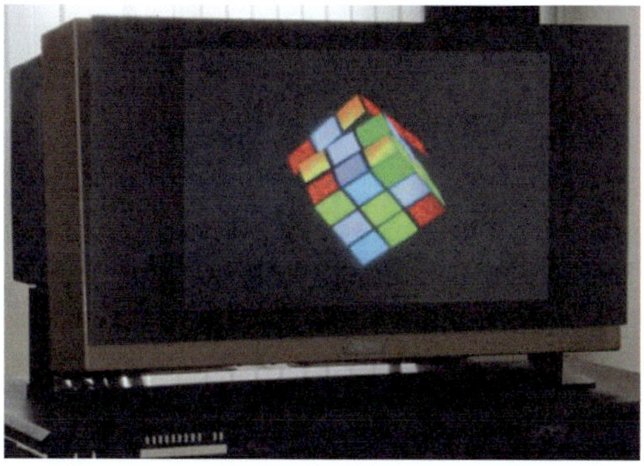

Fig. 16.9 Holografika light field display

16.5.2 Electro-holographic Displays

In the future, 3D displays are likely to be based on holographic technologies that recreate the light field of the 3D scene [11, 35, 36]. The quest for a commercially viable holographic display is still in the early stages of technology readiness. Holographic displays require manipulation of features that are similar in size to the wavelength of light passing through them to enable diffraction. These features may modulate the amplitude and/or the phase of the light, similar to the transmission holograms presented in Sect. 16.3.2.1. It can be shown that phase modulation is much more powerful and efficient than amplitude modulation [37]; it turns out that only eight phase levels are required to attain a theoretical diffraction efficiency of 95%.

Electro-holographic display research has focused on 3D imaging based on high-resolution spatial light modulation (SLM) technology. SLMs are specially constructed micro-displays that provide phase and/or amplitude modulation, thus providing digitally programmable diffractive holographic elements. The diffraction pattern for a scene is computed photon by photon rather than created with laser interference as shown in Sect. 16.3.2, and the pattern is transferred to the SLM either electronically or optically. Computer-generated holography quantizes the hologram or SLM plane, utilising digital Fourier-optical image processing approaches to computation of the interference patterns [38, 39].

Consider a holographic display with 1 μm features and $\lambda = 500$ nm (green), which yields a full diffraction angle of ~30°, from Eq. (16.2). If this display is 50 × 50 mm, then we have a total of 2.5 G 1-μm pixels in the array. If we only have eight phase levels, then three bits of data are required per phase pixel; thus the display requires 937.5 Mb of information to represent a single monochromatic image. If this is running at 25 fps in full RGB colour, then we require a data bandwidth of 70.3 Gb/s for uncompressed video. In terms of computation of the diffraction pattern across the array, first define a voxel size of 1 × 1 × 1 mm or 1 mm^3, as being composed of a number of single-photon emitters. If these emitters are placed 100 μm intervals, then the voxel contains 1000 point sources. If the phase calculation for a single pixel requires just 10 cycles, then we require 25 TFlops of computing power for a volume element the size of a grain of sugar. Larger scenes would require more computation as would real-time video.

It is evident that a holographic display with micron-sized pixel features is a few orders of magnitude beyond the capability current technology. These raw figures appear to be rather daunting in terms of fabrication technology, bandwidth and computation. Nevertheless, there is hope and a number of simplifications can be applied to realise practical displays. A common optimisation is to constrain the parallax of the 3D image to the horizontal plane, which cuts the complexity to the square root of the figures presented here. The same approach is used in light field displays. The following sections discuss different approaches to implementing holographic displays that exploit various optimisation strategies.

16.5.2.1 Rewriteable Holographic Materials

An intuitive extension to the digital holograms discussed in Sect. 16.3.3 is to transform static write-once holograms into rewriteable holograms at video rates. The University of Arizona developed a re-settable photorefractive polymeric material that can be recorded optically by laser interference and erased with a laser under an applied electric field [40]. The first version had monochromatic images that could be erased and rewritten in 4 min. A subsequent version [41] reported in 2010 can rewrite a 100 × 100 mm hologram in just 2 s with 1 mm^2 holographic pixels.

A similar technology utilises a holographic thin film based on a proprietary liquid crystal (LC) mixed with a photosensitive material [42] that can be erased and rewritten in just a millisecond. Unlike the Arizona photopolymer, this photo-LC material is erased and written optically rather than electrically. The photo-LC requires a recording beam at one wavelength, while the holographic interference pattern is read at a different wavelength. The interference pattern is maintained as long as the recording beam is active and it is erased once the recording beam is switched off [43]. This technology is potentially suitable for large-sized real-time dynamic full-colour holographic displays.

The writing of the digital hologram is achieved with colour pulsed lasers similar to writing digital holograms using a holoprinter as described in Sect. 16.3.3. The ultimate goal to reduce this research is to reduce the write time to tens of milliseconds for real-time video. This is very challenging given the amount of information that needs to be written aside from laser safety issues around protection of the viewer during the writing process.

16.5.2.2 MIT Acousto-Optical Modulation

A series of holographic display prototypes were produced at MIT under Benton, starting with the MIT Mark 1 display from 1989, which is an electro-holographic device based on an acousto-optical SLM (AO-SLM) capable of producing 1-in. cubic (25 × 25 × 25 mm) images at 20 frames/s, both monochromatic [44] and colour [45]. The Mark 2 display improves on this in 1994 to achieve a 150 × 75 × 75 mm image. The Mark 2 architecture has better optics, faster electronics to scale the earlier system through tiling hardware and increased parallelism [46, 47]. These displays are some of the best known among the research community. They are horizontal parallax displays and illumination is via a red laser at 632 nm. The third generation includes layered tomographic displays [48] comprising a stack of light-scattering LCDs. Finally, the latest generation is based on a wave-guided acousto-optical modulator in an optical substrate [49].

16.5.2.3 Qinetiq EASLM Array

A CGH display prototype was developed in the mid-2000s by researchers at Qinetiq, a UK military contractor. It was based on arrays of electrically erasable SLMs (EA-SLMs) with a GPU-based computing cluster for computation of the diffraction patterns [50, 51]. Illumination was via RGB lasers at 647, 532, and 457 nm. It was intended for engineering and military visualisation. This display was a proof of concept and while the outcomes were viewed favourably, the R&D has since been discontinued.

16.5.2.4 SeeReal Eye-Tracking System

The SeeReal approach [52, 53] uses a LCD display as a simplified SLM that is combined with eye tracking to present a holographic image within the observer's field of view. This optimisation drastically reduces the required specifications of the holographic display in terms of the resolution, bandwidth and computation requirements. The images are 3D and in full colour. Unfortunately, head or eye tracking has been a difficult technology to implement in practice, and it leads to other problems including timing lags and restricting viewing to just one person.

16.5.2.5 Holoxica Volume Displays

Holoxica has produced three generations of holographic video displays based on volumetric techniques. The first generation demonstrator, presented in 2010, is based on a proprietary holographic screen containing spatially multiplexed interference patterns that can be easily switched by redirecting a pattern of structured illumination [54]. This is suited to simple imagery such as icons, symbols or segmented digits. The second generation display, made in 2013, is based on a large holographic optical element (HOE) and a laser projection system, Fig. 16.10. This enables free-space imaging with arbitrary programmable 3D images visible in mid-air that can change

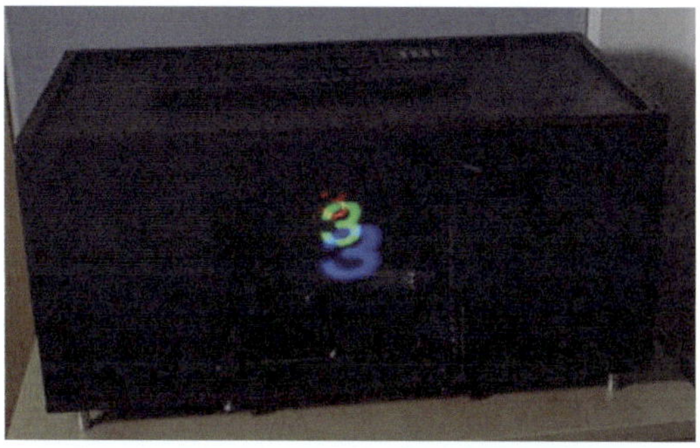

Fig. 16.10 Holoxica second gen display

in real time [55]. Interactivity is added with a motion sensor, which allows the user to 'touch' icons in space and to do things like draw in mid-air. The images are relatively large (70 × 70 mm) and bright enough to be visible under typical office lighting conditions. Holoxica's third generation, display is being designed for volumetric imaging of medical scan data.

The displays are bigger, brighter and better with each generation, for example, the resolution of the first generation was some tens of segments, whereas the second generation is a several 100 k pixels, whereas the third generation will be in the order of millions of voxels. Other key parameters to improve include viewing angle and refresh rate.

16.5.2.6 Emerging Companies

Leia Inc. is a Hewlett Packard spin-out company developing a phone-sized 3D display based on a diffractive light field backlighting architecture. The display is arranged into an array of pixels with each pixel comprising sub-pixels of different grating structures that act as prisms, changing the direction of the incident backlight light. The spatial resolution is 88 pixels/in. Each pixel has 64 independent viewpoints over a 90° field of view [56], i.e. angular resolution of 1.4°. This arrangement yields a ray density of 768 rays/mm^2. A recent startup is the Looking Glass Factory, who offer a horizontal-parallax light field 3D display, with a 50° field of view with an angular resolution of 1.11° (45 views), and display sizes up to 32 inches. This is based on a dense pixel array (8K in the case of 32") with an optical array and combining element to spread and confine the light.

16.5.3 Case Study: Dental Implant Planning

Holoxica collaborated with the Hightech Research Centre for Oral and Cranio-Maxillofacial Surgery of the University of Basel on the 3D visualisation of a procedure around a novel dental implant with a special coronal groove design. The 3D model, Fig. 16.11, visualisation shows the jawbone, teeth, cavity, implant and crown. An animation of the procedure was created, enabling a full 3D view of all of these elements. The titanium implant was created as a mechanical engineering part extracted from a CAD model. The jaw bone and teeth data were extracted semi-automatically from the patient's CT scan via thresholding in slicer. The crown was modelled as a mesh using 3D Studio Max™.

The animated 3D model can be viewed on a light field display (as shown in Fig. 16.11) or a volumetric display (in monochrome) where it can be manipulated, including rotation, zoom as well as pause/stop for the animation. It is even possible to generate a static digital hologram from this model. The visualisation enables a comprehensive appreciation of the angles of entry, constraints within the mouth cavity and freedom of

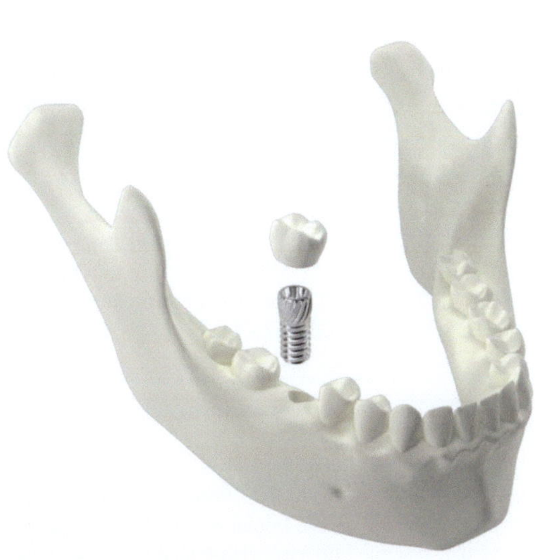

Fig. 16.11 Visualisation for dental implant planning

movement for the surgeon. Especially useful for advanced education programmes and implant training courses, this new technology will open a wide range of unprecedented opportunities to convey state-of-the-art implant dentistry in the future.

16.6 Conclusions

This chapter focused on the creation and visualisation of true 3D images viewed naturally without any form of eye ware, with an emphasis on datasets from medical scanners. The characteristics of human stereoscopic visual perception and potential benefits in medicine were presented. The scientific literature shows that the best methods of creating convincing 3D imagery are holographic and integral imaging techniques. Static imaging with digital holography via holoprinter devices has recently emerged across all medical imaging modalities including ultrasound, CT and MRI. Currently, surface rendering techniques are preferred as the holoprinter workflow leverages computer graphics techniques. Some relevant case studies around forensic archaeology and surgical planning applications were discussed. Dynamic 3D display technologies capable of showing motion video are slowly edging closer to commercial reality, and a review of some popular technologies on the horizon is presented. As ever, a great deal of investment is required to make these displays practical with the military leading the way, followed by the medical community, alongside a few small but innovative high tech companies.

Acknowledgements This work is supported in part by European Union H2020 SME Phase 2 grant number 694328 HoloMedical3D, awarded to Holoxica Limited and EPSRC grant EP/G037523/1.

References

1. Kolb H, Nelson R, Fernandez E, Jones BW. Webvision—The organization of the retina and visual system. http://webvision.med.utah.edu/book/. Accessed 13 Sep 2012.
2. Hoffman DM, Girshick AR, Akeley K, Banks MS. Vergence–accommodation conflicts hinder visual performance and cause visual fatigue. J Vis. 2008;8:33.1–30. https://doi.org/10.1167/8.3.33.
3. Lambooij M, Fortuin M, Heynderickx I, IJsselsteijn W. Visual discomfort and visual fatigue of stereoscopic displays: a review. J Imaging Sci Technol. 2009;53:30201. https://doi.org/10.2352/J.ImagingSci.Technol.2009.53.3.030201.
4. Shibata T, Kim J, Hoffman DM, Banks MS. The zone of comfort: predicting visual discomfort with stereo displays. J Vis. 2011;11(8):11. https://doi.org/10.1167/11.8.11.
5. Khanh TQ, Bodrogi P. Illumination, color and imaging: evaluation and optimization of visual displays. Hoboken, NJ: Wiley; 2012.
6. Maxwell JC. Experiments on colour, as perceived by the eye, with remarks on colour-blindness. Earth Environ Sci Trans R Soc Edinb. 1857;21:275–98. https://doi.org/10.1017/S0080456800032117.
7. McIntire JP, Havig PR, Geiselman EE. Stereoscopic 3D displays and human performance: a comprehensive review. Displays. 2014;35:18–26. https://doi.org/10.1016/j.displa.2013.10.004.
8. Hackett M. Medical holography for basic anatomy training. In: I/ITSEC 2013.
9. The Future of Healthcare in 3D. In: HealthyComms. http://healthycomms.com/2013/07/18/the-future-of-healthcare-in-3d/. Accessed 13 Mar 2014.
10. Fraunhofer P. New opportunities for 3D technology in medicine—Research News March 2013. http://www.fraunhofer.de/en/press/research-news/2013/march/new-opportunities-for-3D-technology-in-medicine.html. Accessed 27 Mar 2013.
11. Bove VM. Display holography's digital second act. Proc IEEE. 2012;100:918–28. https://doi.org/10.1109/JPROC.2011.2182071.
12. Yaras F, Kang H, Onural L. State of the art in holographic displays: a survey. J Disp Technol. 2010;6:443–54.
13. Lippmann G. Epreuves reversibles. photographies integrales. Comptes Rendus. 1908;146:446–51.
14. Jang J-S, Javidi B. Time-multiplexed integral imaging for 3D sensing and display. Opt Photonics News. 2004;15:36–43. https://doi.org/10.1364/OPN.15.4.000036.
15. Dennis G. Improvements in and relating to microscopy. 1947.
16. Gabor D. A new microscopic principle. Nature. 1948;161:777–8. https://doi.org/10.1038/161777a0.
17. Gabor D. Microscopy by reconstructed wave-fronts. Proc R Soc Lond Ser Math Phys Sci. 1949;197:454–87. https://doi.org/10.1098/rspa.1949.0075.
18. Gabor D. Microscopy by reconstructed wave fronts: II. Proc Phys Soc Sect B. 1951;64:449–69. https://doi.org/10.1088/0370-1301/64/6/301.
19. Light 2015 55th anniversary of the laser's invention. In: Int. Year Light Blog. http://light2015blog.org/2015/05/27/55th-anniversary-of-the-lasers-invention/. Accessed 16 Sep 2015.

20. Leith EN, Upatnieks J. Reconstructed wavefronts and communication theory. J Opt Soc Am. 1962;52:1123–8. https://doi.org/10.1364/JOSA.52.001123.
21. Denisyuk Y. On the reflection of optical properties of an object in a wave field of light scattered by it. Dokl Akad Nauk SSSR. 1962;144:1275–8.
22. Saxby G. Practical holography. Boca Raton, FL: CRC Press; 2004.
23. Benton SA, Bove VM. Holographic imaging. Hoboken, NJ: Wiley; 2008.
24. Jurbergs D, Bruder F-K, Deuber F, et al. New recording materials for the holographic industry. Proc SPIE. 2009;7233:72330K.
25. Goodman JW. Introduction to fourier optics. 3rd ed. Greenwood Village, CO: Roberts and Company Publishers; 2005.
26. Kogelnik H. Coupled wave theory for thick hologram gratings. Bell Syst Tech J. 1969;48(9):2909–47.
27. Lorensen WE, Cline HE. Marching cubes: a high resolution 3D surface construction algorithm. In: Proceedings of the 14th annual conference on computer graphics and interactive techniques. New York, NY: ACM; 1987. p. 163–9.
28. Shirley P, Tuchman A. A polygonal approximation to direct scalar volume rendering. In: Proceedings of the 1990 workshop on volume visualization. New York, NY: ACM; 1990. p. 63–70.
29. Levoy M. Display of surfaces from volume data. IEEE Comput Graph Appl. 1988;8:29–37. https://doi.org/10.1109/38.511.
30. Rengier F, Mehndiratta A, von Tengg-Kobligk H, et al. 3D printing based on imaging data: review of medical applications. Int J Comput Assist Radiol Surg. 2010;5:335–41. https://doi.org/10.1007/s11548-010-0476-x.
31. Mironov V, Kasyanov V, Drake C, Markwald RR. Organ printing: promises and challenges. Regen Med. 2008;3:93–103. https://doi.org/10.2217/17460751.3.1.93.
32. Klug MA, Burnett T, Fancello A, et al. A scalable, collaborative, interactive light-field display system. SID Symp Dig Tech Pap. 2013;44:412–5. https://doi.org/10.1002/j.2168-0159.2012.tb05692.x.
33. Balogh T. The HoloVizio system. In: Woods AJ, Dodgson NA, Merritt JO, et al., editors. Proc SPIE. San Jose, CA: SPIE; 2006. p. 60550U.
34. Balogh T. Method and apparatus for displaying three-dimensional images. 1998.
35. Onural L, Yaras F, Kang H. Current research activities on holographic video displays. In: Javidi B, Son J-Y, Thomas JT, Desjardins DD, editors. Three-dimensional imaging, visualization, and display 2010 and display technologies and applications for defense, security, and avionics IV. Proc SPIE. Orlando, FL: SPIE; 2010. p. 769002–10.
36. Hong J, Kim Y, Choi H-J, et al. Three-dimensional display technologies of recent interest: principles, status, and issues [Invited]. Appl Opt. 2011;50:H87–H115. https://doi.org/10.1364/AO.50.000H87.
37. Kress BC, Meyrueis P. Applied digital optics: from micro-optics to nanophotonics. Hoboken, NJ: Wiley; 2009.
38. Voelz DG. Computational fourier optics: a matlab tutorial. Proc SPIE. Orlando, FL: SPIE; 2011.
39. Poon T-C, Kim T. Engineering optics with Matlab. Singapore: World Scientific; 2006.
40. Tay S, Blanche P-A, Voorakaranam R, et al. An updatable holographic three-dimensional display. Nature. 2008;451:694–8. https://doi.org/10.1038/nature06596.
41. Blanche P-A, Bablumian A, Voorakaranam R, et al. Holographic three-dimensional telepresence using large-area photorefractive polymer. Nature. 2010;468:80–3. https://doi.org/10.1038/nature09521.
42. Gao H, Li X, He Z, et al. 59.4: Real-time dynamic holographic display based on a liquid crystal thin film. SID Symp Dig Tech Pap. 2012;43:804–7. https://doi.org/10.1002/j.2168-0159.2012.tb05907.x.
43. Gao H, Li X, He Z, et al. Real-time holographic display based on a super fast response thin film. J Phys Conf Ser. 2013;415:012052. https://doi.org/10.1088/1742-6596/415/1/012052.
44. St-Hilaire P. Scalable optical architectures for electronic holography. Ph.D. Thesis, Massachusetts Institute of Technology. 1994.
45. St-Hilaire P, Benton SA, Lucente ME, Hubel PM. Color images with the MIT holographic video display. Proc SPIE. San Jose, CA: SPIE; 1992. p. 73–84.
46. St-Hilaire P, Benton SA, Lucente ME, et al. Advances in holographic video. Proc SPIE. San Jose, CA: SPIE; 1993. p. 188–96.
47. Lucente ME. Optimization of hologram computation for real-time display. Proc SPIE. San Jose, CA: SPIE; 1992. p. 32–43.
48. Wetzstein G, Lanman D, Heidrich W, Raskar R. Layered 3D: tomographic image synthesis for attenuation-based light field and high dynamic range displays. In: ACM SIGGRAPH 2011 papers. Vancouver, BC: ACM; 2011, p 95:1–95:12.
49. Smalley DE, Smithwick QYJ, Bove VM, et al. Anisotropic leaky-mode modulator for holographic video displays. Nature. 2013;498:313–7. https://doi.org/10.1038/nature12217.
50. Stanley M, Smith MA, Smith AP, et al. 3D electronic holography display system using a 100-megapixel spatial light modulator. Proc SPIE. San Jose, CA: SPIE; 2004. p. 297–308.
51. Slinger C, Cameron C, Stanley M. Computer-generated holography as a generic display technology. Computer. 2005;38:46–53. https://doi.org/10.1109/MC.2005.260.
52. Schwerdtner A, Haussler R, Leister N. Large holographic displays for real-time applications. Proc SPIE. San Jose, CA: SPIE; 2008. p. 69120T.
53. Reichelt S, Leister N. Computational hologram synthesis and representation on spatial light modu-

lators for real-time 3D holographic imaging. J Phys Conf Ser. 2013;415:012038. https://doi.org/10.1088/1742-6596/415/1/012038.
54. Khan J, Underwood I, Greenaway A, Halonen M. A low-resolution 3D holographic volumetric display. In: Schelkens P, Ebrahimi T, Cristobal G, et al., editors. Proc SPIE. Brussels, Belgium: SPIE; 2010. p. 77231B.
55. Khan J, Can C, Greenaway A, Underwood I. A real-space interactive holographic display based on a large-aperture HOE. Proc SPIE. San Francisco: SPIE; 2013. p. 86440M.
56. Fattal D, Peng Z, Tran T, et al. A multi-directional backlight for a wide-angle, glasses-free three-dimensional display. Nature. 2013;495:348–51. https://doi.org/10.1038/nature11972.

Additive Manufacturing and 3D Printing

17

Jan-Michaél Hirsch, Anders Palmquist,
Lars-Erik Rännar, and Florian M. Thieringer

Contents

J.-M. Hirsch
Department of Surgical Sciences, Oral and Maxillofacial Surgery, Medical Faculty, Uppsala University, Uppsala, Sweden

Department of Plastic Surgery and Oral and Maxillofacial Surgery, Uppsala University Hospital, Uppsala, Sweden

A. Palmquist
Department of Biomaterials, Sahlgrenska Academy, University of Gothenburg, Gothenburg, Sweden

L.-E. Rännar (✉)
Sports Tech Research Centre, Mid Sweden University, Östersund, Sweden
e-mail: lars-erik.rannar@miun.se

F. M. Thieringer
Clinic for Oral and Cranio-Maxillofacial Surgery and 3D Print Lab, University Hospital Basel, Basel, Switzerland

Medical Additive Manufacturing Research Group, Department of Biomedical Engineering, Hightech Research Center, University of Basel, Allschwil, Switzerland

S. Stübinger et al. (eds.), *Lasers in Oral and Maxillofacial Surgery*,
https://doi.org/10.1007/978-3-030-29604-9_17

Abstract

This chapter discusses recent applications and findings in additive manufacturing (AM), or 3D printing, applied in oral and maxillofacial surgery. The reader will get an introduction to the basics of AM technology followed by oral and maxillofacial applications like printing of anatomical models and the design and manufacturing of customised implants. Recent research on the biological response of some AM metal alloys is also discussed at the end of the chapter.

Keywords

Additive manufacturing · 3D modelling
Anatomical models · Biological response

17.1 Introduction

Additive manufacturing (AM), or 3D printing, relates to a wide range of technologies where parts are built up by adding material in a layer-wise strategy, which is in contrast with subtractive methods where material is removed. One of the first patents in the area focused on prototyping using UV-curable polymer resins [1], and after that, new technologies were rapidly developed and a variety of materials that could be processed by AM followed. In the mid-1990s, some applications and machines for metal AM were developed, although history shows that these ideas were put on paper already in the 1970s by the French inventor Ciraud [2]. The area of AM has developed from the early days of prototyping to a technology that has begun to compete with traditional methods for serial manufacturing, and it is today seen as an important area for many countries and regions throughout the world for re-industrialisation through the increased competitiveness and sustainability offered by AM. Today, parts manufactured using AM are present in a wide range of different applications, and the technology is broad in the sense that it is applicable to everything from small scale (nanoprinting) to large scale (houses, structural elements for airplanes) and uses a large variety of materials, from food and living cells to electronics.

AM allows for freedom of design, short lead time, flexibility in manufacturing, consolidation of design, minimal material waste, and distributed engineering and manufacturing. These attributes have been shown to be important drivers for AM in general, as well as for medical applications, and AM is today used from individualised and small series manufacturing in order to meet specific needs for patients to serial production where manufacturing cost is the main driver. This chapter explains different technologies available for 3D printing, applications within oral and maxillofacial surgery, and recent findings in the biological response to such applications.

17.2 Technology Overview

Nowadays, a huge variety of 3D printing processes is available on the market. While a few years ago a 3D printer was rather unaffordable for home users, simple 3D printers can now be purchased for just a few hundred dollars (mainly FFF/fused filament fabrication). The considerable cost reduction of printers and printing materials and the increase in user-friendliness of 3D planning and printing software has led to the substantial spread of 3D printers in all areas, especially in industry, design, education, and medicine—however, industrial 3D printers can still cost hundreds of thousands of dollars. Subsequently, more and more medical professionals have become aware of the benefits of 3D printing for use in medicine. Especially in modern dentistry and oral and maxillofacial surgery, 3D printing has become an integral part of the digital medical treatment process (e.g. in the manufacture of sawing or drilling templates, dental models, orthodontic aligners, temporary restorations, or even as a basis for complex final prosthetic restorations or patient-specific implants). Many currently available 3D printing materials are biocompatible and are certified for medical applications and can therefore be used for contact with the human body or even as a substitute material for human tissues. The most widespread 3D printing processes have in common that a printing material (e.g. plastics/polymers, polymer resins, metals, ceramics, or other materials, including biological substances such as living cells) is applied layer by layer to a printing bed and cured by physical and/or chemical processes. These layers can be as thin as only a few micrometres, so the print result can be at a very high resolution and thus correspond exactly to the original computer-aided design (CAD) file. The principle is that the higher the resolution and the larger the building structure, the longer the fabrication time will be. In contrast to the already mentioned subtractive rapid prototyping procedures, which encounter significant limitations compared to the AM processes, 3D printing offers the advantage that almost all geometries can be produced. This offers the advantage that expensive raw material for printing can be saved and that very accurate, light, and resilient bodies that meet biomechanical requirements can be fabricated.

3D printing offers the advantage that engineers, developers, and physicians can segment and design 3D models on the computer and can hold them in their hands in no time at all, thanks to AM. Anatomical physical 3D models and patient-specific 3D-printed implants enable an unprecedented improvement of medical care in many areas. Above all, the fabrication of models with the exact geometry corresponding to the patient's anatomy gives the surgeon or physician the opportunity to plan an invasive procedure in advance and to perform model operations. Taking into account the manufacturing costs of the anatomical biomodels, this leads to cost savings by improving the quality of results and shortening the operating time [3]. The physician can even test different surgical procedures on the basis of preliminary planning and choose the least invasive approach for the patient. 3D printing in medicine enables a cognitive process, which is also called "touch to comprehend" [4].

Increased interest from industry led to the need to categorise different machine technologies and processed materials, so in 2010 an ASTM initiative called "ASTM F42—Additive Manufacturing" formulated a standard where AM was divided into seven different categories—material extrusion, material jetting, binder jetting, vat photopolymerisation, powder bed fusion, sheet lamination, and directed energy deposition. Some of the most common 3D printing technologies are briefly described below.

It must be emphasised that the print result depends mainly on the quality of the digital data set, which typically originates from computed tomography (CT) or magnetic resonance imaging (MRI), and only secondarily on the printing process used. In addition, all AM processes have advantages and disadvantages that must be taken into account when selecting them for appropriate medical applications. For example, the material extrusion process is very well suited for the fabrication of anatomical 3D biomodels but less appropriate for the production of high-precision dental models or splints.

17.2.1 Material Extrusion

Due to its technical simplicity and relatively low purchase costs, material extrusion is widely used for simple 3D printers, and it includes technologies such as FFF and fused deposition modelling (FDM). With this technology, one or more plastic filaments wound on a spool are heated by one or more extruders up to the melting temperature of the material, and the material is then applied to the print bed. There, the material bonds with the layers underneath, cools, and hardens. The print bed is lowered and the next layer is applied in sub-millimetre thickness. The advantage of multi-extruder 3D printers is that different printing materials can be used at the same time. For example, support structures that are necessary for the production of overhangs can be printed with a water-soluble support material such as PVA (polyvinyl alcohol). Some research groups are currently working on FFF printing of high-performance medical polymers such as PEEK (polyether ether ketone). Initial results are very promising and offer a wide range of applications, for example, in the cost-effective production of patient-specific PEEK implants in facial reconstructive surgery [5].

17.2.2 Vat Photopolymerisation

Vat photopolymerisation (often called stereolithography, SLA) is a process in which light (e.g. a UV laser) crosslinks molecules and cures them to solid polymers. Here, too, the building platform is raised and lowered for each cured layer in a vat of liquid polymers and exposed to the laser beam, so that the finished solid 3D model can be removed at the end of the printing process. These methods are especially suitable for very high-resolution structures and exact models. For post-processing, the 3D models often have to be washed in isopropyl alcohol and hardened by UV light to achieve their final strength and durability.

17.2.3 Powder Bed Fusion

This method includes printing processes in which granular materials (polymers, metals, etc.) are evenly distributed on the print bed with a roller and are then selectively fused layer by layer using either a laser or an electron beam. Basically, materials in powder form are melted by heat layer by layer until the model is finished. Laser-based methods include selective laser melting (SLM) and selective laser sintering (SLS), and these can be used for both polymers and metals. Electron beam melting (EBM) has been developed only for metals, and here the raw material (e.g. titanium alloy) is melted in a high vacuum by an electron beam.

17.2.4 Binder Jetting

In the binder jetting process, the powder is selectively bonded by a liquid binding agent sprayed on the powder bed using an inkjet-like technology. By using print heads with many nozzles, many dots can be cured at the same time. In this way, it is possible to fabricate solid models very quickly compared to other methods like FFF/FDM, and typical materials for this process are plastics and metals.

17.2.5 Material Jetting

Here multiple print heads deposit liquid polymers layer wise on a print bed in an inkjet-like fashion. After application of the material, it is cured with UV light. Wax-like, water-soluble, or solvent-soluble structures are used as supports for the printing polymers, and these supports can be easily removed after the printing process. These printing processes enable the processing of a wide variety of polymers with different material properties at very high precision, and some of the technologies are PolyJet and MultiJet printing.

In addition to the printing processes mentioned above, there are also a number of other processes. For the sake of simplicity, and in order not to go beyond the scope of this chapter, the mentioned technologies are discussed only in general terms. Further information can be found in the relevant technical literature.

17.3 From Medical Imaging Data to Manufacturing and Post-processing

Almost all medical three-dimensional 3D printing models used in medical practice or in the clinic begin with a radiological imaging data set. CT data sets, and increasingly cone beam computed tomography (CBCT) data sets, but also MRI and optical surface 3D scans are used to fabricate anatomical models or patient-specific implants. In all radiological imaging modalities, raw data sets of two-dimensional cross-sectional DICOM (Digital Imaging and Communications in Medicine) images are used for further processing. In the first processing step, the images are segmented with the appropriate medical segmentation software. The anatomical region of interest or structure is isolated according to the greyscale values (e.g. Hounsfield units) of the layered medical images and converted (semi-) automatically into a virtual 3D biomodel. This virtual 3D model can now be further processed on the computer. In addition, anatomical defect areas can also be reconstructed virtually, and the resulting structures and geometries serve as the basis for a patient-specific implant. For example, these anatomical defect areas can be supplemented, specific structures can be mirrored and superimposed, or entire virtual surgical procedures can be performed on a workstation. The only limitation is the functionality of the medical modelling software. At the end of the software process chain, the corresponding virtual model is exported as a STL (standard tessellation language) file. This file format can be imported, read, and processed by most 3D printing software packages. Subsequently, the 3D model is prepared for AM and the appropriate layer thickness and model density are selected, the model is orientated on the build platform, and, if necessary, support structures are added (Fig. 17.1).

Depending on the 3D printing technology, the printing process now starts and after several hours' printing time results in an exact representation of the digital anatomical 3D model. In many AM processes, the 3D printed model has to be cleaned during post-processing, freed from support structures, smoothed, and, if necessary, post-hardened. Assuming that biocompatible printing material and a printing process approved for medical applications have been used, the model can be washed and sterilised for intraoperative use.

17.4 Oral and Maxillofacial Applications for Additive Manufacturing

AM has been used for several years for the production of 3D physical models depicting the anatomy of the craniomaxillofacial skeleton [4]. Initially a limiting factor for an accurate model was the slice thickness—the distance between each pair of scans—of the CT scan [6]. Nowadays CT scans are acquired with a slice thickness of 0.65 mm and DICOM volumes of 1 mm and are thus optimal for producing realistic models. The models illustrate complex arrangements of congenital and acquired craniomaxillofacial anomalies, traumatic injuries, tumours, craniosynostoses, and the effects of several syndromes such as facial clefts and dysgnathia. The 3D models are useful in education discussing surgical problems and approaches in complex situations and can be used for model surgery, including the forming of plates and scaffolds. Scanning of an anatomical site and AM can also replace traditional techniques such as impressions to create physical models for the production of maxillofacial prosthesis [7]. The models are a complement to radiology and give the surgical team a realistic 3D picture of the complexity of the case and are valuable for planning and clarifying the need for bone replacement

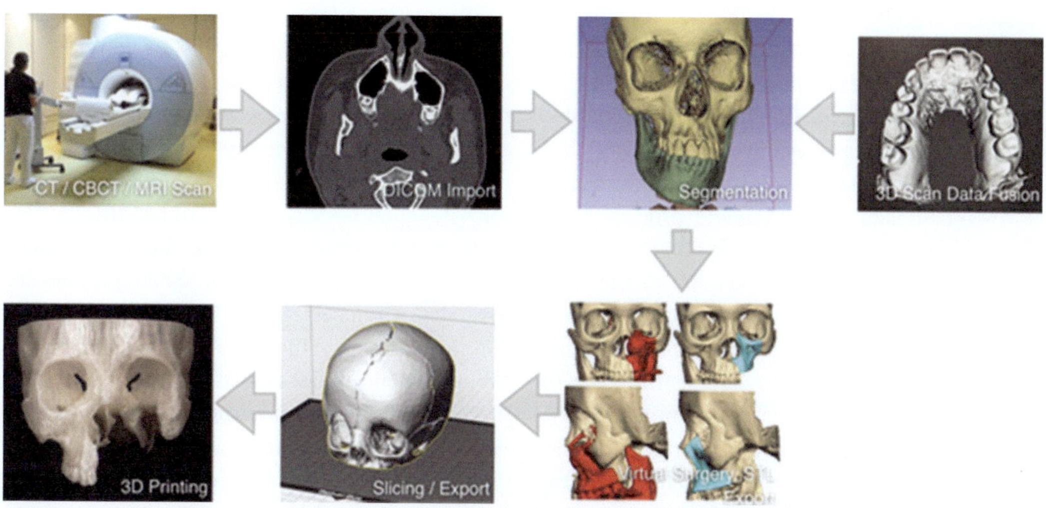

Fig. 17.1 Process workflow from CT scan to 3D physical/AM model (Thieringer)

therapies and patient-specific biomaterial, custom implants, and scaffolds in cases of lost craniofacial tissue. For smaller bony defects, autogenous bone grafts are the standard, while for extensive bone defects following ablative surgery, microvascular reconstructions with osteomyocutaneous flaps are the most versatile and reliable option [8]. Król et al. [9] developed a fully automatic computer-assisted method to find the best donor site for autogenous bone grafts and for the production of templates for harvesting. Nowadays there are commercial software packages available to plan the reconstruction of bone-deficient areas and to design AM guides, which allow for exact harvesting of autogenous grafts and ensure precise bony repositioning to give the desired replacement of lost tissue in terms of both function and aesthetics [10]. When installing osseointegrated dental implants, the use of AM surgical templates is a way to increase predictability, improve cosmetic results, and protect sensitive anatomical structures, thus minimising morbidity. For dental implantology, there are a number of commercially available software packages for virtual planning and AM that can guide the transfer of the plan to real-time surgery [11].

The use of patient-specific guides is partly restricted due to costs and the time required for outsourced manufacturing. Msallem et al. [12] presented an alternative rapid and cost-efficient in-house workflow for craniofacial reconstruction and cranioplasty. A guide is designed using a software package and then manufactured by 3D printing and then a silicone template is moulded manually. The shaped template is then used during surgery to produce a polymethylmethacrylate (PMMA) implant. The complete process takes approximately 2 h. It is concluded that this workflow can be adopted at all hospital centres and can serve underprivileged communities by producing individualised replacements. Performing microvascular-free fibula reconstruction of maxillo-mandibular defects entails mirroring the native jaw in advance of ablative surgery or mirroring the intact contralateral side. The fibula flap is cut in several segments, and plates are used for fixation of the segments to each other and to the native jaw [13]. The graft must be contoured to fit the defect, which is a tedious procedure, and preoperative virtual planning saves time and costs [3]. The earliest systems did not allow for the transfer of the surgical plan to the operating room, but Leiggener et al. [14] developed a method to bring the virtual plan to real-time surgery using an AM cutting guide. The osteotomies were translated into the AM guide, sterilised, and applied during surgery on the fibula allowing for the osteotomies and osteosynthesis to be performed with intact circulation. Planning was conducted using software that simulated the surgery on a workstation. Manufacturing a cutting guide from the computer-based plan speeds up the procedure by several hours [3], thus minimising the ischemic time and increasing precision [14].

Reconstruction plates are usually manually bent by the surgeon perioperatively, which is quite laborious and time-consuming, and the fit is not exact. Dérand et al. [15] developed an algorithm for virtual planning of cutting guides and reconstruction plates that could be transferred for AM in titanium. The workflow has been applied, and the plates have been used in several real-time surgeries and shown to have excellent fit and healing. The virtually planned and EBM-constructed plates also function as guides to guarantee the exact transfer of the plan during surgery. Plate and bone specimens retrieved from a patient nearly 3 years following a mandibular reconstruction were examined morphologically and at the molecular level and showed new bone regeneration and osseointegration except in a minor part where soft tissue ingrowth was present. It was concluded that patient-specific EBM-manufactured plates are well suited for use in microvascular bone reconstructions [16].

It is imperative to analyse the biomechanical requirements of a specific situation to ensure that the produced plate has adequate load-bearing capacity. Huo et al. [17] established a finite-element model from CT data of a mandible reconstructed with autogenous bone and an EBM-produced plate and studied the stresses that developed during mastication. The stress distribution in the load-bearing plate was computed and the location of the main stress concentration in the plate was determined, and it was concluded that finite-element analysis could serve as a tool for optimising the design of mandible implants. The development of the AM technology for the production of patient-specific devices has opened an enormous new field for reconstructive surgery. In oral and craniomaxillofacial surgery, individualised devices needed for all indications can today be manufactured with AM, and new candidate biomaterials have been developed both for hardware and for bone substitutes. Polyetheretherketone (PEEK) is frequently used as an alternative to titanium implants for reconstruction of the cranial vault and for augmentation of facial defects and maxillary or mandibular hypoplasia. The results have been excellent and equivalent to what is achieved with metallic implants. There are now ample opportunities to elaborate and investigate many variables, different materials, systems for production, plate and scaffold designs, surface characteristics, load-bearing capacities, and combinations of bone-replacement therapies. Engstrand et al. [18] developed a bioactive calcium phosphate-based ceramic material that is cast in a mosaic AM titanium scaffold for reconstruction, and this material has been shown to stimulate bone healing in large therapy-resistant defects. An additional attractive alternative to bone grafts and microvascular-free flaps in the future is combining scaffolds and cell therapy, specifically stem cells derived from adipose tissue, or a combination with osteoconductive biomaterials [19]. Martelli et al. [20] reviewed articles on 3D printing and applications published between 2005 and 2015 and concluded that the main advantages were the possibilities for preoperative planning and the accuracy of the planning and manufacturing of devices needed in advance of surgery and the time saved during the reconstructive procedure.

To reduce the time for fabrication of devices and to widen the indications and increase the overall use of AM for patient-specific designs for reconstructive surgery and trauma repair, it is a must that regional centres serve several local hospitals and can design and produce devices quickly. Today there are excellent systems for the virtual planning of reconstructive surgery that in addition to increased precision and reduced morbidity can reduce the time spent in the operating room performing complex procedures by approximately 25% by identifying problems in advance and producing the devices that will be needed prior to the surgery [3, 21]. Nysjö et al. [22] developed a modelling tool that has the potential to be used by surgeons in-house as an alternative to time-consuming outsourcing. It is possible to quickly design models with the help of stereographics, six-degrees-of-freedom input, and haptic feedback using a software package developed at Uppsala University [23] for virtual craniomaxillofacial surgery planning. Surgical guides and plate models can be generated within minutes, with only a few steps, and then can be manufactured using AM [22].

17.5 Biological Response

In order to develop long-lasting AM-based clinical treatment modalities either as customised implants [16, 24, 25] or as mass-produced off-the-shelf implants [26], proper preclinical data are needed. The biological response to AM materials, especially titanium alloy-based powder bed fused material, has been extensively evaluated in a variety of animal models with a variety of implant designs, manufacturing techniques, and surface treatments intended for different clinical applications. This section focuses on the bone formation potential of AM implants with a main focus on preclinical experimental animal studies.

The term "osseointegration"—with reference to the direct bone anchorage of a titanium implant in bone tissue—was coined already in 1977 by P.I. Brånemark [27] long before the introduction of AM. Extensive research in subsequent years led to the global introduction of dental implants in the early 1980s, which is today considered a routine treatment in dentistry. From the research that was conducted, several important material-associated aspects have been pointed out as important for bone healing around implants, with the main aspects being related to the surface structure but also to surface energy, stiffness, and the addition of bioactive coatings. From a bone-regeneration perspective, several hierarchical levels of organisation exist for this nanocomposite material. It is first built up by nanoscale collagen-forming mineralised fibrils (50–100 nm in diameter) together with apatite (plate-shaped, 50 × 20 × 4 nm) as the reinforcement phase, and these fibrils make up fibre bundles (1–2 μm in diameter). In higher organisation of bone, these bundles are laid down in sheets with all of the bundles facing the same direction to form the lamellas. The bundle direction shifts between adjacent lamellas in order to increase the mechanical properties of bone. In cortical bone, the remodelling phase with the coupled action of osteoclasts and osteoblasts creates osteons, which are circular patterns with lamellar bone surrounding a central blood vessel (the typical diameter is about 100 μm). For a bone-anchored implant, these hierarchical levels have been evaluated for improved bone anchorage. With the introduction of AM, the higher degree of design freedom has meant that higher levels of the hierarchy can be accommodated.

Solid EBM material was compared to wrought material to verify the biocompatibility of the materials. No histological differences were seen, but the native roughened surface of the EBM-built cylinder as compared to the machined EBM cylinder and machined wrought material cylinder had a larger surface area allowing for greater contact between the bone and the implant and increased mechanical interlocking [28]. Machined solid EBM material was compared to a macro-porous EBM scaffold, and significantly greater bone ingrowth into the porous region was observed, where more bone was formed in the periphery as compared to the central regions of the scaffold [29]. This was further confirmed in a different animal model with a pore size of approximately 700 μm [30] showing extensive direct bone-implant contact throughout the scaffold, while smaller amounts of bone were found in the centre, indicating bone conduction along the metal struts toward the centre of the implant. The porous region further promoted tissue maturation as evaluated by Raman spectroscopy, and osteocytes made direct contact with the implant [31, 32]. A difference in the ingrowth pattern was observed between trabecular and cortical bone models, where the restitution of the cortical bone and typical endosteal downgrowth was observed in the cortical model, while less total bone area was found in the trabecular model [33]. By changing the design of the porous network, including both the total porosity and the pore size, the stiffness of the constructs could be modified, and more bone ingrowth was observed for the higher porosities [34]. The size of the pores was systematically evaluated using a wire fusion fabrication technique that resulted in well-defined constructs of different pore sizes (approximately 200, 300, and 400 μm), where the largest pore size showed the best bone ingrowth and less bone was formed in the central region as compared to the periphery [35]. Another study evaluated larger pores of 300, 600, and 900 μm in a rabbit model, and the highest biomechanical fixation was seen for the 600 μm sample indicating an upper limit in pore size for effective bone ingrowth [36]. The introduction of porosity will in turn change the global stiffness of the material, where a linear relationship between the relative density to the relative stiffness have been described [37], allowing for mechanical tuning of an implant. It has been shown that a lower stiffness, more similar to the stiffness of natural bone, promotes tissue formation more than an implant with high stiffness [38].

Most of the studies have evaluated the as-produced surface without additional surface treatment, while further improvements in bone growth could be obtained with further surface treatments. The use of anodisation has been evaluated on porous implants, showing an increase in early bone formation and an increase in the biomechanical properties of the implant [39]. The addition of bioactive coatings such as hydroxyapatite [40] or BMP-2-releasing fibrin gels (van der Stok [41]) has been shown to further stimulate healing, and more studies using further refined surface technologies adapted for complexly shaped implants will most likely come in the future.

17.5.1 Other Alloys

Cobalt chromium-based alloys have been evaluated for orthopaedic applications, and these have improved tribological properties compared to titanium-based alloys [42]. EBM has been shown to be a good manufacturing technique allowing complex geometries to be produced, and experiments in rabbits have shown high degrees of osseointegration of EBM-manufactured solid implants with improved biomechanical anchorage when micro-alloyed with 0.04% zirconium [43]. Macro-porous cobalt chromium implants showed similar bone ingrowth compared to titanium alloy implants having similar design, while there was significantly lower bone-implant contact in the porous network [31, 32]. Improved osseointegration of AM cobalt chromium implants could be obtained by the addition of bioactive coatings such as calcium aluminate [44] or hydroxyapatite [45], and the coating procedure is important for porous implants where wet chemistry and the formation of biomimetic coatings allow a uniform coating to be applied throughout the porous network [46].

17.6 Concluding Remarks

Additive manufacturing shows large potential for clinical application, where the modern diagnostic imaging gives patient-specific input, thus enabling preoperative planning, design, and manufacturing of surgical guides as well as implants. The manufacturing technology is in one way still in its infancy, and already there are many promising attempts to use AM to achieve more functional implants, reducing OR time, etc. As the technology evolves, even more application areas will be explored and the technology will certainly be easier and cheaper to use which is a prerequisite before it will be widely used in the area of craniomaxillofacial surgery and planning.

References

1. Hull CW. Apparatus for production of three-dimensional objects by stereolithography. US Patent 4,575,330A, 11 March 1986.
2. Ciraud P. Verfahren und Vorrichtung zur Herstellung beliebiger Gegenstände aus beliebigem schmelzbaren Material. German Patent 2263777, 5 July 1973.
3. Zweifel DF, Simon C, Hoarau R, Pascher P, Broome M. Are virtual planning and guided surgery for head and neck reconstruction economically viable? J Oral Maxillofac Surg. 2015;73(1):170–5.
4. Petzold R, Zeilhofer H-F, Kalender WA. Rapid prototyping technology in medicine—basics and applications. Comput Med Imag Graph. 1999;23(5):277–84.
5. Thieringer FM, Sharma N, Mootien A, Schumacher R, Honigmann P. Patient specific implants from a 3D printer—an innovative manufacturing process for custom PEEK implants in cranio-maxillofacial surgery. In: Meboldt M, Klahn C, editors. Industrializing additive manufacturing—proceedings of additive manufacturing in products and applications—AMPA2017. AMPA 2017. Cham: Springer; 2018. p. 308–15.
6. Sander G, Kärcher H, Gaggl A, Kern R. Stereolithography versus milled three-dimensional models: comparison of production method, indication, and accuracy. Comput Aided Surg. 1998;3(5):248–56.
7. Sykes LM, Parrott AM, Owen CP, Snaddon DR. Applications of rapid prototyping technology in maxillofacial prosthetics. Int J Prosthodont. 2004;17(4):456–9.
8. López-Arcas JM, Arias J, Del Castillo JL, Burgueño M, Navarro I, Morán MJ, Chamorro M, Martorell V. The fibula osteomyocutaneous flap for mandible reconstruction: a 15-year experience. J Oral Maxillofac Surg. 2010;68(10):2377–84.
9. Król Z, Chlebiej M, Zerfass P, Sader R, Zeilhofer HF, Mikołajczak P, Keeve E. Surgery planning tools for the osseous grafting treatment. Biomed Tech (Berl). 2002;47(Suppl 1 Pt 1):97–100.
10. Levine JP, Patel A, Saadeh PB, Hirsch DL. Computer-aided design and manufacturing in craniomaxillofacial surgery: the new state of the art. J Craniofac Surg. 2012;23(1):288–93.
11. Herklotz I, Beuer F, Kunz A, Hildebrand D, Happe A. Navigation in implantology. Int J Comput Dent. 2017;20(1):9–19.
12. Msallem B, Beiglboeck F, Honigmann P, Jaquiéry C, Thieringer F. Craniofacial reconstruction by a cost-efficient template-based process using 3D printing. Plast Reconstr Surg Glob Open. 2017;5(11):e1582.
13. Tarsitano A, Ciocca L, Cipriani R, Scotti R, Marchetti C. Mandibular reconstruction using fibula free flap harvested using a customised cutting guide: how we do it. Acta Otorhinolaryngol Ital. 2015;35(3):198–201.

14. Leiggener C, Messo E, Thor A, Zeilhofer HF, Hirsch JM. A selective laser sintering guide for transferring a virtual plan to real time surgery in composite mandibular reconstruction with free fibula osseous flaps. Int J Oral Maxillofac Surg. 2009;38(2):187–92.
15. Dérand P, Rännar LE, Hirsch JM. Imaging, virtual planning, design, and production of patient-specific implants and clinical validation in craniomaxillofacial surgery. Craniomaxillofac Trauma Reconstr. 2012;5(3):137–44.
16. Thor A, Palmquist A, Hirsch JM, Rännar LE, Dérand P, Omar O. Clinical, morphological, and molecular evaluations of bone regeneration with an additive manufactured osteosynthesis plate. J Craniofac Surg. 2016;27(7):1899–904.
17. Huo J, Dérand P, Rännar LE, Hirsch JM, Gamstedt EK. Failure location prediction by finite element analysis for an additive manufactured mandible implant. Med Eng Phys. 2015;37(9):862–9.
18. Engstrand T, Kihlström L, Neovius E, Skogh AC, Lundgren TK, Jacobsson H, Bohlin J, Åberg J, Engqvist H. Development of a bioactive implant for repair and potential healing of cranial defects. J Neurosurg. 2014;120(1):273–7.
19. Farré-Guasch E, Wolff J, Helder MN, Schulten AJM, Forouzanfar T, Klein-Nulend J. Application of additive manufacturing in oral and maxillofacial surgery. J Oral Maxillofac Surg. 2015;73(12):2408–18.
20. Martelli N, Serrano C, van den Brink H, Pineau J, Prognon P, Borget I, El Batti S. Advantages and disadvantages of 3-dimensional printing in surgery: a systematic review. Surgery. 2016;159(6):1485–500.
21. Nyström I, Olsson P, Nysjö J, Nysjö F, Malmberg F, Seipel S, Hirsch JM, Carlbom IB. Virtual craniomaxillofacial surgery planning with stereo graphics and haptics. In: Ritacco LE, Milano EF, Chao E, editors. Computer-assisted musculoskeletal surgery. Thinking and executing in 3D. AG Switzerland: Springer International Publishing; 2016. p. 29–42.
22. Nysjö F, Olsson P, Filip Malmberg F, Ingrid B, Carlbom IB. Nyström I. Using anti-aliased signed distance fields for generating surgical guides and plates from CT images. J WSCG. 2017;25(1):11–20.
23. Olsson P, Nysjö F, Rodríguez-Lorenzo A, Thor A, Hirsch JM, Carlbom IB. Novel virtual planning of bone, soft-tissue, and vessels in fibula osteocutaneous free flaps with the haptics-assisted surgery planning (HASP) system. Plast Reconstruct Surg Global Open. 2015;3:e479.
24. Jardini AL, Larosa MA, Macedo MF, Bernardes LF, Lambert CS, Zavaglia CAC, Filho RM, Calderoni DR, Ghizoni E, Kharmandayan P. Improvement in cranioplasty: advanced prosthesis biomanufacturing. Procedia CIRP. 2016;49(Supplement C):203–8.
25. Suska F, Kjeller G, Tarnow P, Hryha E, Nyborg L, Snis A, Palmquist A. Electron beam melting manufacturing technology for individually manufactured jaw prosthesis: a case report. J Oral Maxillofac Surg. 2016;74(8):1706 e1701–1706 e1715.
26. Regis M, Marin E, Fedrizzi L, Pressacco M. Additive manufacturing of trabecular titanium orthopedic implants. MRS Bull. 2015;40(2):137–44.
27. Brånemark PI, Hansson BO, Adell R, Breine U, Lindström J, Hallen O, Ohman A. Osseointegrated implants in the treatment of the edentulous jaw. Experience from a 10-year period. Scand J Plast Reconstr Surg Suppl. 1977;16:1–132.
28. Thomsen P, Malmstrom J, Emanuelsson L, Rene M, Snis A. Electron beam-melted, free-form-fabricated titanium alloy implants: material surface characterization and early bone response in rabbits. J Biomed Mater Res B Appl Biomater. 2009;90(1):35–44.
29. Ponader S, von Wilmowsky C, Widenmayer M, Lutz R, Heinl P, Korner C, Singer RF, Nkenke E, Neukam FW, Schlegel KA. In vivo performance of selective electron beam-melted Ti-6Al-4V structures. J Biomed Mater Res A. 2010;92(1):56–62.
30. Palmquist A, Snis A, Emanuelsson L, Browne M, Thomsen P. Long-term biocompatibility and osseointegration of electron beam melted, free-form-fabricated solid and porous titanium alloy: experimental studies in sheep. J Biomater Appl. 2013;27(8):1003–16.
31. Shah FA, Omar O, Suska F, Snis A, Matic A, Emanuelsson L, Norlindh B, Lausmaa J, Thomsen P, Palmquist A. Long-term osseointegration of 3D printed CoCr constructs with an interconnected open-pore architecture prepared by electron beam melting. Acta Biomater. 2016a;36:296–309.
32. Shah FA, Snis A, Matic A, Thomsen P, Palmquist A. 3D printed Ti6Al4V implant surface promotes bone maturation and retains a higher density of less aged osteocytes at the bone-implant interface. Acta Biomater. 2016b;30:357–67.
33. Palmquist A, Shah FA, Emanuelsson L, Omar O, Suska F. A technique for evaluating bone ingrowth into 3D printed, porous Ti6Al4V implants accurately using X-ray micro-computed tomography and histomorphometry. Micron. 2017;94:1–8.
34. Arabnejad S, Burnett JR, Pura JA, Singh B, Tanzer M, Pasini D. High-strength porous biomaterials for bone replacement: a strategy to assess the interplay between cell morphology, mechanical properties, bone ingrowth and manufacturing constraints. Acta Biomater. 2016;30:345–56.
35. Chang B, Song W, Han T, Yan J, Li F, Zhao L, Kou H, Zhang Y. Influence of pore size of porous titanium fabricated by vacuum diffusion bonding of titanium meshes on cell penetration and bone ingrowth. Acta Biomater. 2016;33:311–21.
36. Taniguchi N, Fujibayashi S, Takemoto M, Sasaki K, Otsuki B, Nakamura T, Matsushita T, Kokubo T, Matsuda S. Effect of pore size on bone ingrowth into porous titanium implants fabricated by additive manufacturing: an in vivo experiment. Mater Sci Eng C Mater Biol Appl. 2016;59:690–701.
37. Murr LE, Amato KN, Li SJ, Tian YX, Cheng XY, Gaytan SM, Martinez E, Shindo PW, Medina F,

Wicker RB. Microstructure and mechanical properties of open-cellular biomaterials prototypes for total knee replacement implants fabricated by electron beam melting. J Mech Behav Biomed Mater. 2011;4(7):1396–411.

38. Schouman T, Schmitt M, Adam C, Dubois G, Rouch P. Influence of the overall stiffness of a load-bearing porous titanium implant on bone ingrowth in critical-size mandibular bone defects in sheep. J Mech Behav Biomed Mater. 2016;59:484–96.
39. Xiu P, Jia Z, Lv J, Yin C, Cheng Y, Zhang K, Song C, Leng H, Zheng Y, Cai H, Liu Z. Tailored surface treatment of 3D printed porous Ti6Al4V by micro-arc oxidation for enhanced osseointegration via optimized bone in-growth patterns and interlocked bone/implant interface. ACS Appl Mater Interfaces. 2016;8(28):17964–75.
40. Li X, Feng YF, Wang CT, Li GC, Lei W, Zhang ZY, Wang L. Evaluation of biological properties of electron beam melted Ti6Al4V implant with biomimetic coating in vitro and in vivo. PLoS One. 2012;7(12):e52049.
41. van der Stok J, Koolen MK, de Maat MP, Yavari SA, Alblas J, Patka P, Verhaar JA, van Lieshout EM, Zadpoor AA, Weinans H, Jahr H. Full regeneration of segmental bone defects using porous titanium implants loaded with BMP-2 containing fibrin gels. Eur Cell Mater. 2015;29:141–53.
42. Tkachenko S, Datskevich O, Kulak L, Jacobson S, Engqvist H, Persson C. Wear and friction properties of experimental Ti-Si-Zr alloys for biomedical applications. J Mech Behav Biomed Mater. 2014;39:61–72.
43. Stenlund P, Kurosu S, Koizumi Y, Suska F, Matsumoto H, Chiba A, Palmquist A. Osseointegration enhancement by Zr doping of Co-Cr-Mo implants fabricated by electron beam melting. Addit Manufact. 2015;6:6–15.
44. Palmquist A, Jarmar T, Hermansson L, Emanuelsson L, Taylor A, Taylor M, Engqvist H, Thomsen P. Calcium aluminate coated and uncoated free form fabricated CoCr implants: a comparative study in rabbit. J Biomed Mater Res B Appl Biomater. 2009;91B(1):122–7.
45. Grandfield K, Palmquist A, Goncalves S, Taylor A, Taylor M, Emanuelsson L, Thomsen P, Engqvist E. Free form fabricated features on CoCr implants with and without hydroxyapatite coating in vivo: a comparative study of bone contact and bone growth induction. J Mater Sci Mater Med. 2011;22(4):899–906.
46. Lindahl C, Xia W, Engqvist H, Snis A, Lausmaa J, Palmquist A. Biomimetic calcium phosphate coating of additively manufactured porous CoCr implants. Appl Surf Sci. 2015;353(Supplement C):40–7.

Lasers in the Dental Laboratory

18

Markus Link

Contents

Abstract

For about 30 years, laser technology in all its different forms has been indispensable in the daily laboratory routine of dental technology. In the digital workflow, however, lasers are increasing rapidly. 3D printers are becoming increasingly important just like laser technology too. Resins can be processed easily and inexpensively with simple printers. Metals can already be laser-sintered in acceptable quality. The latest innovations even make it possible to print final sintered ZrO_2 crowns.

Keywords

Laser welding · CAD/CAM · Scanner · ZrO_2 Stereolithography · SLA · Selective laser melting · SLM

M. Link (✉)
Laborlink AG, Basel, Switzerland

18.1 Laser for Joining Metals

The laser first became popular in dental laboratories in the early 1990s. With the broad introduction of titanium as a framework material, a suitable joining option had to be found. Laser welding was the easiest method.

The alternatives at that time were mainly bonding. The typical adhesive materials were plastics and therefore usually not heat-resistant. The temperature-resistant variants made of glass or ceramics were cumbersome and time-consuming to process. In addition, adhesives require a relatively large amount of space to guarantee a high mechanical load-bearing capacity. However, the "passive fit" is better than with all other alternatives.

Some laboratories tried to solder titanium (Fig. 18.1). For this purpose the workpiece was placed under a glass dome, which was first sucked out by a vacuum pump and then flooded

S. Stübinger et al. (eds.), *Lasers in Oral and Maxillofacial Surgery*,
https://doi.org/10.1007/978-3-030-29604-9_18

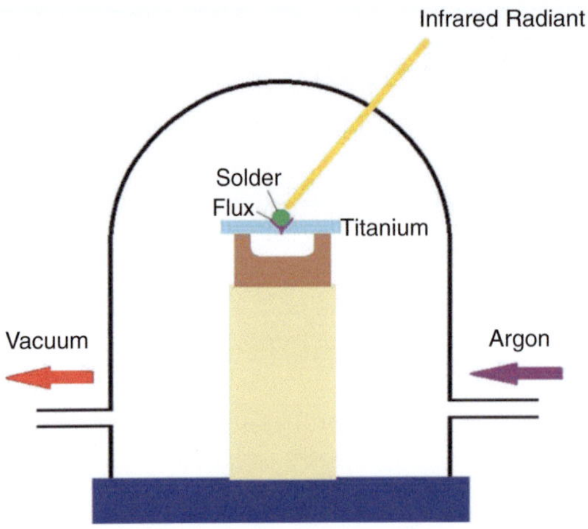

Fig. 18.1 Laborlink AG

with argon. This prevented the embrittlement and formation of the alpha-case layer that occurs when heating titanium in a normal atmosphere. A highly focused infrared beam was now directed through the glass onto the workpiece prepared with solder and flux and heated until the solder began to melt. It was an incredibly complex process, and if the preparations were not perfect, the procedure had to be repeated.

Both joining options, bonding and soldering, were more than questionable, however, as far as the biocompatibility question, which really made titanium "in", was concerned. Laser welding enabled us to join parts together with one and the same material.

Laser welding has remained an indispensable joining method for metal to this day. The laser can be used for almost all metals used in dental technology. Porous surfaces can be sealed with the laser or missing contact points can be created without great effort. Countless ready-made anchors and attachments are lasered onto all possible bases. With extensions, the laser makes it possible to attach retentions to model casted frameworks without destroying the surrounding plastic.

The main risks of laser welding are severe distortion and embrittlement of the material or its destruction (e.g. in titanium, if argon is not flooded enough). The different melting temperatures, thermal conductivity and surface reflection must also be taken into account.

18.2 CAD/CAM Laser as Scanner

At the turn of the millennium, lasers were used in large numbers as scanners, for example, in the Sirona Cerec system. At Sirona, in the early days, a small plaster model was attached to the workpiece holder and optically scanned with a small laser, mounted on one of the grinding motors (Fig. 18.2). Thus, smaller impressions could be digitized and further processed accordingly.

Scanning technologies such as the structured light scan (Fig. 18.3), however, relatively quickly replaced these laser scanners, and they atrophied into barcode readers that determined the shrinkage factor of the ZrO_2 blanks.

Today a lot of modern milling systems use lasers as measuring instruments, for example, to detect the occupancy of tool ports.

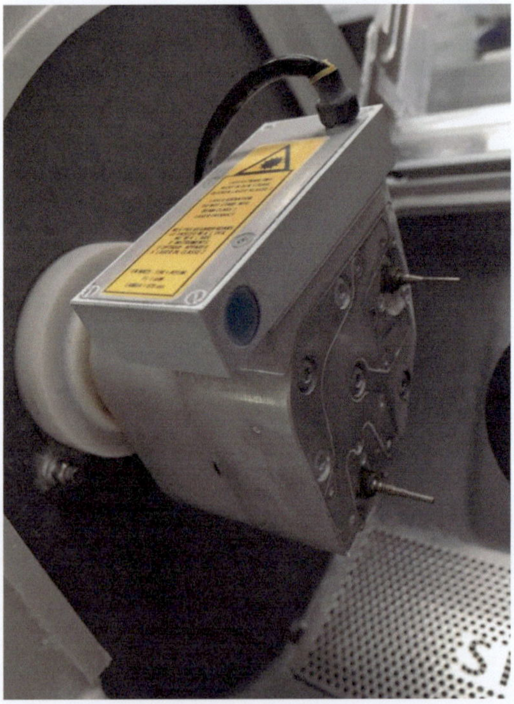

Fig. 18.2 Laborlink AG

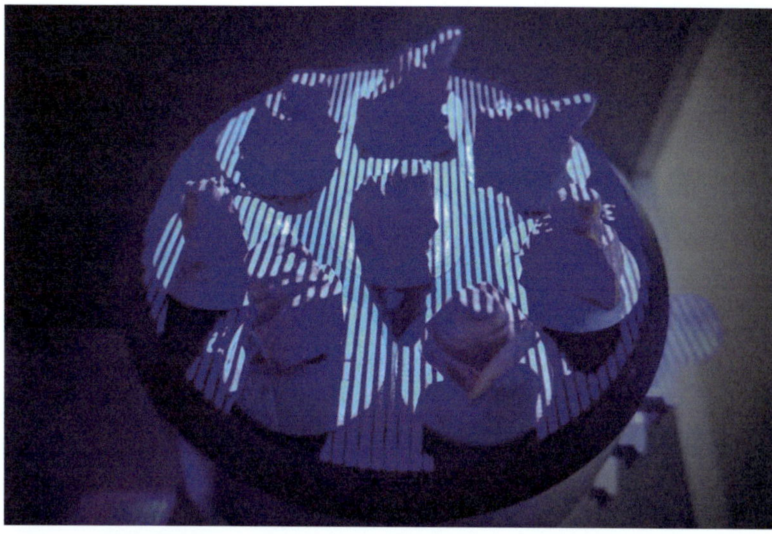

Fig. 18.3 TGF-3D Ltd., Medit/Identica Blue

18.3 CAD/CAM Stereolithography (SLA)

Since some years, the use of 3D printers in dental technology has opened up seemingly endless application possibilities for lasers. Stereolithography printers use laser beams to build the desired shapes layer by layer from a photopolymer resin (Fig. 18.4a, b).

The chemical, biological and physical properties of these light-curing resins currently limit their possible applications. However, research is in progress on materials that can be used specifically for medical applications.

At present, existing materials are used for individual trays or castings. There are already quite good resins that are suitable for model production. Crystal clear splint materials are also available, but unfortunately these are not as colour-fast and also not as stable as the milling blanks made of PMMA or carbides, from which many splints are milled today.

It will also take a while before there are functioning alternatives to the creation of flexible, crystal-clear splints or aligners.

Even if, e.g. for the aligner technology no really usable materials exist yet, in order to print them directly, starting from the digitally generated files, the SLA printers are however an enormous relief.

With 3D programs such as OnyxCeph or Meastro 3D, the corresponding adjustments are planned and then all intermediate steps are printed as a model. Only the corresponding splints have to be deep-drawn.

18.4 Laser Melting of Metals (DMLS) Direct Metal Laser Sintering

The most common method of manufacturing metal CAD/CAM dental frameworks is currently milling from prefabricated blanks. The nature of this subtractive technology means that an enormous number of cutters and metal blanks are worn out. From an economic point of view, doubts about the profitability of components manufactured accordingly are justified.

Additive processes, such as laser melting, seem to be the solution to this problem. Using a focused laser beam, the frameworks are fabricated layer by layer from a bed of metal dust

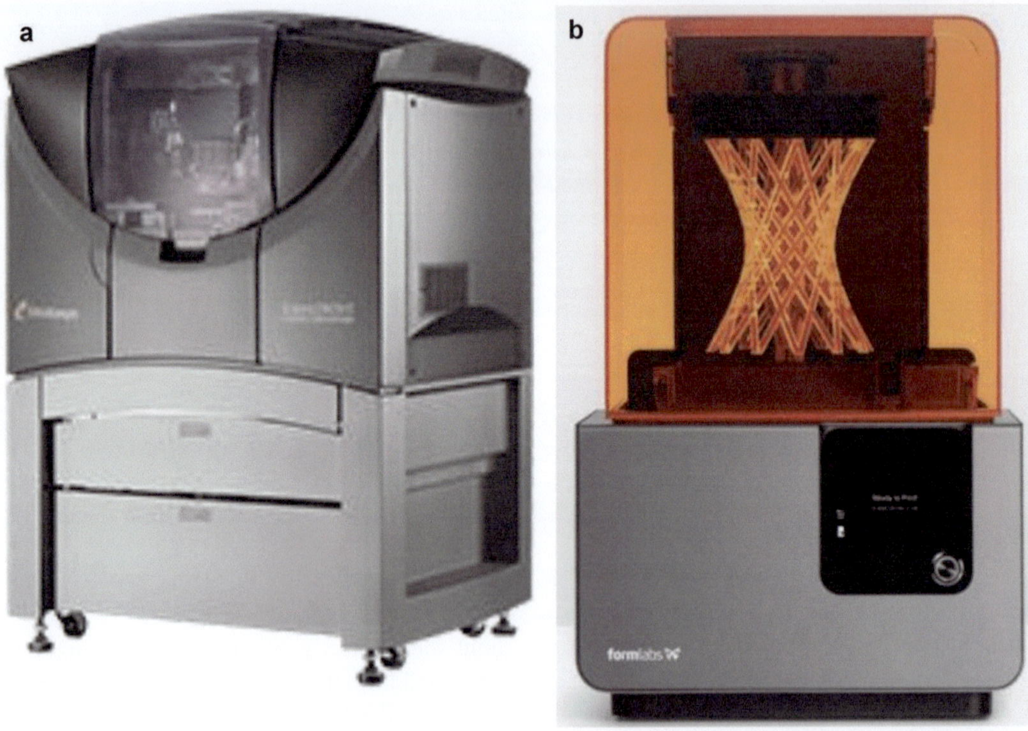

Fig. 18.4 Statasys/Formlabs (Stratasys Ltd. © 2018)

of a specific CoCr alloy or titanium powder (Fig. 18.5). In which individual particles are melted together, almost all shapes can be produced with relative precision (Fig. 18.6).

Cautious it is estimated to be assumed that more than six million units are produced in this way worldwide each year.

Due to the system, however, the same accuracy cannot be achieved with the laser melting process as with milling systems that may even be equipped with linear measuring systems. The melting always causes a distortion in the direction of the beam. An attempt is made to neutralize this effect by subsequent relaxation tempering.

According to some manufacturers, the accuracy of individual caps lies in the range of ±20 μm, but as a bridge becomes bigger, the more the inaccuracies become difficult to control.

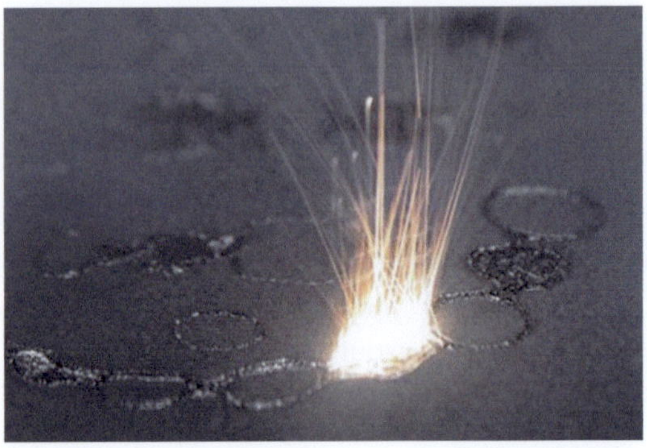

Fig. 18.5 EOS

18.5 Hybrid

For this reason, leading manufacturers of laser melting systems together with their milling machine manufacturers are trying to offer a

Fig. 18.6 EOS

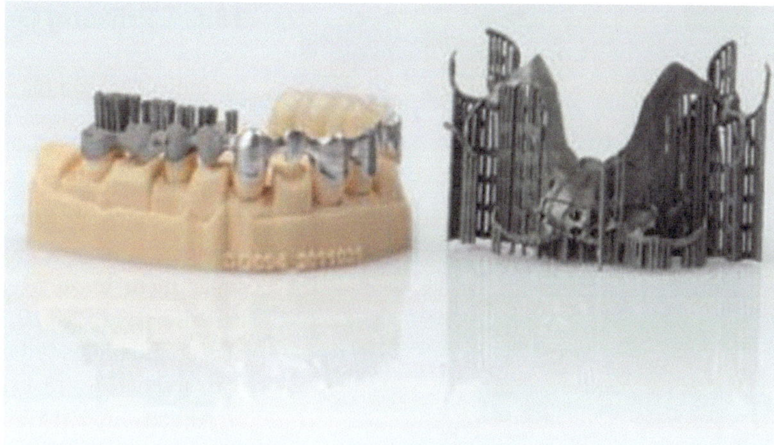

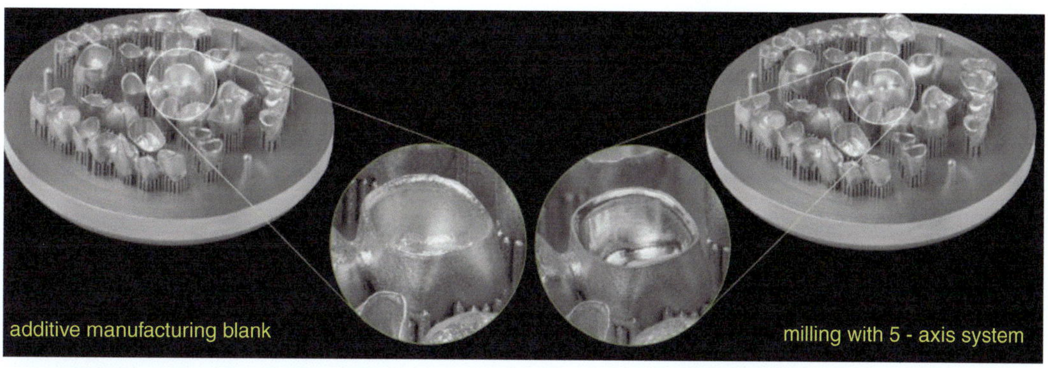

Fig. 18.7 Datron

combination of both technologies. First, the frameworks including a blank, which can then be clamped in a milling system, are generated in the laser melting process using the additive process. However, the size of the offset required for this technology also makes it clear that it will be years before pure laser melting systems will achieve really high precision (Fig. 18.7).

The circular blanks (thermal) passivated according to the manufacturer's specifications are now clamped in a high-precision milling system and milled to a repeat accuracy (over an entire dental arch) of less than 7 μm!

Theoretically, this method makes the most sense. In practice, however, it is still very complex and time-consuming. Only when the combined devices, which are still in the development phase, reach market maturity, an economically and qualitatively optimal production will be possible.

In the extended field of dental technology, bone prostheses are occasionally requested. Holes are also inserted into such parts to make them lighter (Fig. 18.8). The laser melting process makes it possible to produce a hollow form for more complex shapes such as a part of the sphenoid bone (Fig. 18.9). This is impossible with a milling system. Since it is possible to laser melt not only metals but also thermoplastics such as PEEK, these processes will have an important future.

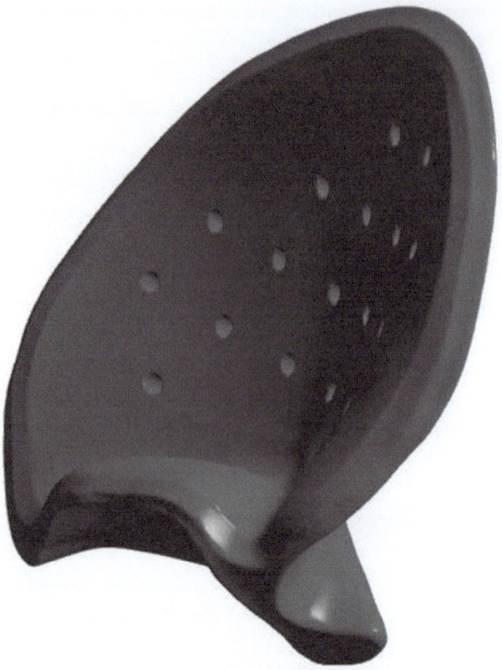

Fig. 18.8 Ad Mirabiles AG

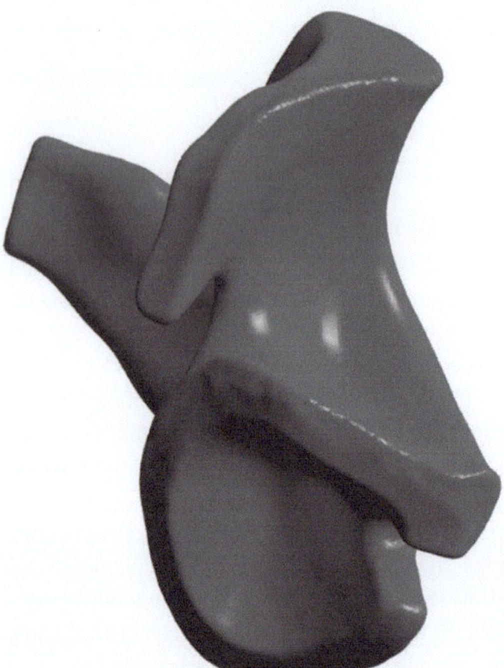

Fig. 18.9 Ad Mirabiles AG

18.6 Printing Ceramics/ZrO_2

In industry, ceramic parts are already being printed in many areas today. Often they are simpler components, crockery or promotional items. Some manufacturers such as Formlabs already offer a material with which anyone can print ceramic parts in a green state and then finally sinter them in an oven without great financial expense (Fig. 18.10). The French company 3DCeram is already busy printing ceramic skull parts today (Fig. 18.11).

Already in 2015 a very interesting study of the University of Wuhan, Hubei, China, was presented, which dealt with the printing of ZrO_2. The

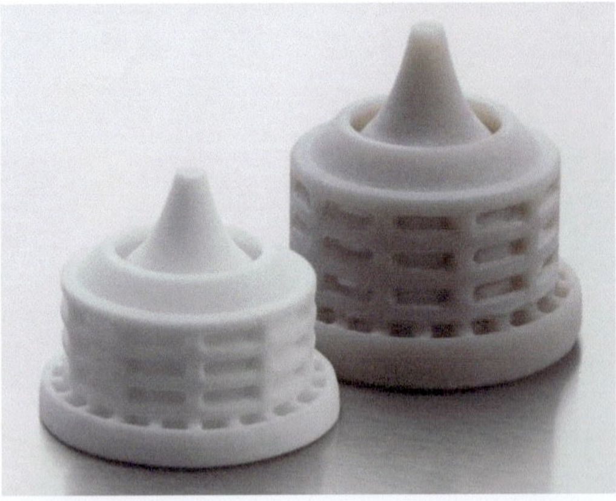

Fig. 18.10 Formlabs

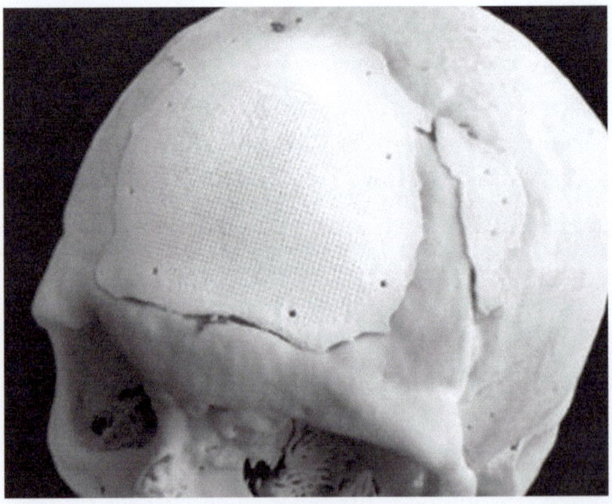

Fig. 18.11 3DCeram

dental market could therefore also be targeted. This study dealt with zircon printing in the green state.

In 2017, the South Korean government invested approx. 37 million dollars in 3D print research, so it is hardly surprising that enormous innovations in this field are currently coming from there. For example, there is a prototype that can already produce the end sintered ZrO_2 product. We will see whether the cosmetics and the fit will be convincing—but we are only just getting started.

The MIRACLE

19

Georg Rauter

Contents

Abstract

Bones in general and human bones in particular are being cut with mechanical tools since thousands of years. Only in the last decades, another technology has evolved that starts challenging the way bone is being cut: lasers. Despite the huge technological effort that is required to guide lasers and make them cut bone without leading to carbonization, laserosteotomes feature several properties that might become a game changer in the medical field and how bones will be cut in the future.

In Basel, Switzerland, the first robot-assisted laserosteotome has been developed that cuts bone in an open surgical process. Due to the promising results with this first device throughout several studies, the MIRACLE project (short for Minimal-Invasive Robot-Assisted Computer-guided LaserosteotomE) has been initiated. MIRACLE is currently on its way of bringing robot-assisted laserosteotomy to the next level.

Keywords

Future of laser osteotomy · MIRACLE Miniature robot · Smart laser osteotome Parallel robot · CARLO · Optical coherence tomograph · Medical robotics

G. Rauter (✉)
Bio-Inspired RObots for MEDicine-Lab (BIROMED-Lab), Department of Biomedical Engineering, University of Basel, Basel, Switzerland
e-mail: georg.rauter@unibas.ch

19.1 The Pathway from Bone Cutting with Mechanical Tools to Lasers

Archaeological findings from the Stone Age show that humans have always used mechanical tools such as saws, scrapers, knives, and drills to

S. Stübinger et al. (eds.), *Lasers in Oral and Maxillofacial Surgery*,
https://doi.org/10.1007/978-3-030-29604-9_19

perform interventions on the human body [1]. These mechanical principles of cutting and drilling have not changed much since then. The surgical instruments have of course become more precise, more sophisticated, and also sterile, but they all work according to simple mechanical principles. Especially in orthopedic surgery and in all interventions in which bone is removed, relatively large forces and torques occur, which also affect the adjacent tissue. For example, sawing and drilling create movements combined with high friction forces that heat up the surrounding tissue. Also, the surface in the cut interface is affected and the porous bone tissue is mechanically flattened. This seems to impair the blood supply to the cells near the interface. In experiments on minipigs, piezoosteotomes flattened the bone surface in the cut. In comparison, cutting bone with a 2.94 [nm] Er:YAG laser produced an open, porous interface. Subsequently, the researchers observed faster healing of bone cuts in the tissues with laser cuts. This finding led the researchers to the conclusion that the way of cutting bone seems to matter for heading [2]. Other positive aspects of laser osteotomy compared to conventional mechanical osteotomy are reduced vibrations [3], reduced heat influence on adjacent tissues [4], as well as higher precision, narrower cuts, arbitrary cut shapes, and faster bone formation in the healing process [5, 6].

19.2 CARLO®, the First Robot for Bone Cutting with Laser

The combination of the many advantages of laser osteotomy over conventional osteotomy has led to the development of the world's first robot for laser osteotomy: CARLO® (short for "Cold Ablation Robot -guided Laser Osteotome" [7], originally patented as "Computer-Assisted and Robot-guided Laser Osteotome" [8]). CARLO® was invented by the founders of Advanced Osteotomy Tools (AOT AG, Basel, Switzerland), a spin-off from the University of Basel. The laser osteotome CARLO® consists of a serial robot and a laser head. The laser head houses the optical components and the nozzles for the irrigating water spray. The robot is basically used as a tool for guiding the laser precisely along the desired cutting paths. Hereby, the movements of the robot are usually pre-planned based on Computed Tomography (CT) data of the respective patient. Registration of the robot, the patient, and the reference CT data set are accomplished via an optoelectronic tracking system.

First studies with CARLO® in human cadavers have been successfully completed and have confirmed positive results from earlier animal studies. In addition to the high cutting accuracy, robot-assisted laserosteotomes can keep up with conventional surgical methods despite the low cutting speed. While mechanical saws cut fast, reconstruction and osteosynthesis take long due to missing planning, incision inaccuracies, and positioning inaccuracies of the implants. Conversely, robot-assisted laser osteotomy takes longer, but the cut bones can be connected quickly and accurately with their counter parts/implants and reveal little possibilities for relative movement. This is only possible since robot-assisted laserosteotomy enables cut execution exactly as planned due to precise depth control using feedback from an optical coherence tomograph and precise laser guidance by the robot under surveillance of an optoelectronical tracking system. Another important novelty that allows simple and precise assembly of bones/implants and bones after robot-assisted laserosteotomy are free cutting geometries such as sine patterns or dovetail profiles. The cut bone parts and implants fit together like puzzle pieces with their counterparts and have functional stability already during mating [7]. For fixation, if any, only a few additional screws are required. Accordingly, a follow-up operation for removing the screws is shorter or not even required. In 2020, CARLO® was successfully applied in the first human patients for maxillofacial surgery. At present, only the relatively high initial costs of the first laser osteotome and the large space requirement in the operating room seem to be limiting factors for laser osteotomy with robots.

19.3 The Future of Laser Osteotomy: The MIRACLE Project

Even if it seems that the end of the technological flagpole has been reached with the invention of CARLO®, there is still a lot more to come. However, the next step in the development of laser osteotomy systems still requires a few more years of work.

Even if it has not been said explicitly until now, laser osteotomy with CARLO® implies that the surgeon opens up the patient to expose the bone to be cut. To overcome the need of opening up the patient, a new research project at the University of Basel has been initiated in 2015. This project aims at turning laser osteotomy into a minimally-invasive procedure. The surgeon should be able to perform the same surgical procedure as with CARLO®, however through a one centimeter wide incision. To reach this new milestone in laserosteotomy, a small miracle is required from the current point of view. However, this miracle seems to turn into reality in a few years from now. According to the researchers around the "MIRACLE project" (short for "Minimally Invasive Robot-Assisted Computer-guided LaserosteotomE") at the Department of Biomedical Engineering (University of Basel, Switzerland), a first functional prototype will be ready in about 3 years from now. Above all, the big challenge in this project is to reduce the size of all components so that the laser can be housed inside a flexible robotic endoscope. At the same time, there should still be room for the actuation of the flexible robotic endoscope itself as well as a working channel, a camera, spray, a suction channel, an optical coherence tomograph (OCT), and other devices for tissue type classification. At the end of surgical procedures with the MIRACLE osteotome, also implants will be introduced into the body in a minimal invasive way to be assembled and fixed like a 3D puzzle. As unsolvable as the task seems, the MIRACLE project can already present first results. The first implants are already distributed via the two spin-offs of the University of Basel "Di Meliora" and "Ad Mirabiles." Also, the planning software, which is used in the MIRACLE project, is already being used at the University Hospital Basel for diagnosis and patient education in selected departments. The planning software is also being used for training purposes with medical students at the Anatomical Institute of the University of Basel. The intriguing novelty of this planning software is that it can display CT data and Magnetic Resonance Imaging data (MRI data) on virtual reality (VR) glasses in 3D immediately after their acquisition. The virtual patient can then be observed at high resolution and with high repetition rates for both eyes for high immersiveness without cyber-sickness. The user of the VR system can easily interact with the virtual 3D data, can see different tissue types in different colors based on automated segmentation, can scale the 3D model, and inspect it from all sides [9]. Soon, also this planning and medical data visualization software will be available as a commercial product.

In total, four research groups are working on the MIRACLE project. These are the "Bio-Inspired RObots for MEDicine-Lab" (BIROMED-Lab) under the lead of Prof. Dr. Georg Rauter, the "Biomedical Laser and Optics Group" (BLOG) under the lead of Prof. Dr. Azhar Zam, the "Planning and Navigation Group" at the Center for Image Analysis and Navigation (CIAN) under the lead of Prof. Dr. Philippe Cattin, and the "Smart Implants Group" at the "Hightech Forschungszentrum" (HFZ) under the lead of Prof. Dr. med. Dr. med. dent. Dr. hc Hans-Florian Zeilhofer. All four groups are located in one building at the Department of Biomedical Engineering of University of Basel. The close vicinity to each other enables short ways to exchange ideas which is one of the most important factors for successful interdisciplinary research.

19.4 The First Application Areas for the MIRACLE Osteotome

At present, the first clinical application is focused on the half-sided replacement of knee joints (unicondylar knee arthroplasty). This first application

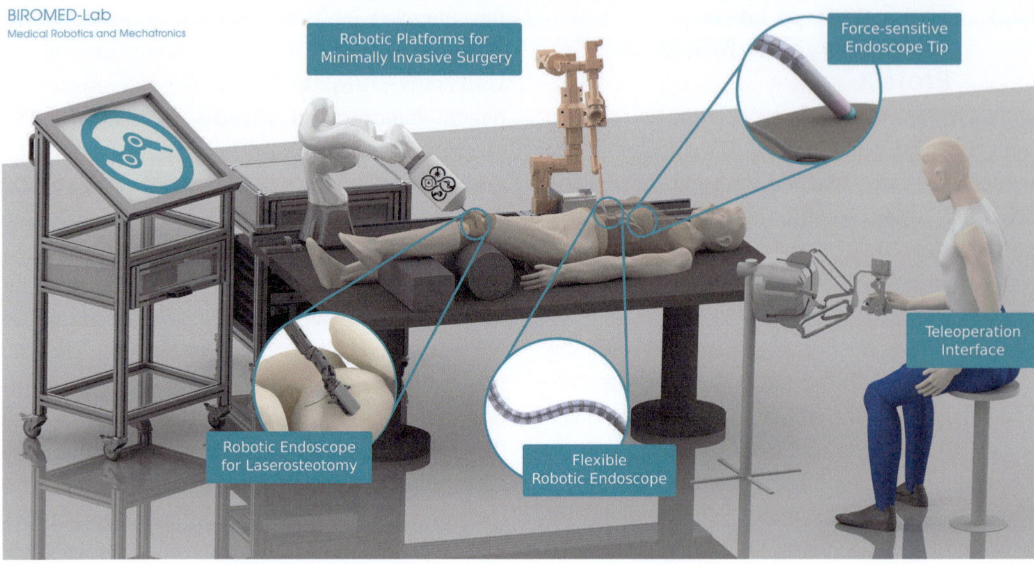

Fig. 19.1 Overview image of various components of the MIRACLE project for unicondylar knee arthroplasty and interventions on the spine with access through the abdomen. The control of the MIRACLE robot is performed by teleoperation on a robotic master device with haptic feedback. (Reproduced with permission from Manuela Eugster, BIROMED-Lab, DBE, University of Basel)

should become a benchmark for the MIRACLE osteotome since the knee joint is one of the bones of largest thickness in the human (about 5 [cm]). The goal is to demonstrate that the MIRACLE osteotome can easily cut the knee joint and thus any other bone in the body. However, there are also other areas of application, such as access to the brain without concussion through mechanical manipulation. Also interventions on the spine that are particularly gentle for the spinal cord and the intervertebral discs are foreseen (see Fig. 19.1). Similar to interventions with the CARLO®, interventions using the MIRACLE osteotome will start with an initial planning phase based on each patient's CT data or MRI data. In the operating room, the surgeon first guides the robotic endoscope manually to the point of entry into the body. The surgeon can then control the robotic MIRACLE osteotome via a robotic master device (a robotic device that allows teleoperation procedures and provides haptic feedback). The movement of the flexible robotic MIRACLE osteotome inside the patient's body will be visualized in real-time by augmented reality glasses since it will be difficult for the surgeon to imagine how the flexible endoscope is shaped inside the patient's body. Once the surgeon has moved the MIRACLE osteotome to the target site, it "attaches" itself to the bone. After successful attachment to the bone, laserosteotomy will be initiated. Since bone tissue retains its shape between the planning and the surgical procedure, the laserosteotomy can be performed autonomously by the robot under supervision of the surgeon.

19.5 The Intelligent Miniature Robot for the MIRACLE Project

A central point for the MIRACLE project is the integration of different technologies in one device, in the MIRACLE osteotome. This integration takes place at the BIROMED Lab, where laser systems from BLOG, own miniature sensors and miniature sensors of the Planning and Navigation Group are combined inside a flexible robotic endoscope. The MIRACLE osteotome needs to be designed so that all components can fit into one robotic endoscope with a diameter of 1 cm. Also the synchronization of the many different components is a major challenge. Standardized interfaces are not necessarily integrated from the beginning in all components. In addition, the components for the laser systems are working at significantly higher sampling rates than robotic hardware, where sampling rates in the kilohertz range are common. Depending on the laser system, sampling rates in the microsecond range and shorter are expected. Another challenge is high data rates. As an example, the OCT system for real-time monitoring of the cut depth can generate gigabytes of data in 1 [s]. This data then has to be processed in real time [10] so that the robotic endoscope can take decisions. For example, the robot has to know whether it is allowed to continue cutting, whether it has already reached the desired depth of the cut, or whether the robot should move the laser to a new location. During laser cutting, also other data can be collected in order to analyze the currently cut tissue type. Tissue differentiation is performed using two different approaches: (1) laser-induced breakdown spectroscopy (LIBS) [11] and (2) acoustic shock wave measurements with Fiber Bragg Gratings (FBG) and miniature microphones [12]. LIBS analyze the reflected light spectrum at the cut; each tissue absorbs a different light spectrum when it is cut by laser light. Accordingly, the reflected light spectrum allows drawing conclusions on the tissue being cut. The same is true for acoustic analysis of the shock waves, which are caused by the short laser pulses during cutting. Depending on the frequency range, the sound waves are either better captured with microphones or FBGs. All analysis methods use methods from the field of machine learning such as neuronal networks, support vector machines, or deep learning to be able to analyze the large amounts of data automatically in the shortest possible time. The results of the data analysis in every time step will be provided to the robot for taking the right decisions and also forward information to the surgeon. The real-time data analysis, classification, and closed-loop real-time control turn the small MIRACLE osteotome into an intelligent miniature robot.

The tip of the robotic endoscope, the so-called end-effector, is a small robot by itself that will incorporate all other technologies accordingly. Once the robotic endoscope has reached the desired position in the body, the end-effector mechanically decouples from the rest of the endoscope and remains connected only via data cables and drive trains (e.g., Bowden cables or flexible shafts). This mechanical decoupling reduces the transmission of mechanical disturbances such as vibrations from the robotic endoscope holder to the robotic endoscope and thus also to the end-effector. It is even expected that the patient can be moved slightly during surgery without affecting the cutting performance since the end-effector is directly attached to the bone and guarantees relative accuracy. The small actuated legs of the end-effector move the housing of the laser together with all other sensing devices along the desired cutting path over the bone (see Fig. 19.2). If the workspace becomes too small, the end-effector can also loosen the legs, fix them in a new position, and drag the end-effector to a new pose. In this way, the endoscope tip can "walk" on the bone. The end-effector of the MIRACLE osteotome is designed as a parallel robot (i.e., a robot, where several actuators connect to one end-effector in parallel). Parallel robots have the advantage over serial robots (i.e., robots where actuated joints are in series one after the other) that they allow high position and orientation accuracy and can realize large forces in comparison to their size. The advantages of parallel robots come with the drawback that they require sophisticated controllers that control the actuators in a synchronized and coordinated way in order to achieve the desired end-effector movement. In case of the MIRACLE osteotome's end-effector, a coordinated movement of four drive trains has to be realized even though the end-effector only moves in 3 degrees of freedom. Since the controller has to actuate more drive trains than degrees of freedom in the robot, a real-time optimization algorithm has to be implemented. This real-time optimization algorithm is able to calculate the commands for the four drive trains based only on a desired 3D end-effector movement. Therefore, not only the real-time data analysis but also the planning and semi-autonomous motion execution of the

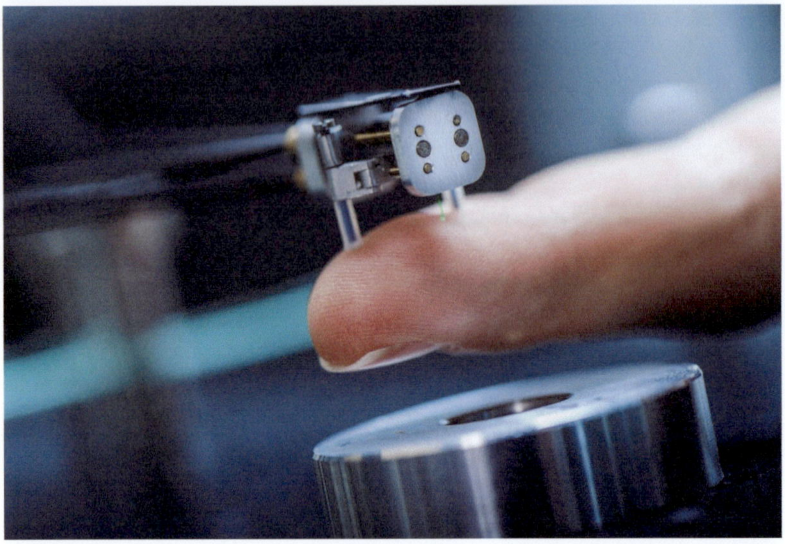

Fig. 19.2 The tip of the MIRACLE osteotome (end-effector) can fix itself on the bone and guide the laser and all sensors over the bone. If the workspace of the end-effector is too small for the planned cuts, the legs can be fixed in a new position and the MIRACLE osteotome can walk on the bone. (Reproduced with permission from Frank Brüderli, Brüderli Longhini AG)

MIRACLE osteotome requires considerable amount of robotic intelligence [13–15].

The individual building blocks for the MIRACLE project are in a promising state. Some individual components are even commercially available. The entire MIRACLE system is expected to be ready for first testing as a medical prototype within 3 years. It is planned to certify the MIRACLE osteotome as a medical device as soon as the desired functionalities are verified.

Acknowledgement The MIRACLE project is financially supported by the Werner Siemens Foundation, Zug, Switzerland.

References

1. Piek J, Lidke G, Terberger T, von Smekal U, Gaab MR. Stone age skull surgery in mecklenburg-vorpommern: a systematic study. Neurosurgery. 1999;45(1):147–51.
2. Baek K-w, Deibel W, Marinov D, Griessen M, Dard M, Bruno A, Zeilhofer H-F, Cattin P, Juergens P. A comparative investigation of bone surface after cutting with mechanical tools and er: Yag laser. Lasers Surg Med. 2015;47(5):426–32.
3. Nguendon Kenhagho HK, Rauter G, Guzman R, Cattin PC, Zam A. Comparison of acoustic shock waves generated by micro and nanosecond lasers for a smart laser surgery system. In: Advanced biomedical and clinical diagnostic and surgical guidance systems XVI, vol. 10484. Bellingham, WA: International Society for Optics and Photonics; 2018. p. 104840P.
4. Stübinger S, Nuss K, Pongratz M, Price J, Sader R, Zeilhofer H-F, von Rechenberg B. Comparison of er: Yag laser and piezoelectric osteotomy: an animal study in sheep. Lasers Surg Med. 2010;42(8):743–51.
5. Augello M, Deibel W, Nuss K, Cattin P, Jürgens P. Comparative microstructural analysis of bone osteotomies after cutting by computer-assisted robot-guided laser osteotome and piezoelectric osteotome: an in vivo animal study. Lasers Med Sci. 2018;33(7):1471–8.
6. Deibel W, Schneider A, Augello M, Bruno AE, Juergens P, Cattin P. A compact, efficient, and lightweight laser head for carlo: integration, performance, and benefits. In: Novel optical systems design and optimization XVIII, vol. 9579. Bellingham, WA: International Society for Optics and Photonics; 2015. p. 957905.
7. Augello M, Baetscher C, Segesser M, Zeilhofer H-F, Cattin P, Juergens P. Performing partial mandibular resection, fibula free flap reconstruction and midfacial osteotomies with a cold ablation and robot-guided er: Yag laser osteotome (carlo)—a study on applicability and effectiveness in human cadavers. J Cranio-Maxillofac Surg. 2018;46(10):1850–5.
8. Bruno AE, Zeilhofer H-F, Jürgens P. Carlo-computer assisted and robot guided laser-osteotome, 30 Aug 30. US Patent App. 13/497,520.
9. Christoph H. Wenn der arzt mit dem ingenieur. Technical report, Basler Zeitung, Wirtschaft, July 2018.
10. Bayhaqi YA, Navarini A, Rauter G, Cattin PC, Zam A. Neural network in tissue characterization of optical coherence tomography (oct) image for smart laser surgery: preliminary study. In: Third international seminar on photonics, optics, and its applications (ISPhOA 2018), vol. 11044. Bellingham, WA:

International Society for Optics and Photonics; 2019. p. 1104402.
11. Abbasi H, Rauter G, Guzman R, Cattin PC, Zam A. Differentiation of femur bone from surrounding soft tissue using laser induced breakdown spectroscopy as a feedback system for smart laserosteotomy. In: Biophotonics: photonic solutions for better health care VI, vol. 10685. Bellingham, WA: International Society for Optics and Photonics; 2018. p. 1068519.
12. Nguendon Kenhagho H, Shevchik S, Saeidi F, Faivre N, Meylan B, Rauter G, Guzman R, Cattin P, Wasmer K, Zam A. Characterization of ablated bone and muscle for long-pulsed laser ablation in dry and wet conditions. Materials. 2019;12(8):1338.
13. Eugster M, Cattin PC, Zam A, Rauter G. A parallel robotic mechanism for the stabilization and guidance of an endoscope tip in laser osteotomy. In: 2018 IEEE/RSJ international conference on intelligent robots and systems (IROS). Piscataway, NJ: IEEE; 2018. p. 1306–11.
14. Eugster M, Weber P, Cattin P, Zam A, Kosa G, Rauter G. Positioning and stabilization of a minimally invasive laser osteotome. In: Proceedings of the Hamlyn symposium on medical robotics. London: Imperial College London and the Royal Geographical Society; 2017. p. 21–2.
15. Eugster M, Weber P, Rauter G. Medical endodevice. European Patent Application, EP 17177760.0, 26. June 2017

Laser Safety

20

Ferda Canbaz and Azhar Zam

Contents

Abstract

Since their invention, lasers have been successfully employed in many applications, ranging from research—in fields such as chemistry, physics, archeology, and medicine—to industry. Lasers are both a practical tool and a potentially dangerous piece of equipment. As users have different educational and experiential backgrounds, common safety rules and regulations must be specified. Currently, safety guidance is provided by international committees (such as the International Commission on Non-Ionizing Radiation Protection, the International Electrotechnical Commission, and the American National Standard). According to the regulations, users should be trained before working with lasers in order to provide a safe environment. Safety regulations focus mainly on protection of the human eye and skin, which are the organs most vulnerable to laser exposure. To protect these organs, it is important to know maximum exposure levels and the class of laser being used. This chapter offers some insight into working with lasers, highlighting the biological aspects underlying injury risks for different parts of the human body, laser classification details, and basic rules for laser safety.

Keywords

Lasers · Laser safety · Laser exposure
Maximum permissible emission (MPE)

F. Canbaz (✉) · A. Zam
Department of Biomedical Engineering, University of Basel, Basel, Switzerland
e-mail: ferda.canbaz@unibas.ch; azhar.zam@unibas.ch

S. Stübinger et al. (eds.), *Lasers in Oral and Maxillofacial Surgery*,
https://doi.org/10.1007/978-3-030-29604-9_20

20.1 Lasers

Lasers are optical oscillators that produce spatially and temporally coherent light. Laser light is directional, monochromatic, and intensely bright. The output of a laser beam spreads due to diffraction, but it does not spread as much as the beam of a flashlight. Hence, even after propagating over long distances, a laser beam can still be hazardous to the human eye and skin. With regard to color, lasers produce light with a very narrow spectrum. The narrow spectral width and the limited cross-sectional area of the beam gives some indication of how bright laser output can be, even with modest output power [1, 2]. Compared to incoherent light sources, these properties make direct viewing of lasers dangerous, even at low power levels. When it comes to laser safety, irradiance must be taken into account. Irradiance is defined as the radiant flux per unit area ($d\varphi/dA$, where $d\varphi$ is the unit flux and dA is the unit area). Lasers can produce continuous-wave or time-dependent output. In the case of pulsed lasers, it is possible to generate high peak power levels at low average output power levels. Since the peak power of a pulsed laser can be more than a million times higher than the average power, users must be more careful when using pulsed lasers. The maximum permissible exposure (MPE) of a laser depends on its operation wavelength, operation type (pulsed or continuous wave), and duration of exposure. MPE levels for skin and eyes are specified in specific laser safety standards [3, 4].

20.2 Why We Need to Avoid Laser Exposure

The eye is the part of the body most sensitive to light exposure. The human eye is formed by a cornea, pupil, iris, focusing lens, retina, and optical nerves. A detailed image of the human eye can be seen in Fig. 20.1. Figure 20.2 illustrates how the eye sees. For example, light from a candle passes through the cornea and the pupil. The image is reversed and projected to the retina. The retina then converts the image to an electrical signal. With the help of optical nerves, the electrical signal is transferred to the brain. The brain, in turn, interprets the electrical signal so as to reproduce the image.

Laser radiation reaches different parts of the human eye, depending on its wavelength [3, 4]. The range of light from 100 to 315 nm (Ultraviolet-B and Ultraviolet-C) is absorbed by the cornea. As a result of this absorption, a photochemical process occurs in the cornea. This process is known as photokeratitis. Corneal damage resulting from exposure to light in the range of 100–315 nm is generally temporary. Corneal regeneration is a quick process; it takes less than

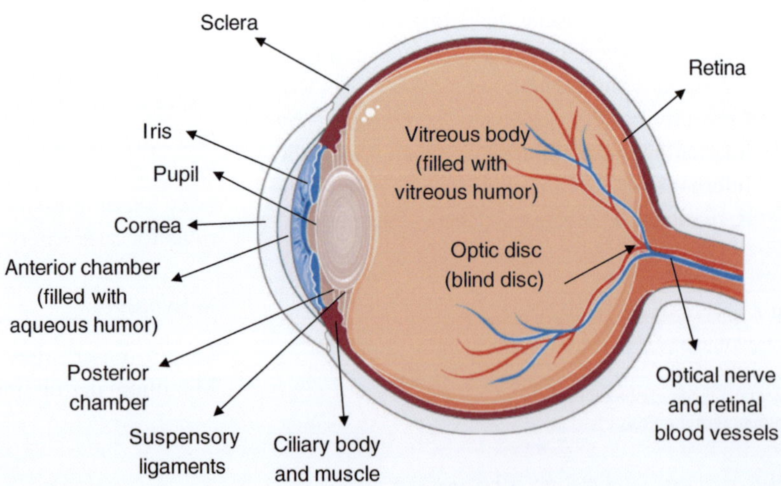

Fig. 20.1 A schematic representation of parts of the human eye

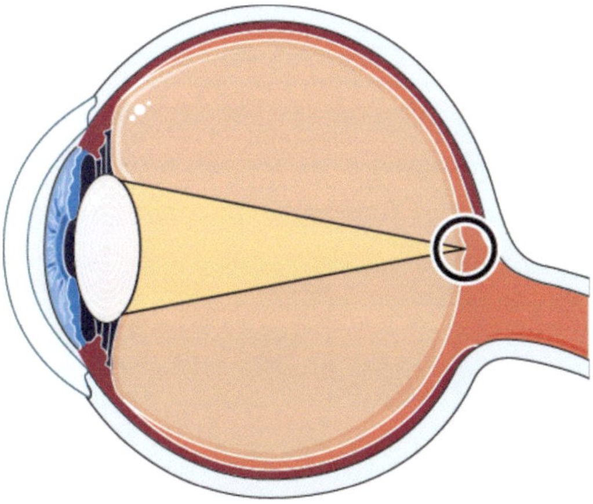

Fig. 20.2 Schematic of the formation of images on the retina

24 h. From 315 to 400 nm (Ultraviolet-A), the cornea and aqueous humor let the light in, but it is absorbed by the focusing lens. This kind of absorption, in particular, leads to denaturation of the proteins in the lens, resulting in the formation of cataracts. In the light ranges 400–800 nm (visible) and 800–1400 nm (infrared-A), light can reach the retina. Retinal tissue damage occurs due to absorption, similar to the other parts. Generation of heat bases on either melanin granules in the pigmented epithelium or photochemical reaction in the photoreceptor. The aversion reflex can prevent damage in the retina only if the light intensity is lower than that which affects the retina in 0.25 s. However, in the wavelength region of 700–1400 nm, the human eye remains insensitive; thus lasers may cause damage to the retina. An additional problem with the visible and infrared-A wavelength region pertains to the focusing effect of the cornea and lens. These parts can increase retinal irradiance by a factor of 100,000 just by focusing light onto the retina, leading to possible retinal damage even with low power levels. Above 1400 nm (infrared-B and infrared-C), the cornea absorbs the light and does not let it propagate further. The resulting heat causes protein denaturation on the cornea surface.

Light exposure can be dangerous not only to the human eye but also for the skin. In terms of functionality, damage to the eye is much more significant than that to the skin. However, since the surface area of the skin is much larger than that of the human eye, the possibility of light exposure is higher. Figure 20.3a shows the layers that make up human skin. The epidermis is the outmost part of the skin and is formed of five different layers: stratum basale, stratum spinosum, stratum granulosum, stratum lucidum, and stratum corneum. Stratum corneum is the outer layer of the epidermis, and it is made of flat dead cells (Fig. 20.3, inset). Next comes the dermis, which includes different types of tissues such as collagen, elastic tissue, and reticular fibers. The subcutaneous tissue lies beneath the dermis layer; here, fat and connective tissues are present. As in the case of the human eye, different wavelengths penetrate the skin at different depths [3, 4]. For example, light with a wavelength of 800 nm can penetrate the subcutaneous layer of the skin (Fig. 20.3b). Damage thresholds for the human eye and skin are comparable. Depending on the penetration depth, a temperature increase occurs at different levels of the skin. For example, deep heating can be caused by exposure to light in the infrared-A region. If skin damage is isolated in a small area, it can be painful, but it will be temporary. The recovery process may be long; however, it does not impair functionality. Damage to a large area of the skin is not common in laser laboratories but could cause severe injury, due to the extensive loss of body liquid.

20.3 Maximum Permissible Exposure (MPE)

Maximum permissible exposure (MPE) or exposure limit (EL) is the maximum threshold level at which one can avoid damage to the eye or skin [6]. MPE depends on the target organ, type of laser, operation wavelength, source size, pulse duration, and repetition rate. MPE is not a constant value; it must be calculated by the laser safety officer for each laser, depending on its operational parameters. There are set levels, however, based on experimental studies and determined by the International Commission on Non-Ionizing Radiation Protection (ICNIRP) [7],

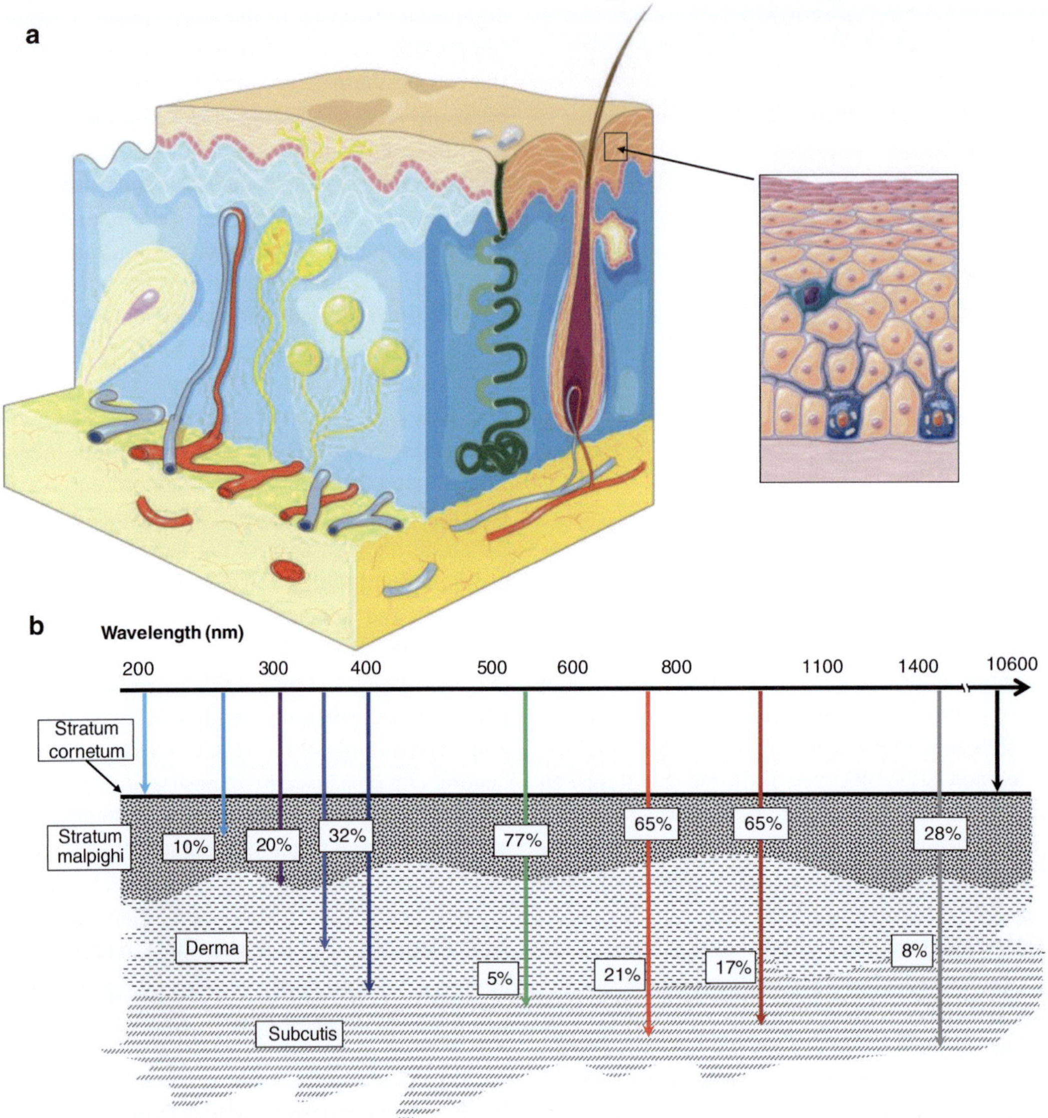

Fig. 20.3 (**a**) A schematic of the layers of the human skin. Inset shows the layers of the epidermis. (**b**) Penetration depth varies as a function of wavelength layers under light exposure. Depending on the center wavelength of the light beam, absorbed radiation is also shown as a fraction at each layer. (Adopted from Ref. [5])

the International Electrotechnical Commission (IEC) [6], and the American National Standard (ANSI) [8]. The MPE values for eyes and skin published by the three committees are nearly identical, except in some special cases. The laser safety standards are listed in IEC 60825-1 and ANSI Z136.1. MPE calculations are useful for understanding safety limits. However, these levels should not be considered as a stringent line, precisely differentiating between a safe level and a dangerous one.

Pulsed lasers are used in laboratories for a multitude of applications. As stated above, MPE values vary with the pulse width and pulse repetition frequency. Hence, setting MPE values for a pulsed laser is complex [6]. Furthermore, the MPE value depends on the wavelength, complicating MPE estimates for a broadband light source. In the case of repetitively pulsed or modulated lasers:

1. The exposure level of a single pulse that is part of a pulse train should not be higher than the MPE level for a single pulse.
2. In a given time interval, *T*, the average exposure level of a train of pulses should not exceed the exposure level for a single pulse with a duration of *T*.
3. The average exposure of multiple pulses belonging to a particular train of pulses should not be higher than the MPE level for a single pulse, multiplied by the correction factor C_5.

The reduced MPE for any single pulse in the pulse train (MPE_{train}) is calculated from:

$$MPE_{train} = MPE_{single} \times C_5$$

where MPE_{single} is the MPE for a single pulse and C_5 is calculated from minus one fourth power of the number of pulses expected in the exposure ($C_5 = N^{-1/4}$, N: the number of pulses) [6]. In the calculations, C_5 can only be used for pulse durations shorter than 0.25 s. If the resulting MPE value is similar to that obtained from a continuous wave (cw) exposure time, then cw MPE values can be used instead. In the case of multi-pulsing, each pulse needs to be considered as an independent single pulse. If pulse widths change over a time interval, total-time-on-pulse (TOTP) needs to be considered in order to calculate MPE. TOTP is simply a summation of the pulse durations within the exposure time. To check the MPE values for eyes and skin, consult the tables provided by the IEC.

To determine a realistic exposure level, MPE values must be averaged over a circular aperture and in consideration of the angle of acceptance of the retina. In the case of ocular exposure in the visible wavelength range, 100 mm distance should be used as a minimum measurement distance. To establish the angle of acceptance from a particular source, one can follow the details published in IEC 60825-1.

20.4 Classification of Laser

Lasers are classified depending on their operational parameters, but in the field of laser safety, it is not easy to say that a laser is safe or not. As explained in part 3, MPE calculations for different sources can be complicated. No single chart reflects every possible condition, such as exposure duration or viewing scheme. For example, a laser source may be safe for viewing with the naked eye but unsafe for viewing with binoculars. Hence it is not easy to succinctly classify a particular laser as "safe" or "hazardous." The classification standards are determined by the international laser safety standards (IEC 60825-1, ANSI Z136.1). A laser or an LED is usually classified by the manufacturer, based on the radiation emission. The manufacturer usually does not have much information about how the product will be used. Instead of discussing exposure levels for the eye or skin, they refer to the energy or power at a given diameter and distance. As a result, the classification has an upper limit for the power or energy values at a given diameter and distance, known as Accessible Emission Limit (AEL) values. The laser safety class determined by the manufacturer depends on the direct exposure to the laser beam [6]. Laser safety classifications are defined as follows:

- Class 1: Lasers belonging to this class are safe both for direct exposure and for use with optical instruments. Output power of a Class 1 laser should be lower than 0.39 mW.
- Class 1M: Lasers operating in the wavelength range of 300–4000 nm are safe for direct exposure to the eye or skin. However, using optical components such as binoculars may be harmful to the eye.
- Class 1C: Lasers used for cosmetic applications related to the skin such as hair removal, acne treatment, and tattoo removal are recently established as a new class in IEC60825 version 07-2015. A clear objective is assigned for this class of lasers and they usually have a protection measure which ensures safety for the case of a user error.
- Class 2: Hazard depends on the exposure time of the eye to the particular lasers. For lasers operating in the visible range of light (400–700 nm), the aversion response (t = 0.25 s) guarantees the

exposure time for bright light, meaning that visible Class 2 lasers are safe for the naked for eye, even with the use of optical components. If staring into the laser beam intentionally, these lasers can be hazardous and cause flash blindness. Lasers in this class are not hazardous for the skin.

- Class 2M: This class is similar to Class 2 except that in the case of using eye loupes or binoculars, these lasers may harm the human eye.
- Class 3R: Lasers in the wavelength above 300 nm fall into this category. The risk level for accidental exposure of the eye is low with lasers belonging to this class. With exposure to the laser light, there is no risk for the skin. However, intentional staring at the light beam may cause eye injury. Trained personnel are required to operate this class of lasers.
- Class 3B: Even in the case of accidental exposure, the risk level for the eye and for the skin are medium and low, respectively. Direct viewing is hazardous, but viewing diffusive reflections is safe. For skin, if the beam is focused on a tiny spot, the feeling would be similar to a pinprick.
- Class 4: The most dangerous class of lasers poses a high risk of injury for both eye and skin. Even diffusive reflections can be hazardous. Interaction with the lasers causes temperature increases, which may result in a fire.

In the classification, M and R stand for Magnifying and Relaxed or Reduced [6]. Hence M is used for laser classes that cannot be used safely with magnifying optics. When R is used to define the class of a laser, it means there is no need to use an interlock or key switch. It also means that wearing protective goggles is not mandatory. The use of B to classify a laser has a meaning similar to M; it changed from A to B after the publication of the 2001 edition of the laser safety regulations [6].

20.5 Manufacturer Responsibilities

Depending on the class of a laser, there are many safety requirements that must be fulfilled by the manufacturer during production. Classification of the laser must be specified by the manufacturer. The requirements will be discussed in the following paragraphs.

First, the manufacturer needs to ensure that the user has the proper training to use the laser. After selling the product, if the user modifies the laser in a way that requires a new classification, the manufacturer would not be responsible for the new classification. Reclassification and relabeling must be done by the user, in this case.

Laser products, in general, must have a protective housing in order to avoid direct viewing of laser radiation, unless the user must see the inner parts of the product. A safety interlock would protect the user by stopping the laser operation whenever the housing is opened. During maintenance, the access panel needs to be removed intentionally and the user needs to be able to make changes inside the housing.

A remote interlock connector and a key control must be provided by the manufacturer for Class 3B and Class 4 lasers. An audible or a visible warning must be placed in the laser housing of Class 3B (operation wavelength below 400 nm or above 700 nm), 3R, and 4 lasers to alert the user, for example, when it is switched on. If the safety warning is only visible, then it must be visible through protective goggles. If there is more than one output aperture from a laser, a visible warning should clearly show the aperture in use. A beam stop or an attenuator must further be included at the output of a Class 3B or Class 4 laser to reduce laser radiation exposure. Control of the laser should be placed in such a way as to protect the user from exposure to laser radiation for all Class 3R, Class 3B, or Class 4 lasers [6].

As a final remark, non-optical hazards during laser operation must also be addressed. These can include electrical hazards, fire ignition, excessive temperature or an explosion due to a fault, etc. the manufacturer should describe non-optical hazards in the product safety standard; however, if it is not provided, then the relevant instructions in IEC 61010-1 can be considered [6].

20.6 Ensuring Safety

This section introduces some recommendations for staying safe while using lasers. The safety precautions are offered to avoid hazardous accidents. For example, a laser safety officer (LSO) must be employed to install and to operate a Class 3R, Class 3B, or Class 4 laser. Before installation, the LSO needs to follow up the safety regulations and take initial control measurements as per IEC 60825-1 [6]. If any laser is modified by the user, reclassification must be done and communicated by the user.

- Use a remote interlock connector for Class 3B and Class 4 lasers. The interlock should be connected to the entrance in such a way so as to avoid light exposure. If trained personnel declare no probability for optical hazard, the interlock can be overridden.
- Remove the key on the control panel after use, to prevent unauthorized use of Class 3B and Class 4 lasers.
- Prevent accidental exposure of eyes and skin to Class 3B or Class 4 lasers by using beam attenuators or beam stops during operation. Beam stops should be placed even for the reflected light beam from any surface.
- Place warning signs to entrances, especially on Class 3B and Class 4 lasers, to avoid accidental damage.
- Carefully align the laser beam, especially for the Class 3B and Class 4 lasers. The beam paths should be as short as possible without any crossing ways. The beam should be blocked at the end of the path (for Class 3B and Class 4 lasers). The beam paths of Class 3R lasers should also be as short as possible, except for those operating in the visible region. Open laser beam paths must be below or above eye level for all classes of lasers. Using beam tubes in the beam paths offers another way to avoid beam exposure.
- Rigidly mount optical elements reflecting or transmitting light beams from Class 3R, 3B, and 4 lasers. Carefully align by following the reflected light beam. To avoid damaging the surfaces of the optical elements, keep them as clean as possible. For Class 1M and Class 2M lasers, focus optics carefully; beam blocks may be used behind the mirrors to block transmitted light beams.
- Use of protective goggles while operating Class 3R (except for the visible wavelength region of operation), Class 3B, and Class 4 lasers is mandatory. Exceptions may be made (1) during engineering or administrative controls and (2) during experiments (that have been approved by the laser safety officer) where wearing goggles is not practical. The choice of goggles is important to ensure safety. Goggles need high optical density (for lower transmission) relative to the operation wavelength of the laser(s). Radiant exposure and MPE must be considered in order to prevent eye damage. The damage threshold of the eyewear must be known and indicated. Comfort and ventilation of the goggles are important, as the user may wear them for the whole day. The design of the goggles must be chosen to provide as wide a field of view as possible. Strength and degradation of the material may vary and should be considered. The goggles must be designed to block peripheral vision as well, as shown in Fig. 20.4.
- Label protective eyewear properly including the information of the wavelength range and optical density at the wavelength range. The spectral optical density (D_λ) of the protective eyewear can be calculated from

$$D_\lambda = \log_{10}\frac{H_0}{\text{MPE}}.$$

Here, H_0 is the expected exposure level of the unprotected eye. D_λ depends on the wavelength. The minimum value of D_λ for the particular wavelength range needs to be indicated on the protective eyewear.

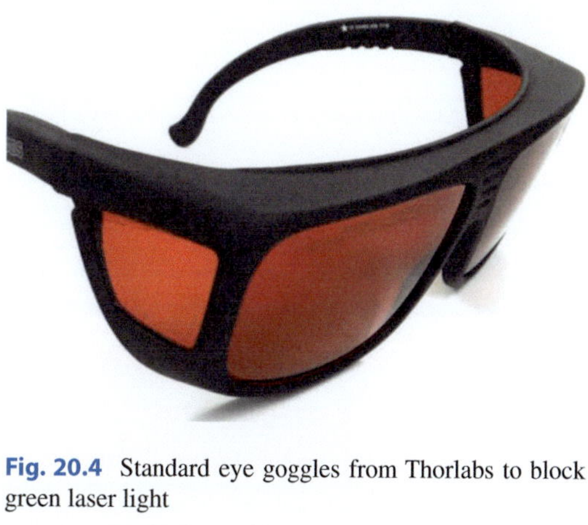

Fig. 20.4 Standard eye goggles from Thorlabs to block green laser light

- Provide suitable clothing for use during experiments with Class 4 lasers that have radiation levels higher than stated MPE values for skin. Clothing material must be resistant to heat as this class of laser can start fires.
- Ensure that only trained personnel are in charge of operating or aligning Class 1M, Class 2M, Class 3R, Class 3B, and Class 4 lasers; these lasers may cause a hazard not only to the users but also to the people standing further away. The training can be given by the manufacturer, the laser safety officer, and certified external organization. Training should include (1) system operating procedures, (2) hazard control procedures, (3) personal protection requirements, (4) accident procedures, and (5) information about interactions between the laser and eye or skin.
- Provide pre-, interim-, and post-employment ophthalmic examinations for users of the Class 3B and Class 4 lasers. Upon suspicion of injury, the user must see a specialist.

In addition to the safety regulations listed above, users must not take any risk, especially while working with Class 3B or Class 4 lasers.

References

1. Siegman AE. Lasers. Sausalito, CA: University Science Books; 1986. p. 1283.
2. Sennaroglu A. Photonics and laser engineering: principles, devices, and applications. New York: McGraw-Hill; 2010.
3. Barat K. Laser safety management. Boca Raton, FL: CRC Press; 2006.
4. Henderson R, Schulmeister K. Laser safety. Boca Raton, FL: CRC Press; 2003.
5. Sliney D, Wolbarsht M. Optical radiation hazards to the skin. In: Safety with lasers and other optical sources. New York: Springer; 1980. p. 161–85.
6. IEC 60825-1. Safety of laser products—Part 1: Equipment classification, requirements and user's guide. Geneva: IEC; 2001.
7. ICNIRP. Guidelines. Health Phys. 2000;79:431–40.
8. LIA Z136.1. American National Standard for safe use of lasers. FL: LIA; 2000.

Index

S. Stübinger et al. (eds.), *Lasers in Oral and Maxillofacial Surgery*,
https://doi.org/10.1007/978-3-030-29604-9

M

MIX
Papier aus verantwortungsvollen Quellen
Paper from responsible sources
FSC® C105338
FSC
www.fsc.org

If you have any concerns about our products,
you can contact us on
ProductSafety@springernature.com

In case Publisher is established outside the EU,
the EU authorized representative is:
Springer Nature Customer Service Center GmbH
Europaplatz 3, 69115 Heidelberg, Germany

Printed by Libri Plureos GmbH
in Hamburg, Germany